MORGAN AND MIKHAIL'S CLINICAL ANESTHESIOLOGY CASES

a LANGE medical book

MORGAN AND MIKHAIL'S CLINICAL ANESTHESIOLOGY CASES

EDITED BY

JOHN F. BUTTERWORTH IV, MD
Professor and Chairman, Department of Anesthesiology, Virginia Commonwealth University School of Medicine VCU Health System, Richmond, Virginia

DAVID C. MACKEY, MD
Professor, Department of Anesthesiology and Perioperative Medicine, University of Texas MD Anderson Cancer Center, Houston, Texas

JOHN D. WASNICK, MD, MPH
Steven L. Berk Endowed Chair for Excellence in Medicine, Professor and Chair Department of Anesthesia, Texas Tech University Health Sciences Center, School of Medicine, Lubbock, Texas

New York   Chicago   San Francisco   Athens   London   Madrid   Mexico City
Milan   New Delhi   Singapore   Sydney   Toronto

1 2 3 4 5 6 7 8 9   DSS   25 24 23 22 21 20

ISBN 978-0-07-183612-8
MHID 0-07-183612-8
ISSN 2641-1105

This book was set in Minion Pro by Cenveo® Publisher Services.
The editors were Jason Malley and Christie Naglieri.
The production supervisor was Richard Ruzycka.
Project management was provided by Tania Andrabi, Cenveo Publisher Services.
The cover designer was W2 Design.

This book is printed on acid free paper.

McGraw-Hill Education books are available at special quantity discounts to use as premiums and sales promotions or for use in corporate training programs. To contact a representative, please visit the Contact Us pages at www.mhprofessional.com.

CONTENTS

SECTION 1   ANESTHETIC EQUIPMENT & MONITORS

SECTION 2   CLINICAL PHARMACOLOGY

SECTION 3   ANESTHETIC MANAGEMENT

CONTENTS

CONTENTS

CONTRIBUTORS

SALAHADIN ABDI, MD, PhD
Professor and Chair
Department of Pain Medicine
University of Texas MD Anderson Cancer Center
Houston, Texas

CLAYTON ADAMS, MD
Former Resident
Department of Anesthesiology
Texas Tech University Health Sciences Center
Lubbock, Texas

SHADY ADIB, MD
Assistant Professor
Department of Anesthesiology
University of Missouri-Columbia
Columbia, Missouri

SARAH ARMOUR, MD
Assistant Professor
Department of Anesthesiology
Mayo Clinic
Rochester, Minnesota

BENJAMIN ARNOLD, MD
Associate Professor
Department of Anesthesiology and Perioperative Medicine
University of Texas MD Anderson Cancer Center
Houston, Texas

ARPITA D. BADAMI, MD
Attending Anesthesiologist
Downeast Surgery Center
Bangor, Maine

RON BANISTER, MD
Associate Professor of Anesthesiology
Texas Tech University Health Sciences Center
Lubbock, Texas

SHREYAS BHAVSAR, MD
Associate Professor
Department of Anesthesiology and Perioperative Medicine
University of Texas MD Anderson Cancer Center
Houston, Texas

JOHN F. BUTTERWORTH IV, MD
Professor and Chairman
Department of Anesthesiology
Virginia Commonwealth University School of Medicine
VCU Health System
Richmond, Virginia

MATTHEW T. CHAROUS, MD
Attending Anesthesiologist
Midwest Anesthesia Partners, LLC
Chicago, Illinois

KALLOL CHAUDHURI, MD, PhD
Professor and Vice Chair
Department of Anesthesiology
Texas Tech University Health Sciences Center
Lubbock, Texas

SWAPNA CHAUDHURI, MD, PhD
Professor and Vice Chair
Department of Anesthesiology
Texas Tech University Health Sciences Center
Lubbock, Texas

CHASE CLANTON, MD
Former Resident
Department of Anesthesiology
Texas Tech University Health Sciences Center
Lubbock, Texas

LYDIA CONLAY, MD, PhD, MBA
Former Professor
Department of Anesthesiology
Texas Tech University Health Sciences Center
Lubbock, Texas

CHARLES E. COWLES, JR., MD, MBA, FASA
Associate Professor/Assistant Clinical Director
Department of Anesthesiology and Perioperative Medicine
Divisional Safety Officer
Division of Anesthesiology, Critical Care, and Pain Medicine
University of Texas MD Anderson Cancer Center

LORI A. DANGLER, MD, MBA
Associate Professor
Department of Anesthesiology and Perioperative Medicine
University of Texas MD Anderson Cancer Center
Houston, Texas

RYAN DERBY, MD, MPH
Clinical Assistant Professor
Department of Anesthesiology, Perioperative, and Pain Medicine
Stanford University School of Medicine
Palo Alto, California

CONTRIBUTORS

JOHANNES DERIESE, MD
Former Assistant Professor
Department of Anesthesiology
Texas Tech University Health Sciences Center
Lubbock, Texas

ANISH I. DOSHI, MD
Attending Anesthesiologist
Rancocas Anesthesiology PA
Jefferson Health–New Jersey
Mount Laurel, New Jersey

LARRY C. DRIVER, MD
Professor
Department of Pain Medicine
The University of Texas MD Anderson Cancer Center
Houston, Texas

ASHRAF N. FARAG, MD
Associate Professor
Department of Anesthesiology
Texas Tech University Health Sciences Center
Lubbock, Texas

JOEL FEINSTEIN, MD
Assistant Professor
Department of Anesthesiology and Perioperative Medicine
University of Alabama at Birmingham
Birmingham, Alabama

MICHAEL A. FRÖLICH, MD, MS
Professor and Associate Vice Chair for Clinical Research
Department of Anesthesiology
The University of Alabama at Birmingham
Birmingham, Alabama

NISCHAL K. GAUTAM, MD
Associate Professor
Department of Anesthesiology
McGovern Medical School | UT Health Houston
Houston, Texas

MARINA GITMAN, MD
Assistant Professor
Department of Anesthesia
University of Illinois
Champaign, Illinois

CONTRIBUTORS

DAN S. GOMBOS, MD, FACS
Professor and Section Chief
Section of Ophthalmology
Department of Head and Neck Surgery
Division of Surgery
University of Texas MD Anderson Cancer Center
Clinical Co-Director
The Retinoblastoma Center of Houston
MD Anderson Cancer Center, Texas Children's Hospital, Houston Methodist Hospital &
Baylor College of Medicine
Houston, Texas

JAGTAR SINGH HEIR, DO
Professor
Department of Anesthesiology and Perioperative Medicine
University of Texas MD Anderson Cancer Center
Houston, Texas

BRIAN HIRSCH, MD
Former Resident
Department of Anesthesiology
Texas Tech University Health Sciences Center
Lubbock, Texas

DENNIS HO, DO
Former Assistant Professor
Department of Anesthesiology
Texas Tech University Health Sciences Center
Lubbock, Texas

ERIK HUSTAK, MD
Assistant Professor
Department of Anesthesiology
University of Texas Medical Branch
Galveston, Texas

BRIAN M. ILFELD, MD, MS
Professor in Residence
Department of Anesthesiology
Division of Regional Anesthesia and Acute Pain Medicine
University of California San Diego
San Diego, California

CARRIE JOHNSON, MD
Attending Anesthesiologist
Carolinas Pain Institute
Winston-Salem, North Carolina

ROBERT JOHNSTON, MD
Associate Professor
Department of Anesthesiology
Texas Tech University Health Sciences Center
Lubbock, Texas

RAVISH KAPOOR, MD
Assistant Professor
Department of Anesthesiology and Perioperative Medicine
University of Texas MD Anderson Cancer Center
Houston, Texas

SABRY KHALIL, MD
Former Assistant Professor
Department of Anesthesiology
Texas Tech University Health Sciences Center
Lubbock, Texas

BAHAREH KHATIBI, MD
Associate Clinical Professor
Department of Anesthesiology
Division of Regional Anesthesia and Acute Pain Medicine
University of California San Diego
San Diego, California

CHRISTIN KIM, MD
Assistant Professor
Department of Anesthesiology
Virginia Commonwealth University
Richmond, Virginia

KATRINA VON KRIEGENBERGH, MD
Former Resident
Department of Anesthesiology
Texas Tech University Health Sciences Center
Lubbock, Texas

JAVIER LASALA, MD
Associate Professor
Department of Anesthesiology and Perioperative Medicine
University of Texas MD Anderson Cancer Center
Houston, Texas

DAVID C. MACKEY, MD
Professor
Department of Anesthesiology and Perioperative Medicine
University of Texas MD Anderson Cancer Center
Houston, Texas

TONI MANOUGIAN, MD
Assistant Professor
Department of Anesthesiology
New York Medical College
Valhala, New York

CONTRIBUTORS

EDWARD R. MARIANO, MD, MAS (CLINICAL RESEARCH)
Chief
Anesthesiology and Perioperative Care Service
Associate Chief of Staff for Inpatient Surgical Services
VA Palo Alto Health Care System
Professor of Anesthesiology, Perioperative, and Pain Medicine
Stanford University School of Medicine
Palo Alto, California

BRIAN McCLURE, DO
Former Resident
Department of Anesthesiology
Texas Tech University Health Sciences Center
Lubbock, Texas

THOMAS McHUGH, MD
Former Resident
Department of Anesthesiology
Texas Tech University Health Sciences Center
Lubbock, Texas

GLORIMAR MEDINA-RIVERA, MD, MBA
Executive Vice President/Administrator for Ambulatory Care Services
Harris Health Systems
Houston, Texas

MONICA RICE MURPHY, MD
Attending Anesthesiologist
North American Partners in Anesthesiology
Affiliate Faculty
Virginia Commonwealth University Department of Anesthesiology
Richmond, Virginia

LINH T. NGUYEN, MD
Associate Professor
Department of Anesthesiology and Perioperative Medicine
University of Texas MD Anderson Cancer Center
Houston, Texas

JASON NOBLE, MD
Assistant Professor
Department of Anesthesiology
Virginia Commonwealth University
Richmond, Virginia

SUZANNE NORTHCUTT, MD
Assistant Professor
Department of Anesthesiology
Texas Tech University Health Sciences Center
Lubbock, Texas

CONTRIBUTORS

PASCAL OWUSU-AGYEMANG, MD
Associate Professor
Department of Anesthesiology and Perioperative Medicine
University of Texas MD Anderson Cancer Center
Houston, Texas

NITIN PARIKH, MD
Assistant Professor
Department of Anesthesiology
Texas Tech University Health Sciences Center
Lubbock, Texas

COOPER W. PHILLIPS, MD
Assistant Professor
Department of Anesthesiology
Texas Tech University Health Sciences Center
Lubbock, Texas

MARK POWELL, MD
Associate Professor
Department of Anesthesiology and Perioperative Medicine
University of Alabama at Birmingham
Birmingham, Alabama

MICHAEL RAMSAY, MD, FRCA
Chairman
Department of Anesthesiology
Baylor University Medical Center
Dallas, Texas

ELIZABETH REBELLO, MD
Associate Professor
Department of Anesthesiology and Perioperative Medicine
University of Texas MD Anderson Cancer Center
Houston, Texas

ANGELO RICCIONE, DO
Resident
Department of Anesthesiology
Texas Tech University Health Sciences Center
Lubbock, Texas

ELIZABETH R. RIVAS, MD
Assistant Professor
Department of Anesthesiology
Texas Tech University Health Sciences Center
Lubbock, Texas

MADHUMANI RUPASINGHE, MBBS, FRCA
Associate Professor
Department of Anesthesiology
The University Health Science Center at Houston
Houston, Texas

BETTINA SCHMITZ, MD
Assistant Professor
Department of Anesthesiology
Texas Tech University Health Sciences Center
Lubbock, Texas

SPENCER THOMAS, MD
Former Resident
Department of Anesthesiology
Texas Tech University Health Sciences Center
Lubbock, Texas

CHRISTIANE VOGT HARENKAMP, MD, PhD
Assistant Professor
Department of Anesthesiology
Texas Tech University Health Sciences Center
Lubbock, Texas

MUKESH WADHWA, DO
Former Assistant Professor
Department of Anesthesiology
Texas Tech University Health Sciences Center
Lubbock, Texas

CHARLOTTE WALTER, MD
Former Resident
Department of Anesthesiology
Texas Tech University Health Sciences Center
Lubbock, Texas

JOHN D. WASNICK, MD, MPH
Steven L. Berk Endowed Chair for Excellence in Medicine
Professor and Chair
Department of Anesthesia
Texas Tech University Health Sciences Center
School of Medicine
Lubbock, Texas

GARY WELCH, MD
Former Assistant Professor
Department of Anesthesiology
Texas Tech University Health Sciences Center
Lubbock, Texas

JOHN WELKER, MD
Former Resident
Department of Anesthesiology
Texas Tech University Health Sciences Center
Lubbock, Texas

CONTRIBUTORS

JENNIFER WU, MD, MBA
Associate Professor
Department of Anesthesiology
McGovern Medical School at UT Houston Science Center
Houston, Texas

SHIRAZ YAZDANI, MD
Assistant Professor
Department of Pain Medicine and Anesthesiology
Texas Tech University Health Sciences Center
Lubbock, Texas

GANG ZHENG, MD
Associate Professor
Department of Anesthesiology and Perioperative Medicine
University of Texas MD Anderson Cancer Center
Houston, Texas

CONTRIBUTORS

PREFACE

Adult learners acquire new knowledge in a variety of ways, and there has never been a greater variety of modes of learning as is available today. For example, how many of our readers would have used podcasts, YouTube videos, or online resources as their primary ways to keep up with the advances in medicine? Nevertheless, reflecting the overwhelming conservatism of the medical profession, one of the least effective mechanisms for transmission of new knowledge, the 50-minute lecture, remains prominent in formal undergraduate, graduate, and continuing medical education.

Some will claim that books are passé. We agree that the 4-kg, multiauthor monstrosities so often recommended when we were in medical school are on the way out. On the other hand we believe that primers that studiously avoid esoterica, however interesting, will always be valuable to learners. Studies consistently show that adults are more likely to retain new knowledge when it connects directly with what they do each day. Thus, we have launched this book of clinical case vignettes to accompany our primer, *Morgan & Mikhail's Clinical Anesthesiology*, Sixth Edition. In both these books we have tried to emphasize the common medical issues we face in anesthetic practice, rather than the esoteric ones. In this textbook, we have also tried to illustrate how clinicians use critical thinking in medical decision-making. We would expect experienced clinicians to find most of the clinical decision-making relatively easy and straightforward. If that happens, then we have succeeded in our task!

Unlike those who write standardized examination questions, we recognize that there is no need for physicians to memorize, say, the citric acid cycle or the exact values of MAC for commonly used anesthetics. However, clinicians must know how the differences between aerobic and anaerobic metabolism relate to metabolic acidosis and the relative potencies of volatile agents. With that in mind, we have provided cases that, whenever possible, address the "big picture" rather than the minutiae. When we dig in and provide seemingly arcane facts or measurements, it is because we believe they illustrate important "big picture" concepts.

We hope that our readers will agree with our assessment. We greatly appreciate how our thoughtful, sharp-eyed readers have helped us address errors in the past. If you find typographical or other errors within this text, please email us at mm6ed@gmail.com. We will also appreciate your suggestions regarding topics and cases that you think should be included in our next edition.

John F. Butterworth IV, MD
David C. Mackey, MD
John D. Wasnick, MD, MPH

CHAPTER 1

The Practice of Anesthesiology

CASE 1 | Responsibility and Authority in the Operating Room

Jason Noble, MD

1. During an elective laparoscopic colectomy for adenocarcinoma, the patient, with a history of drug-controlled hypertension and 40 years of smoking one pack of cigarettes per day, experiences some unexpected blood loss that is now under control. Starting hemoglobin was 11.5 g/dL. Vital signs have remained stable throughout the anesthetic. The surgeon demands that you give 2 units of packed red cells immediately. The best response would be:

   A. Do as the surgeon demands, as the surgeon is the "captain of the ship" in the operating room and his or her commands should be obeyed.
   B. Tell the surgeon to worry about what happens on his or her side of the drapes and you will take care of the issues on your side.
   C. Measure the hemoglobin in a new blood sample, and then make a considered medical decision with the surgeon based on evidence.
   D. Tell the surgeon that you will give the blood as soon as it arrives, and then delay infusing it until you think it's appropriate.

The correct answer is C. First introduced into malpractice law in 1949, the idea of the surgeon as "captain of the ship" was the legal argument that just as a ship's captain has complete charge of all those on board, so too was the surgeon in the operating room expected to be in charge of all health care providers present and, therefore, be responsible and liable for their actions as well as his or her own. Since that time, there has been considerable evolution of this concept. At present, in most jurisdictions, unless the surgeon exerts specific control over the anesthesia provided, he or she is not liable for untoward anesthesia complications. Instead, the surgeon is entitled (and expected) to depend on the expertise of the anesthesiologist.

In the given scenario, the question is whether or not the surgeon has the right to exert control over the anesthesia provider. Nowadays, this is no longer considered a valid notion when an anesthesiologist is present, as he or she is to be considered a fellow specialist not under the direct control of the surgeon. Rather, the surgeon and anesthesiologist should function together as an effective team with clear lines of communication between them. The best response would be option C.

2. Nevertheless, you decide that you would rather avoid a confrontation with the surgeon. You assume that the surgeon will just give the blood anyway in the postanesthesia care unit, so you administer 2 units of packed RBCs. The patient subsequently develops transfusion-related acute lung injury (TRALI) and, as a result, has an unplanned and prolonged stay in the ICU. Which of the following is the most accurate statement?

   A. Because the blood was given at the demand of the surgeon, the anesthesiologist is not liable.
   B. Because the blood was given at the demand of the surgeon, both the surgeon and the anesthesiologist are liable.
   C. Even though the blood was given at the demand of the surgeon, the anesthesiologist remains liable.
   D. Provided the patient signed an informed consent for blood transfusion, neither physician is liable.

The correct answer is C. Nowadays, unless it can be shown that the surgeon was able to actively exert control over the administration of the anesthesia, he or she does not take on the liability of anesthesia mishaps. It must be demonstrated that the surgeon had actual control of the means rather than control of the ends. If the blood was given without any evidence that it was medically indicated, the anesthesia provider—as an independent specialist—is responsible for its complications. TRALI is a cause of transfusion-related deaths and, in this scenario, may be considered an unwarranted complication secondary to an unnecessary transfusion. The most correct response would be option C.

3. Somehow, you get a "do over." You have appropriately waited until a repeat hemoglobin returns at 9.3 g/dL. The patient remains stable, with no change in vital signs, and an arterial blood gas analysis shows no metabolic acidosis, increased lactate, or any other signs of inadequate tissue perfusion. The surgeon demands that you transfuse the patient immediately because the hemoglobin is below 10 g/dL. The surgeon notes that the patient is *her* patient, and therefore, *she* has the right to order you to give the transfusion. Which of the following is the most correct statement?

   A. Because the surgeon is now exerting control over her patient, you give the transfusion, as you are no longer liable.
   B. Because this confrontation is becoming difficult, you give the transfusion.

C. Because you are an independent specialist, despite this being the surgeon's patient, you postpone giving the transfusion until you decide it is appropriate.
D. Because you can no longer take this kind of abuse, you ask for another anesthesia provider to take over supervision of this case.

The correct answer is C. Although confrontations in the operating room are rarely necessary or helpful, they are sometimes unavoidable. However, you are also the patient's advocate for the best possible quality of anesthesia care. If the available evidence demonstrates that a transfusion is unnecessary, then no transfusion should be given. A hemoglobin <10 g/dL was formerly considered an indication for transfusions; however, it is no longer considered a valid reason in and of itself. Despite the surgeon claiming "ownership" of the patient, as an independent specialist, your decision to transfuse any blood products should be based on best medical evidence. The best answer is option C.

DID YOU LEARN?

- Legal and professional obligations of anesthesia staff.
- Doctrine of "captain of the ship."

Recommended Readings

American Board of Anesthesiology Primary Certification Policy Book (Booklet of Information), 2017. http://www.theaba.org/ABOUT/Policies-BOI. Accessed January 19, 2018.

Bacon DR. The promise of one great anesthesia society. The 1939–1940 proposed merger of the American Society of Anesthetists and the International Anesthesia Research Society. *Anesthesiology.* 1994;80:929.

Bergman N. *The Genesis of Surgical Anesthesia.* Schaumberg, IL: Wood Library-Museum of Anesthesiology; 1998.

Butterworth IV JF, Mackey DC, Wasnick JD, eds. The practice of anesthesiology. In: *Morgan & Mikhail's Clinical Anesthesiology.* 6th ed. New York, NY: McGraw-Hill Education; 2018:1-8.

Eger EI II, Saidman L, Westhorpe R, eds. *The Wondrous Story of Anesthesia.* New York, NY: Springer; 2014.

Keys TE. *The History of Surgical Anesthesia.* Tulsa, OK: Schuman Publishing; 1945.

Reves JG, Greene NM. Anesthesiology and the academic medical center: Place and promise at the start of the new millennium. *Int Anesthesiol Clin.* 2000;38:iii.

Shepherd D. *From Craft to Specialty: A Medical and Social History of Anesthesia and Its Changing Role in Health Care.* Bloomington, IN: Xlibris Corporation; 2009.

Sykes K, Bunker J. *Anaesthesia and the Practice of Medicine: Historical Perspectives.* London, United Kingdom: Royal Society of Medicine Press; 2007.

SECTION I

Anesthetic Equipment & Monitors

CHAPTER 2
The Operating Room Environment

CASE 1 Fire in the Operating Room

Charles E. Cowles, MD, MBA, FASA

You are asked to provide anesthetic care for a 66-year-old man in an ambulatory surgery center. The surgeon has posted the case as needing monitored anesthesia care (MAC) for removal of a nevus on the lateral aspect of the cheek using a Nd:YAG laser. The patient is 180 cm tall (5′11″) and weighs 122 kg (270 lb), with a body mass index (BMI) of 37.7. The patient states that he snores quite a bit at night and was advised to use a continuous positive airway pressure (CPAP) device, but he rarely does so because he does not like the noise or the fit of the mask. He admits to occasional daytime somnolence.

1. Optimally, when and where should this case be scheduled?

   A. Early in the day and only in the main operating room of a general hospital.
   B. Early in the day and either at the ambulatory or main operating room.
   C. Later in the day and only in the main operating room of a general hospital.
   D. Later in the day and either at the ambulatory or main operating room.

The correct answer is B. If an obstructive sleep apnea (OSA) patient undergoes a surgical procedure under local anesthesia in an ambulatory setting, no special planning is needed. However, for such patients undergoing sedation or general anesthesia, the outpatient surgery facility should have difficult airway and respiratory care equipment immediately available, as well as radiology and clinical laboratory facilities. Prior to discharge, the patient should be observed to be free of hypoxemic or airway obstruction episodes in the recovery area. Most experts agree that recovery of patients with OSA takes an average of 3 h longer than in patients without OSA. Monitoring should take place for a median of 7 h after the last episode of airway obstruction or desaturation while breathing room air. Patients with OSA can safely undergo procedures in any setting appropriate for non-OSA patients, provided that the above support systems exist. Given the amount of time needed for recovery and monitoring, the procedure would most conveniently be performed earlier in the day.

2. What factor makes this case a high risk for a surgical fire?

A. The surgical site is anatomically above the level of the xiphoid, and the patient is scheduled for MAC.
B. The patient has a BMI greater than 30 and a procedure scheduled in an ambulatory surgery center.
C. The patient is having facial surgery performed at an ambulatory surgery center versus at an inpatient facility.
D. The patient will likely require CPAP during the course of care.

The correct answer is A. Fire risk is increased when the anatomic site is superior to the xiphoid or the fifth thoracic vertebra, when there is open delivery of oxygen, and when an ignition source is used. Although more fires are reported at ambulatory care facilities, this is related to the open delivery of oxygen during MAC cases and not to the facility itself. Neither CPAP use nor increased BMI is a specific fire risk; however, the use of open delivery of oxygen is more common for OSA and ambulatory surgery patients, and the open delivery of oxygen increases the risk of fire in any population.

3. What entity establishes the standards for operating room laser safety in the United States?

A. U.S. Food and Drug Administration (FDA).
B. National Fire Protection Agency (NFPA).
C. Association for the Advancement of Medical Instrumentation (AAMI).
D. American National Standards Institute (ANSI).

The correct answer is D. The ANSI establishes the standards for laser safety for all laser devices in the United States. The U.S. FDA enforces laws relating to medical devices and regulates the design of certain laser devices that could be harmful if used improperly. The NFPA is an international trade organization that establishes fire and life-safety codes for facilities, including health care facilities. The AAMI is a private organization that assists both developers and end-users in the development, management, and safe and effective use of medical technology. Although each of the listed organizations addresses medical lasers, only the ANSI establishes safety standards for operating room lasers in the United States.

4. The wavelength of the laser must be listed on which of the following?

A. On signs posted at the entryway to the operating room.
B. On laser goggles.

C. On the laser device.

D. All of the above.

The correct answer is D. To ensure protection specific to the type and wavelength of the laser used, signage that includes the laser wavelength must be present on the device, on each entryway to the room where the laser will be in use, and on the goggles/glasses used for laser protection. Laser-associated eye injury can be avoided by always confirming that the protective goggles provided are appropriate for the laser type being used.

You and the surgeon agree that the optimal anesthetic is sedation with local anesthesia under MAC, given the superficial nature of the lesion and the patient's marked obesity and OSA. Standard American Society of Anesthesiologists (ASA) monitors are applied, including end-tidal carbon dioxide ($ETCO_2$) monitoring via an integrated port in the nasal cannula. Oxygen at 4 L/min is initiated.

The circulating nurse uses a 26-mL chlorhexidine/alcohol applicator to prepare the surgical site, taking great care not to introduce the solution into the patient's eye or ear. Three minutes of drying time elapse before the surgical drapes are applied. The applicator is discarded in the trash pail in the operating room (OR).

5. Which of the following statements is true concerning the use of alcohol-based prep solutions?

A. Any size of prefilled surgical skin preparation applicator is appropriate for head-and-neck surgery cases.

B. A total of 3 min is adequate drying time for all alcohol-based surgical skin preparation agents.

C. A 26-mL chlorohexidine/alcohol applicator is specifically prohibited by the FDA for use in head-and-neck cases.

D. Iodine-based and alcohol-based surgical skin preparation agents are equally flammable, especially when a high concentration of oxygen is present.

The correct answer is C. The FDA package insert for alcohol-based skin preparation agents prohibits the use of the 26-mL-size applicator for head-and-neck surgical cases. Although a total of 3 min is usually sufficient for drying time, longer drying times are recommended when excess skin folds, large surface areas, or excessive hair are present. Iodine-based skin preparation solutions, such as betadine, are not flammable.

The surgeon infiltrates the surgical site with a local anesthetic, and you administer 100 mcg of fentanyl IV and initiate a propofol infusion at 100 mcg/kg/min IV. The patient moves on incision, so you administer an additional 50 mcg of fentanyl IV and increase the propofol infusion rate to 125 mcg/kg/min. Subsequently, the oxygen saturation drops to 91%; you increase the oxygen flow to 6 L/min and initiate a jaw thrust. SpO_2 increases to 98%, and the snoring stops.

6. Which of the following is the best course of action with regard to this patient's airway, considering the surgical fire risk?

A. Switch to a nonrebreather-style mask and continue with the case.
B. Abort the procedure and awaken the patient.
C. Control the airway by placement of an endotracheal tube or supraglottic airway device.
D. Continue with nasal cannula oxygen administration, but lower the flow to less than 2 L/min.

The correct answer is C. Options A and D both create a high risk for surgical fire due to the open delivery of 100% oxygen. Although option B would eliminate fire risk, the patient still has other anesthesia-related risks, and by aborting the procedure, the patient has assumed those risks without the benefit of the therapy being completed. In addition, the patient requires additional airway maneuvers that may need to be continued into the recovery period. Oxygenation and ventilation will be improved by controlling the airway with a supraglottic airway device or endotracheal tube, and the risk of fire will be greatly decreased because oxygen will be delivered via a closed system.

When the surgeon activates the laser, there is a loud "pop" followed by a visible flash over the patient's face, and flames erupt and begin to burn the surgical drapes, melting the nasal cannula to the patient's face and nose. In less than 3 s, the patient has sustained second- and third-degree burns to the face, nose, mouth, trachea, and back of the head. The OR smells like burnt plastic, and the patient is in significant pain. You intubate the patient, give more IV opiates, and arrange to transfer the patient to a burn unit for further evaluation.

While you continue to attend to the patient, the surgeon speaks to the patient's family, and they became irate and leave before you can finish speaking with them. Six months later, the patient's attorney sends you a notice of intent to sue. The letter states that the basis of the patient's injury was the failure of the anesthesiologist to communicate with the surgeon with respect to the concentration of oxygen in the surgical field. They also imply that there were no documented steps to mitigate the fire risk by you or the OR team.

7. One of the most effective means of disclosing a medical error to the family is by which of the following?

A. Beginning with a heartfelt apology, telling the family or patient you are sorry for what happened.
B. Discussing first with a risk-management or legal representative how to disclose this event to the patient and family.
C. Allowing only one involved provider to interact and engage with the patient or family.
D. Avoiding any admission of error that could be documented and used in the litigation process.

The correct answer is A. Apology and conveyance of empathy have been shown to place victims of medical error and their families at ease and hasten the acceptance and resolution of issues surrounding the event. Many states have created statutes protecting medical providers who offer sincere apologies, deeming such an apology a gesture of empathy and not an admission of negligent behavior. Although early consultation with risk-management and legal personnel is nearly always a good idea (and indeed may be a requirement of your liability policy), risk managers may advise practices that place care providers in a defensive position against the patient and their family. One of the best approaches for conveying bad news is to approach the family as a team, introducing each member of the team and describing their specific role in the care of the patient. Often, the patient and family members are surprised by the number of individuals who have actually provided care for the patient in the time of crisis. Also, a team-based review of the event with the patient and family may avoid a shift of blame to a party who may not be present. Often the underlying reason for medical litigation is that the patient or family never felt that the health care institution or provider(s) ever admitted error or acknowledged the adverse effects of the event. Many plaintiffs state that the motivation for their suit is to prevent such errors from being repeated.

DID YOU LEARN?

- The anesthetic and perioperative implications for caring for the patient with OSA.
- Risk factors for surgical fires, and how to mitigate the risk of fire by recognition of these factors.
- The agencies and organizations responsible for laser safety and their standards regarding the use of medical lasers in the United States.
- The recommendations for the safe use of alcohol-based surgical prep solutions.
- The hazards of the open delivery of oxygen related to surgical fire risk.
- The importance of disclosure of errors to patients and family members, and how including an apology may affect the patient and their family.

Recommended Reading

Cowles CE. The operating room environment. In: Butterworth IV JF, Mackey DC, Wasnick JD, eds. *Morgan & Mikhail's Clinical Anesthesiology*. 6th ed. New York, NY: McGraw-Hill Education; 2018:9-32.

References

Apfelbaum JL, Caplan RA, Barker SJ; American Society of Anesthesiologists Task Force on Operating Room Fires. Practice advisory for the prevention and management of operating room fires: An updated report by the American Society of Anesthesiologists Task Force on Operating Room Fires. *Anesthesiology*. 2013;118(2):271-290.

Boothman RC. Apologies and a strong defense at the University of Michigan Health System. *Physician Exec*. 2006;32(2):7-10.

Gallagher T, Studdert D, Levinson W. Disclosing harmful medical errors to patients. *N Engl J Med*. 2007;356:2713-2719.

Gross JB, Bachenberg KL, Benumof JL; American Society of Anesthesiologists Task Force on Perioperative Management of Patients with Obstructive Sleep Apnea. Practice guidelines for the perioperative management of patients with obstructive sleep apnea. *Anesthesiology*. 2006;104(5):1081-1093.

Kelz RR, Freeman KM, Hosokawa PW, et al. Time of day is associated with postoperative morbidity: An analysis of the National Surgical Quality Improvement Program Data. *Ann Surg*. 2008;247(3):544-552.

Kraman SS, Hamm G. Risk management: Extreme honesty may the best policy. *Ann Int Med*. 1999;131(12):963-967.

Stoelting RK, Feldman JM, Cowles CE, Bruley ME. Surgical fire injuries continue to occur: Prevention may require more cautious use of oxygen. *APSF Newsletter*. 2012;26(3):41-43.

Wojcieszak D, Banda J, Houk C. The sorry works! Coalition: Making the case for full disclosure. *J Qual Pt Safety*. 2006;32:344-450.

CHAPTER 3

Breathing Systems

CASE 1 | Child for Myringotomy

Clayton Adams, MD, and Mukesh Wadhwa, DO

A 15-kg, 3-year-old boy who was born at 38 weeks' gestation presents for bilateral myringotomy tube placement for treatment of chronic ear infections. An inhalational induction with sevoflurane and spontaneous ventilation are planned.

1. Which breathing circuit would be optimal?

   A. Mapleson A type.
   B. Bain.
   C. Mapleson D type.
   D. None of the above.

The correct answer is A. The relative location of the components in Mapleson circuits determines circuit performance. The Mapleson A circuit is the method of choice for inhalation induction with spontaneous ventilation. The adjustable pressure-limiting (APL) valve in the Mapleson A circuit is located near the face mask, and the reservoir bag is located at the opposite end of the circuit. During spontaneous ventilation, alveolar gas containing carbon dioxide (CO_2) will be exhaled into the breathing tube or directly vented through an open APL valve. Before the next inhalation occurs, if the fresh gas flow equals or exceeds alveolar minute ventilation, the inflow of fresh gas will force the alveolar gas remaining in the breathing tube to exit from the APL valve. Changing the position of the APL valve and the fresh gas inlet transforms a Mapleson A into a Mapleson D circuit. The Mapleson D circuit is efficient during controlled ventilation, since fresh gas flow forces alveolar air away from the patient and toward the APL valve. The Bain circuit is a coaxial version of the Mapleson D circuit that incorporates the fresh gas inlet tubing inside the breathing tube. Its advantage is better conservation of heat and humidity than a conventional Mapleson D circuit as a result of partial warming of the inspiratory gas by countercurrent exchange.

2. Which of the following is *not* an advantage of Mapleson circuits over a circle system?

A. Mapleson circuits allow for increased portability.
B. The unidirectional valves of a Mapleson system decrease resistance.
C. Mapleson circuits are less expensive.
D. Mapleson circuits provide a lower work of breathing.

The correct answer is B. Mapleson circuits provide the benefits of portability and cost-effectiveness when compared to circle systems. The disadvantage of Mapleson circuits is that high fresh gas flows are required to prevent rebreathing. Circle systems allow low fresh gas flows, resulting in less waste of anesthetic agent, less pollution of the environment, and minimal loss of patient heat and humidity. The disadvantages of circle systems include unidirectional valves and CO_2 absorbers, which increase flow resistance and the work of breathing.

3. Which of the following is the most reliable ventilation management to prevent rebreathing of exhaled CO_2?

A. Controlled ventilation through a circle system with fresh gas flow equal to half of minute ventilation.
B. Controlled ventilation through a Mapleson A circuit with fresh gas flow equal to minute ventilation.
C. Spontaneous ventilation through a Mapleson D circuit with fresh gas flow equal to half of minute ventilation.
D. Spontaneous ventilation through a Mapleson A circuit with fresh gas flow equal to half of minute ventilation.

The correct answer is A. Circle systems can use very low flow states safely without concern for rebreathing of CO_2 gas because they actively scavenge CO_2 using CO_2 absorbers. Mapleson circuits require relatively high fresh gas flows to prevent rebreathing. The relative location of the components in Mapleson circuits determines circuit performance. The Mapleson A circuit is the method of choice for inhalation induction with spontaneous ventilation. During spontaneous ventilation, if the fresh gas flow equals or exceeds alveolar minute ventilation, the inflow of fresh gas will force the alveolar gas remaining in the breathing tube to exit from the APL valve. Positive pressure during controlled ventilation, however, requires a partially closed APL valve. Thus, high fresh gas flows (greater than three times minute ventilation) are required to prevent rebreathing with a Mapleson A circuit during controlled ventilation. Changing the position of the APL valve and the fresh gas inlet transforms a Mapleson A into a Mapleson D circuit. The Mapleson D circuit is efficient during controlled ventilation, since fresh gas flow forces alveolar air *away* from the patient and *toward* the APL valve. Spontaneous ventilation in Mapleson D circuit requires two to three times the rate of minute ventilation rate to prevent rebreathing.

Classification and Characteristics of Mapleson Circuits

Mapleson Class	Other Names	Configuration[1]	Required Fresh Gas Flows		Comments
			Spontaneous	Controlled	
A	Magill attachment	FGI → Breathing tube / APL valve / Breathing bag / Mask	Equal to minute ventilation ($\approx$ 80 mL/kg/min)	Very high and difficult to predict	Poor choice during controlled ventilation. Enclosed Magill system is a modification that improves efficiency. Coaxial Mapleson A (Lack breathing system) provides waste gas scavenging.
B		FGI / APL valve	2 × minute ventilation	2–2½ × minute ventilation	
C	Waters' to-and-fro	FGI / APL valve	2 × minute ventilation	2–2½ × minute ventilation	
D	Bain circuit	APL valve / FGI	2–3 × minute ventilation	1–2 × minute ventilation	Bain coaxial modification: fresh gas tube inside breathing tube.
E	Ayre's T-piece	FGI	2–3 × minute ventilation	3 × minute ventilation (I:E =1:2)	Exhalation tubing should provide a larger volume than tidal volume to prevent rebreathing. Scavenging is difficult.
F	Jackson-Rees[1] modification	APL valve / FGI	2–3 × minute ventilation	2 × minute ventilation	A Mapleson E with a breathing bag connected to the end of the breathing tube to allow controlled ventilation and scavenging.

[1]FGI, fresh gas inlet; APL, adjustable pressure-limiting (valve).

Reproduced with permission from Butterworth JF, Mackey DC, Wasnick JD: *Morgan and Mikhail's Clinical Anesthesiology*, 6th ed. New York, NY: McGraw-Hill Education; 2018.

DID YOU LEARN?

- Advantages/disadvantages of Mapleson circuits and circle circuit system.
- Relationship between minute ventilation and fresh gas flow in Mapleson circuits.
- Use of Mapleson circuits in spontaneous versus controlled ventilation.

CASE 2   Hypercapnia during Laparoscopy

Chase Clanton, MD

A healthy 30-year-old woman weighing 60 kg undergoes a laparoscopic cholecystectomy. She has undergone general anesthesia previously for arthroscopic knee surgery. There are no previous issues involving anesthesia either with her or in her family.

1. The patient is ventilated using volume control mode set at a respiratory rate of 12 breaths/min, tidal volume of 450 mL, I:E ratio of 1:2, and no positive end-expiratory pressure (PEEP). Twenty minutes after the start of surgery, a sustained increase in end-tidal CO_2 to 48 mm Hg is seen on the capnograph. Vital signs are stable. What is the *most* likely cause?

    A. Hyperalimentation.
    B. Malignant hyperthermia (MH).
    C. Hyperthyroidism.
    D. Increased absorption of CO_2 from CO_2 insufflation.

The correct answer is D. Based on the history that this is a healthy patient with stable vital signs, the most likely cause of a sustained increase in end-tidal CO_2 is increased CO_2 absorption from CO_2 insufflation utilized to create a pneumoperitoneum for the laparoscopic procedure. An increase in end-tidal CO_2 suggests either an increase in metabolic rate that exceeds ventilation or a decrease in CO_2 elimination. Febrile state, MH, hyperalimentation, and hyperthyroidism increase CO_2 production. Extreme hypermetabolism from uncontrolled muscle contraction occurs during MH. Tachycardia, acidosis, and rigidity are additional signs of MH in susceptible patients following administration of an MH-triggering agent such as a halogenated anesthetic. An increase in patient temperature is a late sign of MH. There is no indication of other signs of MH in this patient; however, MH should not be immediately dismissed from the differential diagnosis. There is no history of hyperalimentation resulting in an increased production of CO_2. Likewise, the patient does not have a history of hyperthyroidism or sepsis.

Hypoventilation decreases CO_2 elimination. Failure to adequately eliminate CO_2 (due to a depleted CO_2 absorber) from the breathing circuit results in rebreathing of CO_2. Rebreathing occurs when there is insufficient fresh gas flow or incompetent unidirectional valves in the breathing circuit, as well as when the capacity of the CO_2 absorber is exhausted.

2. Looking at the capnograph below, what is the *most* likely cause of the increased inspired CO_2 40 min after the start of surgery?

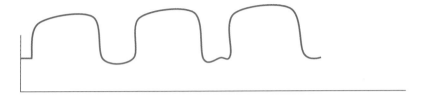

A. Exhausted CO_2 absorber.
B. Fresh gas flow at 2 L/min in circle system.
C. Capnograph artifact (water in sampling cell).
D. Leak in inspiratory limb of circle system.

The correct answer is A. The most likely cause of an increase in inspiratory CO_2 is an exhausted CO_2 absorber or a malfunctioning unidirectional valve. In a circle system, a fresh gas flow of 2 L/min is adequate to prevent rebreathing CO_2. A capnogram displays a patient's CO_2 concentration sampled at the airway during ventilation on a continuous concentration versus time plot. The first phase represents the initiation of expiration, which reflects the anatomic dead space that contains no CO_2. Alveolar gas then enters the airway shown by the upstroke. An expiratory plateau is reached and the end-tidal CO_2 concentration is taken at the peak. In the final phase, inspiration occurs, and fresh gas washes away the CO_2. Adding 5 mm Hg to the end-tidal CO_2 to account for alveolar dead space ventilation provides a good estimate of $PaCO_2$ assuming no pulmonary pathology.

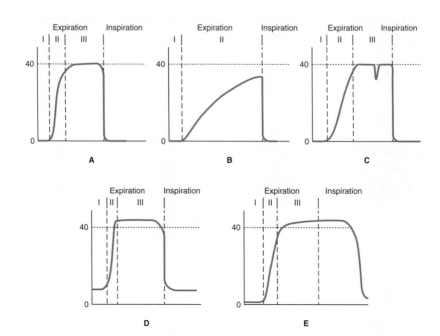

A. Normal capnograph demonstrating the three phases of expiration: phase I—dead space; phase II—mixture of dead space and alveolar gas; phase III—alveolar gas plateau. **B.** Capnograph of a patient with severe chronic obstructive pulmonary disease. No plateau is reached before the next inspiration. The gradient between end-tidal CO_2 and arterial CO_2 is increased. **C.** Depression during phase III indicates spontaneous respiratory effort. **D.** Failure of the inspired CO_2 to return to zero may represent an incompetent expiratory valve or exhausted CO_2 absorbent. **E.** The persistence of exhaled gas during part of the inspiratory cycle signals the presence of an incompetent inspiratory valve.

3. Next day, you arrive in the morning to prepare for the scheduled cases. You check the anesthesia machine and it passes all tests. Twenty minutes into a case involving general anesthesia, the CO_2 absorber's color changes from white to mostly purple. What are some of the changes seen on capnograph?

    A. Decreased end-tidal CO_2.
    B. Increased inspiratory CO_2.
    C. A decrease in both end-tidal CO_2 and inspiratory CO_2.
    D. None of the above.

The correct answer is B. The CO_2 absorber is exhausted, which results in the rebreathing of CO_2. Rebreathing will cause an increase, not a decrease, in end-tidal CO_2 and inspiratory CO_2. A pH indicator dye such as ethyl violet changes color from white to purple as the absorber is exhausted and hydrogen ion concentration increases.

4. Which of the following is true of Compound A?

A. It has been proven to cause nephrotoxicity in humans.
B. Compound A results from the degradation of desflurane.
C. It is found to be harmful in rats.
D. All of the above.

The correct answer is C. Dry barium hydroxide lime, increased respiratory gas temperatures, low-flow anesthesia, high sevoflurane concentrations, and anesthetics of long duration are known to favor Compound A formation, a sevoflurane by-product that is nephrotoxic in rats. Desflurane, more than any other volatile anesthetic, undergoes degradation by dry CO_2 absorbents to produce carbon monoxide (CO). CO has a very high affinity for hemoglobin, potentially producing CO poisoning.

DID YOU LEARN?

- Factors responsible for increased end-tidal CO_2.
- Factors responsible for increased inspiratory CO_2.
- Physiologic basis of color change for CO_2 absorbent dye indicators and its significance.
- Factors leading to Compound A and CO formation from volatile anesthetics.

Recommended Readings

Butterworth IV JF, Mackey DC, Wasnick JD, eds. Breathing systems. In: *Morgan & Mikhail's Clinical Anesthesiology.* 6th ed. New York, NY: McGraw-Hill Education; 2018:33-46.
Dobson MB. Anaesthesia for difficult locations—developing countries and military conflicts. In: Prys-Roberts C, Brown BR, eds. *International Practice of Anaesthesia.* Oxford, United Kingdom: Butterworth Heinemann; 1996.
Dorsch JA, Dorsch SE. *Understanding Anesthesia Equipment.* 5th ed. Philadelphia, PA: Lippincott, Williams & Wilkins; 2008.
Gegel B. A field expedient Ohmeda Universal Portable Anesthesia Complete Draw-over vaporizer setup. *AANA J.* 2008;76:185.
Rose G, McLarney JT. *Anesthesia Equipment Simplified.* New York, NY: McGraw-Hill; 2014.

CHAPTER 4

The Anesthesia Workstation

CASE 1 Anesthesia for Trauma Surgery

Ashraf N. Farag, MD, and Cooper W. Phillips, MD

A 45-year-old man requires emergent surgery for multiple stab wounds to the abdomen. Past medical history is significant for placement of a drug-eluting stent in the left anterior descending coronary artery. Vital signs include blood pressure 80/50 mm Hg, heart rate 120 beats/min, and respiratory rate 30 breaths/min. The patient is uncooperative and combative. One IV catheter remains functional.

1. Rapid sequence induction is successful with ketamine and succinylcholine. However, after connecting the patient to the anesthesia machine, the anesthetist cannot generate positive pressure. The differential diagnosis of the leak includes:

   A. A low-pressure circuit disconnect.
   B. Adjustable pressure-limiting valve closed.
   C. A torn endotracheal cuff.
   D. Both A and C.
   E. Both B and C.

The correct answer is D. Failure to adequately check the anesthesia machine is an all-too-common error that constitutes a breach in the standard of care. Whenever fresh gas flow is insufficient to replace the volume of gas lost through a leak and through gas uptake, the breathing bag will collapse and positive-pressure ventilation will not be possible. When there is a leak, the circuit should be traced from the endotracheal tube back to the anesthesia machine. Leaks often occur at connections in the breathing circuit or as a consequence of an inadequately inflated tracheal tube cuff. Machine leaks routinely occur at the base plate of the carbon dioxide (CO_2) absorber when the absorbent canisters are incorrectly seated in the machine. In patients with bronchopleural fistulae treated by thoracostomy tube, anesthetic gases may escape through the chest tube during positive-pressure ventilation. A closed, adjustable pressure-limiting valve will not contribute to gas loss and is not included in the differential diagnosis of an anesthetic gas leak.

2. The source of the leak cannot be found. The next most appropriate course of action is to:

A. Call for help and wake up the patient.
B. Remove the endotracheal tube and mask ventilate.
C. Provide a 100% oxygen concentration at maximal flow and use apneic oxygenation while another anesthesia machine is located.
D. Disconnect the anesthesia machine, and use a resuscitation breathing bag to ventilate the patient with 100% oxygen.

The correct answer is D. All anesthetizing locations should be equipped with a resuscitation breathing bag to provide positive-pressure ventilation in the event of machine failure. Calling for help is always a good suggestion, but there is no immediate need to awaken the patient. A replacement anesthesia machine can be identified, or the procedure can continue using total intravenous anesthesia (TIVA) if medically acceptable. Apneic oxygenation is oxygen insufflation at a rate greater than oxygen consumption. Ultimately, apneic oxygenation is inadequate as CO_2 tension continues to rise. Moreover, if there is a leak in the system, it is unclear if 100% oxygen would be available to the patient, depending upon the unidentified source of the system leak. Mask ventilation is not necessary assuming the endotracheal tube is intact. Although a replacement anesthesia machine is required, delivery would likely take too long to be a first course of action in this setting.

3. A replacement anesthesia machine is obtained and fluid resuscitation is instituted. The surgeon reports that the abdomen is distended and there is likely a requirement for mass blood transfusion. This patient likely manifests which hemorrhage classification according to the American College of Surgeons (ACS)?

A. Class I hemorrhage.
B. Class II hemorrhage.
C. Class lll hemorrhage.
D. Class IV hemorrhage.

The correct answer is C. The ACS identifies four classes of hemorrhage. Class I hemorrhage is the volume of blood that can be lost without hemodynamic consequence. This is generally less than 15% of the blood volume. Class II hemorrhage is the blood volume that, when lost, prompts a sympathetic response (15–30% blood-volume loss). Heart rate and diastolic pressure increase as a consequence of compensatory vasoconstriction. Class III hemorrhage represents the loss of up to 40% of the blood volume, resulting in inadequate oxygen delivery to tissues and metabolic acidosis. Class IV hemorrhage represents a life-threatening loss of more than 40% of the blood volume. The patient is profoundly hypotensive and unresponsive. This patient remains responsive and is not profoundly hypotensive. Nonetheless, activation of massive transfusion protocol is indicated.

4. A thromboelastograph (TEG) is employed to assist in management of blood component therapy. Of the TEG graphs below, which is consistent with hypocoagulation?

A. Graph A.
B. Graph B.
C. Graph C.
D. Graph D.

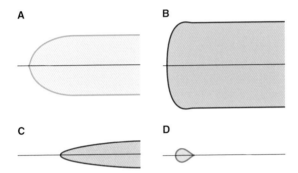

(Reproduced with permission from Johansson PI, Stissing T, Bochsen L, et al. Thrombelastography and thromboelastometry in assessing coagulopathy in trauma. *Scand J Trauma Resusc Emerg Med.* 2009 Sep 23:17:45.)

The correct answer is C. Tissue hypoperfusion leads to the development of a trauma-induced coagulopathy. During hypoperfusion, the endothelium releases thrombomodulin and activated protein C to prevent microcirculation thrombosis. Thrombomodulin binds to thrombin, thereby preventing thrombin from cleaving fibrinogen to fibrin. Protein C inhibits the extrinsic coagulation pathway and likewise inhibits plasminogen activator inhibitors, resulting in increased fibrinolysis. TEG provides a quick assessment of the patient's coagulation state. Graph A is a normal tracing; graph B represents hypercoagulation; graph C indicates a hypocoagulable state; and graph D represents fibrinolysis. The TEG begins as a straight line until clot is formed, reflecting the enzymatic stage of clotting. As the clot develops, the pattern of the graph identifies the components of the clot. The *alpha angle* is reflective of fibrinogen and the maximum amplitude (MA) of platelet contribution to the clot.

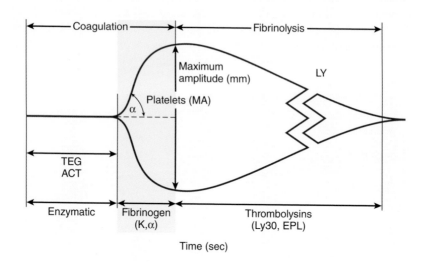

(Reproduced with permission from Kashuk JL, Moore EE, Sawyer M, et al. Postinjury coagulopathy management: Goal directed resuscitation via POC thrombelastography. *Ann Surg.* 2010 Apr;251(4):604-614.)

5. The patient requires transfusion before typed blood can be identified. Which antibodies/antigens are present in type O negative blood?

   A. Anti-A, anti-B antibody.
   B. A antigen, B antigen.
   C. RhD antigen.
   D. A antigen and RhD antigen.

The correct answer is A. Blood is typed according to the presence or absence of A or B red cell-surface antigens. Type A blood has A antigen. Type B blood has B antigen. Type AB blood has both surface antigens, and type O blood has neither. Antibodies are produced against those antigens that are missing. Hence, type O blood would contain anti-A and anti-B antibodies in the serum. The majority of patients are RhD-positive, meaning they possess the RhD surface antigen. Rh-negative patients lack the surface antigen. Unlike the ABO groups, patients missing the Rh surface antigen do not form antibodies spontaneously to antigens that they do not possess. Only after Rh-positive transfusion or sensitization (where an Rh-negative mother develops antibodies against an Rh-positive baby) do antibodies form. After multiple units (>8) of O blood are administered, it is advised to continue resuscitation with this blood type and not return to the patient's actual typed blood as it becomes available.

The patient undergoes damage-control surgery and the abdominal cavity is packed under a wound vacuum. The patient is transported to the ICU and develops the following vital signs: blood pressure 50/20 mm Hg and heart rate 30 beats/min. The patient is on mechanical ventilation. Oxygen saturation is undetected. An ECG is obtained while epinephrine is administered.

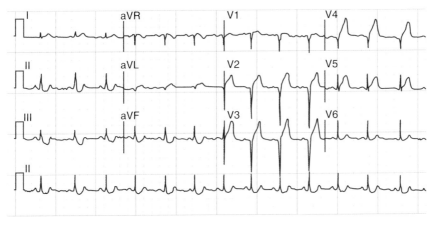

(Reproduced from Jameson JL, Fauci AS, Kasper DL, et al: *Harrison's Principles of Internal Medicine*, 20th ed. New York, NY: McGraw-Hill Education; 2018.)

6. The patient's ECG demonstrates:

A. Atrial fibrillation.
B. Myocardial infarction.
C. Wolff–Parkinson–White syndrome.
D. Ventricular tachycardia.

The correct answer is B. This patient had a previous drug-eluting stent in the left anterior descending artery. During the course of resuscitation, he received numerous agents to improve coagulation. Unfortunately, the stent may have occluded, now producing left ventricular dysfunction and cardiogenic shock. Options are limited. Catheterization could open the occluded vessel; however, the anticoagulation required might further increase postoperative bleeding. Inotropic support and balloon counterpulsation could be employed to improve ventricular function. Ultimately, revascularization is the ideal treatment for the patient with acute myocardial infarction perioperatively, assuming that the patient can survive the anticoagulation necessary to perform the procedure.

DID YOU LEARN?

- Response to anesthesia machine failure.
- Classes of hemorrhage.
- Identification of TEG.

Recommended Readings

Baum JA, Nunn G. *Low Flow Anaesthesia: The Theory and Practice of Low Flow, Minimal Flow and Closed System Anaesthesia*. 2nd ed. Oxford, United Kingdom: Butterworth Heinemann; 2001.

Block FE, Schaff C. Auditory alarms during anesthesia monitoring with an integrated monitoring system. *Int J Clin Monit Comput*. 1996;13:81.

Butterworth IV JF, Mackey DC, Wasnick JD, eds. The anesthesia workstation. In: *Morgan & Mikhail's Clinical Anesthesiology*. 6th ed. New York, NY: McGraw-Hill Education; 2018:47-80.

Caplan RA, Vistica MF, Posner KL, Cheney FW. Adverse anesthetic outcomes arising from gas delivery equipment: A closed claims analysis. *Anesthesiology*. 1997;87:741.

Dorsch JA, Dorsch SE. *Understanding Anesthesia Equipment*. 5th ed. Philadelphia, PA: Lippincott, Williams & Wilkins; 2008.

Eisenkraft JB, Leibowitz AB. Ventilators in the operating room. *Int Anesthesiol Clin*. 1997;35:87.

Klopfenstein CE, Van Gessel E, Forster A. Checking the anaesthetic machine: Self-reported assessment in a university hospital. *Eur J Anaesthesiol*. 1998;15:314.

Mehta S, Eisenkraft J, Posner K, Domino K. Patient injuries from anesthesia gas delivery equipment. *Anesthesiology*. 2013;119:788.

Rose G, McLarnery J, eds. *Anesthesia Equipment Simplified*. New York, NY: McGraw-Hill Education; 2014.

Somprakit P, Soontranan P. Low pressure leakage in anaesthetic machines: Evaluation by positive and negative pressure tests. *Anaesthesia*. 1996;51:461.

CHAPTER 5
Cardiovascular Monitoring

CASE 1 Echocardiographic Evaluation of a Patient with Ischemic Bowel

Elizabeth R. Rivas, MD

A 75-year-old man presents for emergent resection of ischemic bowel. His past medical history includes systolic heart failure (ejection fraction 20%) assessed during a recent transesophageal echocardiography (TEE) examination. At the time, he was noted to have left ventricular anterior wall akinesis.

1. In the diagram below, which ventricular walls are primarily supplied by branches of the left anterior descending artery?

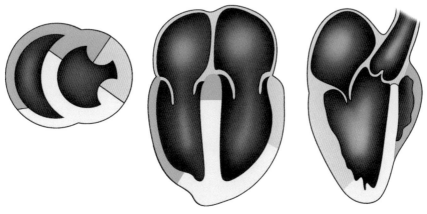

(Reproduced with permission from Butterworth JF, Mackey DC, Wasnick JD: *Morgan and Mikhail's Clinical Anesthesiology*, 6th ed. New York, NY: McGraw-Hill Education; 2018.)

   A. Green-shaded walls.
   B. Blue-shaded walls.
   C. Pink-shaded walls.
   D. No walls displayed are supplied by the left anterior descending artery.

The correct answer is B. The left anterior descending artery supplies blood primarily to the blue-shaded areas. Areas of ischemia can appear hypokinetic, akinetic, or dyskinetic on echocardiographic examination.

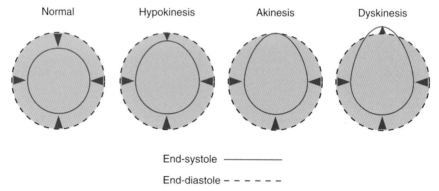

| Normal | Hypokinesis | Akinesis | Dyskinesis |

End-systole ————————

End-diastole – – – – – –

(Reproduced with permission frm Butterworth JF, Mackey DC, Wasnick JD: *Morgan and Mikhail's Clinical Anesthesiology,* 6th ed. New York, NY: McGraw-Hill Education; 2018.)

Upon further review of the previous TEE examination, pulse-wave Doppler of the mitral valve inflow was completed, as shown in the next figure.

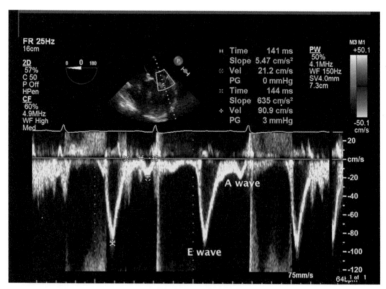

(Reproduced with permission from Wasnick J, Hillel Z, Kramer D, et al. *Cardiac Anesthesia & Transesophageal Echocardiography.* New York, NY: McGraw-Hill; 2011.)

2. This pattern is most consistent with:

A. Normal diastolic filling.
B. Pseudonormal diastolic filling.
C. Restrictive diastolic filling.
D. Impaired diastolic relaxation.

The correct answer is C. Systolic heart failure is characterized by low ejection fraction (stroke volume/end-diastolic volume). Diastolic *dysfunction* routinely occurs in association with hypertension, aortic stenosis, or systolic heart *failure*; however, diastolic heart *failure* can also occur despite preserved ventricular systolic function. When the heart fails to relax, early filling, characterized by the E-wave, predominates. Atrial contraction fails to significantly augment diastolic filling in late diastole because of impaired ventricular compliance. Patterns of diastolic impairment progress from normal, impaired relaxation, pseudonormal, up to restrictive. When left-ventricular relaxation is delayed initially, the initial pressure gradient between the left atrium and left ventricle is reduced, resulting in a decline in early filling and consequently a reduced peak E-wave velocity. The E/A ratio is reduced. As diastolic dysfunction advances, the left-atrial pressure increases, restoring the gradient between the left atrium and the left ventricle with an apparent restoration of the normal E/A ratio of 0.8 to 1.2. As diastolic dysfunction continues to worsen, the pressure in the atrium builds, resulting in a dramatic peak in early filling with an E/A ratio of greater than 2:1.

Tissue Doppler studies examine the movement of the myocardium at the lateral annulus of the mitral valve. During systole, the heart contracts toward the apex, away from the TEE probe in the esophagus. Movement away from the probe is usually characterized as a negative deflection below the baseline. During diastolic filling, the heart moves toward the probe in the esophagus, resulting in a positive deflection. The e′ and a′ waves reflect the movement of the lateral annulus during early and late diastolic filling, respectively. The pseudonormal pattern is not seen in tissue Doppler. The e′ velocity continues to decrease as diastolic dysfunction progresses. These patterns are demonstrated in the below figure.

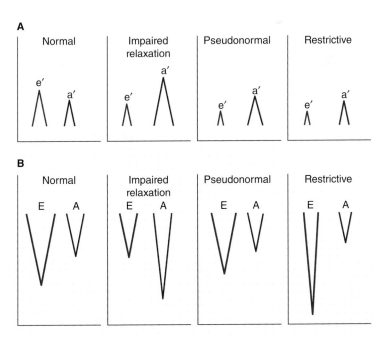

(Reproduced with permission from Wasnick JD, Hillel Z, Kramer D, et al. *Cardiac Anesthesia & Transesophageal Echocardiography.* New York, NY: McGraw-Hill Education; 2011.)

The following finding was also noted on color Doppler.

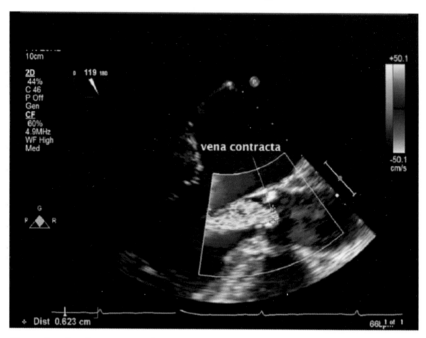

(Reproduced with permission from Wasnick J, Hillel Z, Kramer D, et al. *Cardiac Anesthesia & Transesophageal Echocardiography*. New York, NY: McGraw-Hill; 2011.)

3. This image is most consistent with the diagnosis of:

A. Severe aortic stenosis.
B. Severe mitral stenosis.
C. Severe aortic insufficiency.
D. Mild aortic insufficiency.

The correct answer is C. This is the aortic valve long-axis view. Color-flow Doppler is employed, demonstrating a regurgitant jet during diastole. The vena contracta represents the narrow part of the jet, which here is measured at 0.623 cm, consistent with severe aortic regurgitation. The normal views on TEE can be found in the following figure.

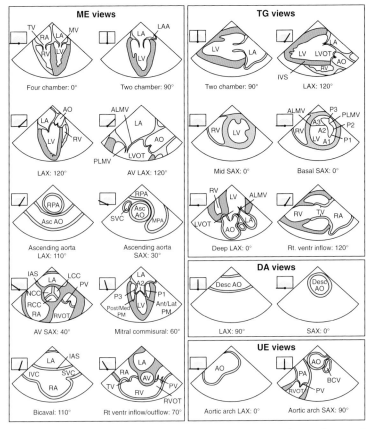

The views have been grouped together based upon the location in the esophagus where they are obtained, upper esophageal (UE), middle esophageal (ME), transgastric (TG), and descending aortic (DA). Major cardiac structures are labeled including:

right atrium (RA)
left atrium (LA)
mitral valve (MV)
tricuspid valve (TV)
right ventricle (RV)
left ventricle (LV)
left atrial appendage (LAA)
aorta (AO)
anterior leaflet of the mitral valve
  (ALMV)
posterior leaflet of the mitral valve
  (PLMV)
ascending aorta (Asc AO)
right pulmonary artery (RPA)
superior vena cava (SVC)
main pulmonary artery (MPA)
intra atrial septum (IAS)

pulmonic valve (PV)
right ventricular outflow tract (RVOT)
non-coronary cusp of the aortic valve (NCC)
right coronary cusp of the aortic valve (RCC)
left coronary cusp of the aortic valve (LCC)
posterior scallops of the mitral valve P1, P2, P3
anterior scallops of the mitral valve A1, A2, A3
posterior medial papillary muscle
  (Post/Med PM)
anterior scallops of the mitral valve A1, A2, A3
posterior medial papillary muscle
  (Post/Med PM)
anterolateral papillary muscle (Ant/Lat PM)
inferior vena cava (IVC)
descending aorta (Desc AO)
left brachiocephalic vein (BCV)

(Reproduced with permission from Wasnick J, Hillel Z, Kramer D, et al. *Cardiac Anesthesia & Transesophageal Echocardiography.* New York, NY: McGraw-Hill; 2011.)

4. Of the pressure–volume loops shown in the below figure, which is most likely consistent with chronic severe aortic insufficiency?

A. Loop A.
B. Loop B.
C. Loop C.
D. Loop D.
E. Loop E.

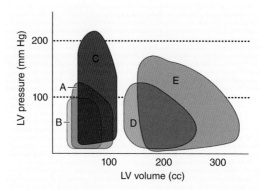

(Reproduced with permission from Jackson JM, Thomas SJ, Lowenstein E. Anesthetic management of patients with valvular heart disease. *Semin Anesth.* 1982;1:239.)

The correct answer is E. Pressure–volume loops are useful to understand the compensatory mechanisms of the heart in response to various hemodynamic challenges. Valvular lesions that lead to volume overload such as mitral regurgitation (D) and aortic regurgitation (E) result in dilatation of the heart to accommodate increased volume. Curve A is the normal pressure volume for a normal heart. Loop C reflects a heart with severe aortic stenosis subject to increased pressure work. Increased pressures are needed to facilitate ventricular ejection. Lastly, loop B reflects an underloaded left ventricle secondary to severe mitral stenosis.

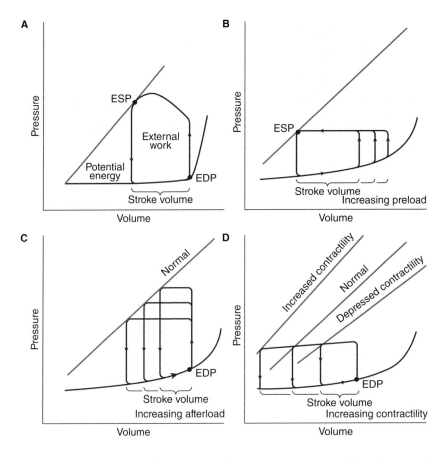

(Reproduced with permission frm Butterworth JF, Mackey DC, Wasnick JD: *Morgan and Mikhail's Clinical Anesthesiology*, 6th ed. New York, NY: McGraw-Hill Education; 2018.)

The above figure presents ventricular pressure–volume diagrams illustrating the adaptive responses to increased afterload (eg, aortic stenosis), increased preload (eg, aortic insufficiency), and decreased ventricular compliance (eg, cardiomyopathy). Panel A demonstrates a single ventricular contraction. The stroke volume represents change in volume on the x-axis (difference between end-systolic volume and end-diastolic volume), and the circumscribed area represents the external work performed by the ventricle. Panel B demonstrates the response to increasing preload, as seen in regurgitant valvular lesions. Panel C reflects the effects of increased afterload. Higher pressures are required to overcome the increased afterload to eject the stroke volume. Lastly, panel D demonstrates the response to increasing or decreasing ventricular contractility. ESP = end-systolic point, EDP = end-diastolic point.

DID YOU LEARN?

- Vascular supply of the heart.
- Patterns of diastolic dysfunction.
- Basic TEE views.
- Pressure–volume loops and valvular heart disease.

CASE 2 — Value of Focused Transthoracic Echocardiographic Exam of a Patient with Colonic Perforation

Ashraf N. Farag, MD

A 78-year-old patient is scheduled for emergent exploratory celiotomy for suspected colonic perforation secondary to diverticulitis. Vital signs include blood pressure 80/62 mm Hg, respiratory rate 32 breaths/min, and heart rate 120 beats/min. The patient has no immediate family; however, a friend reports that the patient was told in the past that he needed heart surgery, which the patient declined. Physical examination is noteworthy for patient distress, bilateral rales, and a systolic heart murmur. In the holding area, the anesthesiologist performs a focused assessed transthoracic echo (FATE) examination. The FATE examination provides a method to rapidly and noninvasively assess heart function and structure perioperatively.

1. Identify the chambers of the heart demonstrated in the schematic below.

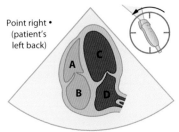

Point right •
(patient's
left back)

Apical 4-chamber

(Reproduced with permission from UltraSound Airway Breathing Circulation Dolor (USabcd) and Prof. Erik Sloth. http://usabcd.org/node/35.)

   A. A = right ventricle (RV), B = right atrium (RA), C = left ventricle (LV), D = left atrium (LA).

   B. A = right atrium (RA), B = right ventricle (RV), C = left ventricle (LV), D = left atrium (LA).

   C. A = right ventricle (RV), B = right atrium (RA), C = left atrium (LA), D = left ventricle (LV).

   D. None of the above.

The correct answer is A. A = right ventricle, B = right atrium, C = left ventricle, and D = left atrium.

2. What heart valve(s) is/are seen in this parasternal long-axis FATE view? What cardiac chambers are visualized?

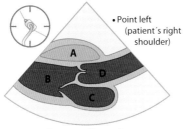

Parasternal long axis

(Reproduced with permission from UltraSound Airway Breathing Circulation Dolor (USabcd) and Prof. Erik Sloth. http://usabcd.org/node/35.)

A. Tricuspid valve.
B. Mitral valve.
C. Pulmonic valve.
D. Aortic valve.
E. Mitral and pulmonic valves.
F. Mitral and aortic valves.

The correct answer is F. The mitral and aortic valves can be examined in this long-axis view. The chambers seen are A = right ventricle, B = left ventricle, C = left atrium, and D = ascending aorta.

3. The patient has a systolic heart murmur likely secondary to aortic stenosis. Of the following schematics, which are most likely associated with aortic stenosis? With dilated cardiomyopathy? With pericardial effusion?

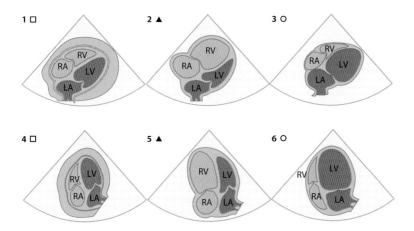

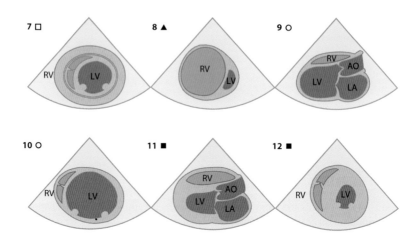

(Reproduced with permission from UltraSound Airway Breathing Circulation Dolor (USabcd) and Prof. Erik Sloth. http://usabcd.org/node/35.)

A. Aortic stenosis: images 11 and 12; dilated cardiomyopathy: images 3, 6, 9, and 10; pericardial effusion: images 1 and 7.

B. Dilated cardiomyopathy: images 11 and 12; aortic stenosis: images 3, 6, 9, and 10; pericardial effusion: images 1 and 7.

C. Pericardial effusion: images 11 and 12; dilated cardiomyopathy: images 3, 6, 9, and 10; aortic stenosis: images 1 and 7.

D. Aortic stenosis: images 11 and 12; pericardial effusion: images 3, 6, 9, and 10; dilated cardiomyopathy: images 1 and 7.

The correct answer is A. Images 11 and 12 are associated with aortic stenosis, arterial hypertension, left-ventricular outflow tract obstruction, hypertrophic cardiomyopathy, and myocardial deposit diseases. Images 3, 6, 9, and 10 are associated with dilated cardiomyopathy, aortic insufficiency, and other conditions. Images 1 and 7 are consistent with findings of a pericardial effusion.

4. After reviewing the patient's records, it is found that a previous echocardiographic examination demonstrated that the patient had an aortic valve area of less than 1 cm^2. Hemodynamic management should center upon:

A. Keeping the heart rate greater than 100 beats/min and reduced systemic vascular resistance.

B. Keeping the heart rate greater than 100 beats/min and increased systemic vascular resistance.

C. Keeping the heart rate less than 100 beats/min and increased systemic vascular resistance.

D. Keeping the heart rate less than 100 beats/min and reduce systemic vascular resistance.

The correct answer is C. The patient is hypotensive, tachycardic, and likely septic secondary to colonic perforation. The presence of tight aortic stenosis further complicates patient management. In addition to aortic stenosis, the patient will have diastolic dysfunction secondary to concentric left-ventricular hypertrophy. The patient already manifests signs of pulmonary congestion (bilateral rales). The best answer is to support blood pressure by increasing systemic vascular resistance and attempt to reduce the heart rate through volume administration (option C). Intraoperative echocardiography can be useful to guide volume administration and monitor cardiac function.

5. Which of the following parameters is or are necessary to estimate this patient's cardiac output using echocardiography?

   A. The peak velocity of flow across the stenotic aortic valve.
   B. The peak velocity of flow across the tricuspid valve.
   C. The diameter of the left-ventricular outflow tract.
   D. The velocity-time integral of the left-ventricular outflow tract.
   E. A and B.
   F. C and D.

The correct answer is F. Knowledge of the diameter of the left-ventricular outflow tract (LVOT) and the velocity-time integral of the LVOT permits calculation of the patient's stroke volume.

The velocity-time interval reflects the distance blood moves during a single beat (stroke distance). The diameter of the LVOT is used to calculate the area through which the blood passes assuming that the LVOT is a cylinder:

$$\text{Area} = \pi r^2 = 0.785 \times \text{diameter}^2$$

Knowing the area through which the blood moves and the distance it travels (the stroke distance), it is possible to calculate a volume:

$$\text{Area} \times \text{length} = \text{volume}$$

The volume calculated is the stroke volume (SV = left-ventricular end-diastolic volume – left-ventricular end-systolic volume).

Cardiac output (CO) is determined by multiplying the SV by the heart rate (HR):

$$\text{SV} \times \text{HR} = \text{CO}$$

It is possible to calculate the peak pressure gradient across the stenotic aortic valve by knowing the velocity of flow across the valve using continuous-wave Doppler and the Bernoulli equation:

$$\text{Pressure gradient} = 4V^2$$

Knowledge of the peak velocity of the jet of the tricuspid valve can be used to estimate pulmonary artery systolic pressures. Assuming the patient has no pulmonic valvular disease, right-ventricular systolic pressure equals pulmonary artery systolic pressure:

Pressure gradient = Right ventricular systolic pressure − right atrial pressure

$4V^2$ = Right ventricular systolic pressure − right atrial pressure

$4V^2$ + right atrial pressure = Right ventricular systolic pressure

where

Right ventricular systolic pressure = pulmonary artery systolic pressure
V = Peak velocity (m/s) of the jet of tricuspid regurgitation

DID YOU LEARN?

- Elements of the FATE examination.
- Hemodynamic calculations using echocardiography.

Recommended Readings

Beaulieu Y, Marik P. Bedside ultrasonography in the ICU: Part 1. *Chest.* 2005;128:881.

Beaulieu Y, Marik P. Bedside ultrasonography in the ICU: Part 2. *Chest.* 2005;128:1766.

Butterworth IV JF, Mackey DC, Wasnick JD, eds. Cardiovascular monitoring. In: *Morgan & Mikhail's Clinical Anesthesiology.* 6th ed. New York, NY: McGraw-Hill Education; 2018:81–118.

Chatterjee K. The Swan Ganz catheters: Past, present, and future. A viewpoint. *Circulation.* 2009;119:147.

Funk D, Moretti E, Gan T. Minimally invasive cardiac monitoring in the perioperative setting. *Anesth Analg.* 2009;108:887.

Geisen M, Spray D, Fletcher S. Echocardiography-based hemodynamic management in the cardiac surgical intensive care unit. *J Cardiothorac Vasc Anesth.* 2014;28:733.

Marik P. Noninvasive cardiac output monitors: A state of the art review. *J Cardiovasc Thorac Anesth.* 2013;27:121.

Ramsingh D, Alexander B, Cannesson M. Clinical review: Does it matter which hemodynamic monitoring system is used. *Crit Care.* 2013;17:208.

Shanewise J, Cheung A, Aronson S, et al. ASE/SCA guidelines for performing a comprehensive intraoperative multiplane transesophageal echocardiography examination: Recommendations of the American Society of Echocardiography Council for Intraoperative Echocardiography and the Society of Cardiovascular Anesthesiologists Task Force for Certification in Perioperative Transesophageal Echocardiography. *Anesth Analg.* 1999;89:870.

CHAPTER 6
Noncardiovascular Monitoring

CASE 1 Patient for Laparoscopic Cholecystectomy

Christiane Vogt Harenkamp, MD, PhD, and Charlotte Walter, MD

A 45-year-old woman presents for a laparoscopic cholecystectomy. She admits to smoking a pack of cigarettes a day for 20 years but denies any medical problems other than gallstones. Her vital signs in the holding area reveal a heart rate of 74 beats/min, blood pressure of 134/77 mm Hg, temperature of 97.6°C, and oxygen saturation pulse oximetry of 95%. Physical exam is unremarkable. She proceeds to the operating room, where after a smooth induction, vital signs remain stable. However, it is noted that her capnogram has a slow upstroke (see below).

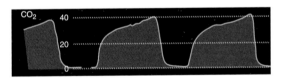

1. What is the diagnosis?

   A. Aspiration.
   B. Esophageal intubation.
   C. Chronic obstructive pulmonary disease (COPD).
   D. Normal variant.

The correct answer is C. Capnography is an indispensable monitor of ventilation during anesthesia. Normal capnography demonstrates the three phases of expiration: phase I, which represents dead space; phase II, which represents the mixture of dead space and alveolar gas; and phase III (alveolar gas plateau), which represents the alveolar carbon dioxide (CO_2) concentration. In patients with severe COPD, the alveolar gas plateau is never reached, leading to an up-sloping capnogram.

The diagnosis of COPD should be made preoperatively. Preoperative assessment includes a focused history and physical examination to identify signs and symptoms related to COPD such as history of tobacco abuse, dyspnea, chronic productive cough, frequent pulmonary infections, cyanosis, a barrel chest, clubbing of the nails, cachexia, and wheezes and distant breath sounds. An arterial blood gas may show a decrease in arterial PO_2, an increase in $PaCO_2$, and a compensatory increase in serum bicarbonate. Spirometry may be used to assess the severity of COPD.

A decrease in the FEV_1/FVC ratio results from the decrease in peak expiratory flows through obstructed airways. Although in mild disease the FEV_1/FVC ratio may be near normal, a decrease in the FEV_{25-75} (maximum mid-expiratory flow) will reveal disease of the small airways. Chest x-rays may show hyperinflation (2), flattening of the diaphragms (1), slender heart silhouette, and later a prominent right atrium (cor pulmonale).

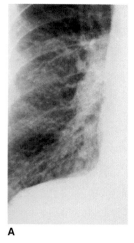

A

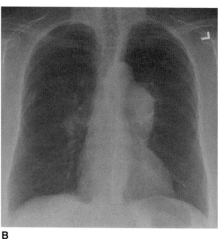

B

(Reproduced with permission from Grippi MA, Elias JA, Fishman JA, et al: *Fishman's Pulmonary Diseases and Disorders*, 5th ed. New York, NY: McGraw-Hill Education; 2008.)

Finally, ECG findings in severe COPD may include right axis deviation, right-ventricular hypertrophy (secondary to pulmonary hypertension), a right bundle branch block, and multifocal atrial tachycardia.

2. In the preceding case, the airway pressures continue to rise and chest auscultation reveals bilateral expiratory wheezes. An arterial blood gas is drawn. What is the gradient between end-tidal CO_2 and arterial CO_2 in this patient?

   A. Increased.
   B. Decreased.
   C. Normal.
   D. No gradient exists.

The correct answer is A. In severe COPD (FEV_1 <30% predicted), the alveolar gas plateau may not be reached during a normal breathing cycle. Due to a decreased elastic recoil and gas trapping, expiration may be very prolonged and incomplete, leading to an increase in end-tidal to arterial CO_2 gradient. Although other disease processes can also cause a decrease in end-tidal CO_2 and increased alveolar–arterial CO_2 gradient, they will not show the up-sloping of the capnogram. Any process that decreases cardiac output and lung perfusion (eg, hypovolemia, shock, pulmonary embolism, increased intraabdominal pressure from pneumoperitoneum, and reversed Trendelenburg position, as in laparoscopic cholecystectomy) will lead to a relative increase in dead space ventilation (West Zone 1) and a relative decrease of West Zone 2 and will increase V/Q mismatch. Auscultation of the lungs, increased airway pressures (may occur with pulmonary embolism too due to reflex broncho-constriction), capnography, and arterial blood gas evaluations will help to discern acute airway obstruction from these other causes of decreased end-tidal CO_2.

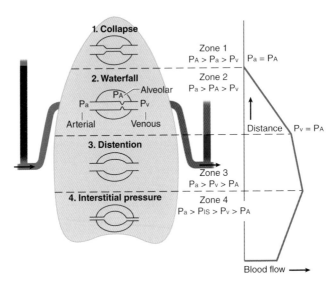

Classic West zones of blood flow distribution in the upright position. (Modified with permission from West JB. *Respiratory Physiology: The Essentials*. 6th ed. Philadelphia, PA: Williams and Wilkins; 2000.)

3. After the diagnosis of acute airway obstruction from COPD is made in the patient, which change in ventilator management should be made?

A. Increase FiO_2.
B. Increase inspiration time.
C. Increase expiration time.
D. Increase respiratory rate.

The correct answer is C. Patients with COPD require increased expiration time to allow the plateau phase of expiration to be reached and their lungs to fully deflate. An increased respiratory rate and subsequent decrease of breath cycle duration may lead to "stacking," intrinsic positive end-expiratory pressure, and potential barotrauma. A decrease in respiratory rate is aimed to avoid this phenomenon. External positive end-expiratory pressure (PEEP) may be employed carefully so as to avoid overinflation of the lungs, which may increase intrathoracic pressure, decrease venous return, and worsen a V/Q mismatch.

Pharmacological treatments mainly rely on inhaled bronchodilators and anticholinergic agents. Albuterol is a β-agonist and ipratropium is an anticholinergic agent, and both cause bronchodilation. Steroids decrease pulmonary inflammation; however, due to their delayed action, steroids have little or no value in treating acute exacerbations. Patients with severe disease may be on chronic steroid medication preoperatively and may require stress doses in the perioperative period.

DID YOU LEARN?

- To evaluate the severity of COPD and its associated comorbidities preoperatively.
- To recognize COPD and active airway obstruction during a general anesthetic.
- To develop a differential diagnosis for acute airway obstruction intra- and postoperatively.
- To understand and correctly employ the various treatments for acute airway obstruction.

CASE 2   Patient for Cervical Laminectomy

Ashraf N. Farag, MD, and Shiraz Yazdani, MD

A 110-kg, 46-year-old woman is scheduled to undergo a cervical laminectomy and fusion. She has a history of hypertension, fibromyalgia, asthma, and gastroesophageal reflux disease. Her home medications include pregabalin, atenolol, hydrochlorothiazide, and oxycodone. She has not taken her metoprolol for several days. On interview, she reports no complications with her sole previous surgery, which was a cesarean section performed with spinal anesthesia. She reports an exercise capacity of greater than four METs. She does admit to having occasional palpitations, although she denies syncopal episodes. Physical examination reveals a Mallampati class III airway, micrognathia, poor dentition, clear breath sounds, and a regular heart rhythm without murmur. Her preoperative temperature is 37.1°C, heart rate is 68 beats/min, blood pressure is 134/65 mm Hg, respiratory rate is 18 breaths/min, and oxygen saturation is 96% while breathing room air. While examining the patient, she reports numbness in her thumb and index finger upon neck extension. Upon speaking with the surgeon, you learn that somatosensory evoked potentials are to be monitored intraoperatively.

1. Upon entering the operating room, you place the patient on standard American Society of Anesthesiologists (ASA) monitors. She is placed on 100% oxygen for 5 min. The most appropriate approach for airway management is:

    A. Rapid-sequence induction with direct laryngoscopy.
    B. Awake fiber-optic intubation.
    C. Placement of a laryngeal mask airway.
    D. Mask induction with sevoflurane.

The correct answer is B. This patient has signs of cervical instability as evidenced by neurologic symptoms upon neck manipulation. While securing the airway, it is of utmost importance to maintain the cervical spine neutrality in order to avoid the risk of cord compromise. Appropriate methods for securing the airway in this patient include awake fiber-optic intubation. Intubation under general anesthesia using video laryngoscopy or a fiberoptic technique with in-line stabilization would be another possible option; however, her obesity and micrognathia make awake fiber-optic intubation the best choice among the options offered. Option A does not mention the need for in-line stabilization in this patient with cervical spine instability. In a trauma resuscitation situation, rapid-sequence intubation with in-line stabilization would be an appropriate approach with video laryngoscopy. Placement of a laryngeal mask airway may be appropriate as a rescue strategy in a "can't intubate, can't ventilate" situation; however, it risks gastric aspiration, as this patient has untreated gastroesophageal reflux disease. The same risk is present for mask induction. Additionally, the patient's airway anatomy could make mask ventilation difficult.

2. During the case, the patient has been maintained on a remifentanil infusion at 0.2 mcg/kg/min, 50% nitrous oxide in 50% oxygen, and propofol at 100 mcg/kg/min. The patient's mean arterial pressure is 100 mm Hg. The surgeon reports significant intraoperative bleeding and requests that the patient's blood pressure be reduced. The most appropriate next step is to:

    A. Administer labetalol intravenously.
    B. Add sevoflurane to the inspired gases.
    C. Deepen anesthetic with intravenous ketamine.
    D. Begin clevidipine infusion.

The correct answer is D. Management of intraoperative hemodynamics can be complex, with many factors to take into account. Although maintaining an adequate perfusion pressure is essential, the effects of intraoperative hypertension on blood loss must be taken into consideration. In patients with chronic hypertension, the autoregulation curve may be shifted to the right. Although these patients may need a higher than normal mean arterial pressure to maintain perfusion, keeping the pressure within 20% of their baseline is generally considered safe. Reducing this patient's blood pressure can be achieved in a variety of ways, but the most appropriate is by beginning a clevidipine infusion. Labetalol administration will decrease the blood pressure, but is relatively contraindicated in this patient due to her history of asthma. The potential for concomitant bronchoconstriction exists because labetalol is a nonselective β-adrenergic antagonist, whereas esmolol is selective for β_1 receptors. Deepening the anesthetic may reduce the mean arterial pressure. However, adding sevoflurane may adversely affect the monitoring of somatosensory evoked potentials. Somatosensory evoked potentials are sensitive to many anesthetic agents. Nitrous oxide, opioids, and neuromuscular blocking agents cause minimal changes, whereas volatile agents cause more significant changes and are best avoided. Administering ketamine may deepen the anesthesia, but may increase the patient's blood pressure due to its inherent sympathomimetic activity.

3. Your next patient is to undergo the same procedure. The surgeon requests motor evoked potential monitoring. Which of the following accurately describes the difference between motor evoked potentials and somatosensory evoked potentials?

   A. Somatosensory evoked potentials are more sensitive to volatile anesthetics.
   B. Motor evoked potentials measure impulses through the corticospinal tract.
   C. Even minimal degrees of twitch depression are contraindicated when measuring motor evoked potentials.
   D. Somatosensory evoked potentials are useful in detecting anterior spinal artery compromise.

The correct answer is B. Although all evoked potentials are sensitive to volatile anesthetics, motor evoked potentials are affected the most, followed by somatosensory evoked potentials, followed by brainstem auditory evoked potentials. Motor evoked potentials are useful in monitoring the corticospinal tract, whereas somatosensory evoked potentials travel through the dorsal columns. Neuromuscular blockade during motor evoked potential monitoring must be closely monitored and reported to the neurophysiologist. Although high-dose neuromuscular blockers may adversely affect such monitoring, maintaining steady, low-dose neuromuscular relaxation may be performed. Somatosensory evoked potentials do not measure the integrity of the ventral spinal cord and are therefore not useful in detecting anterior spinal artery compromise.

DID YOU LEARN?

- Airway management techniques for the unstable cervical spine.
- Management of intraoperative hypertension in the setting of evoked potential monitoring.
- Effects of various anesthetic agents on evoked potentials.
- Differences between somatosensory and motor evoked potentials.

CASE 3   Oximetry

John D. Wasnick, MD, MPH

A 78-year-old patient is scheduled for coronary artery bypass surgery. As a part of routine monitoring, near-infrared spectroscopy is employed

1. Which of the following statements regarding oximetry is/are correct?

   A. Pulse oximetry is dependent on the difference in absorption of red and infrared light between oxygenated and reduced hemoglobin.
   B. Oxygenated hemoglobin absorbs more red light.
   C. Deoxygenated hemoglobin absorbs more infrared light.
   D. Carboxyhemoglobin and oxyhemoglobin absorb light at 660 nm similarly.
   E. Methemoglobin has the same absorption coefficient at both red and infrared wavelengths.
   F. A, D, and E are correct.

The correct answer is F. Oximetry depends on the observation that oxygenated and reduced hemoglobin differ in their absorption of red and infrared light (Lambert-Beer Law). Specifically, oxyhemoglobin absorbs more infrared light (940 nm), whereas deoxyhemoglobin absorbs more red light (660 nm), and thus appears blue or cyanotic. The change in light absorption during arterial pulsation is the basis of oximetric determination and infrared wavelengths. The greater the ratio of red to infrared absorption, the lower the arterial hemoglobin oxygen saturation. Arterial pulsations are identified by plethysmography, allowing corrections for light absorption by nonpulsating venous blood and tissue. The figure below demonstrates the differing absorption of red and infrared light by oxygenated and deoxygenated hemoglobin.

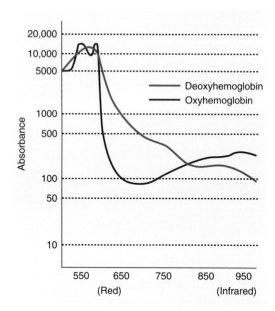

(Reproduced with permission from Butterworth JF, Mackey DC, Wasnick JD: *Morgan and Mikhail's Clinical Anesthesiology*, 6th ed. New York, NY: McGraw-Hill Education; 2018.)

Carboxyhemoglobin and oxyhemoglobin absorb light at 660 nm similarly, and thus, pulse oximeters that compare only two wavelengths of light will register a falsely high reading in patients with carbon monoxide poisoning. Methemoglobin has the same absorption coefficient at both red and infrared wavelengths, resulting in a 1:1 absorption ratio and a saturation reading of 85%.

2. Unlike pulse oximetry, which of the following statements regarding cerebral oximetry is/are true?

A. Cerebral oximetry is dependent upon reflectance rather than transmittance of light.
B. Cerebral oximetry measures arterial saturation like pulse oximetry.
C. Cerebral oximetry oxygen saturation represents the average oxygen saturation of all regional microvascular hemoglobin.
D. None of the above are true.
E. A and C are true.

The correct answer is E. Noninvasive brain oximetry monitors regional oxygen saturation of hemoglobin in the brain. A sensor placed on the forehead emits light of specific wavelengths and measures light reflected back to the sensor. Unlike pulse oximetry, brain oximetry measures venous and capillary blood oxygen saturation in addition to arterial blood saturation. Thus, its oxygen saturation readings represent the average oxygen saturation of all regional microvascular saturation (~60–70%).

3. Upon the initiation of cardiopulmonary bypass, the cerebral oxygen saturation falls from 45% to 35%. Possible etiologies of this decrease include all of the following *except*:

A. Reduced hemoglobin concentration.
B. Reduced arterial oxygen concentration.
C. Reduced cerebral perfusion.
D. Increased $PaCO_2$.
E. Increased cerebral oxygen consumption.

The correct answer is D. Reduced cerebral blood flow, anemia, reduced arterial oxygen content, increased cerebral vascular resistance, and increased cerebral oxygen consumption can all reduce cerebral oxygen saturation. Increased $PaCO_2$ generally improves cerebral blood flow and, as such, would likely not contribute to a decrease in cerebral oxygen saturation. Clinically, changes in cerebral oxygen saturation are often multifactorial and are of concern when values fall below 40%. Conversely, adverse neurological outcomes can occur during heart surgery irrespective of normal cerebral oxygen saturations during the perioperative period.

DID YOU LEARN?

- The difference between pulse and cerebral oximetry.
- The differential diagnosis of decreased cerebral saturation during cardiac surgery.

Recommended Readings

Avidan M, Zhang L, Burnside B, et al. Anesthesia awareness and bispectral index. *N Engl J Med.* 2008;358:1097.

Bergeron EJ, Mosca MS, Aftab M, Justison G, Reece TB. Neuroprotection strategies in aortic surgery. *Cardiol Clin.* 2017;35:453.

Butterworth IV JF, Mackey DC, Wasnick JD, eds. Noncardiovascular monitoring. In: *Morgan & Mikhail's Clinical Anesthesiology.* 6th ed. New York, NY: McGraw-Hill Education; 2018:119-138.

Kertai M, White W, Gan T. Cumulative duration of "triple low" state of low blood pressure, low bispectral index, and low minimum alveolar concentration of volatile anesthesia is not associated with increased mortality. *Anesthesiology.* 2014;121:18.

Lien CA, Kopman AF. Current recommendations for monitoring depth of neuromuscular blockade. *Curr Opin Anaesthesiol.* 2014;27:616.

SECTION II

Clinical Pharmacology

CHAPTER 7

Pharmacological Principles

| CASE 1 | Double Trouble: Identical Twin Trauma Victims |

Jason Noble, MD

Identical twins are involved in a motor vehicle accident that results in multiple orthopedic injuries requiring surgery. Although genetically identical, the twins' differing lifestyles have brought about major physiological differences. One is 80% above ideal body weight, but otherwise healthy. The other is a cachexic alcoholic with portal hypertension and ascites. The decision is made to take both twins directly to the operating room (OR) for open reduction and internal fixation.

1. Because fewer than 6 h have passed since the accident and because there are concerns regarding increased risk of aspiration in both obese patients and those with ascites, the decision is made to perform a rapid-sequence induction with propofol and succinylcholine for both twins. Which of the following is the best answer regarding the dosing for these patients?

   A. The dosing (mg/kg) should be the same for both patients.
   B. The dosing (mg/kg) of propofol should be increased and the succinylcholine decreased in the obese patient as compared to the alcoholic patient.
   C. The dosing (mg/kg) of propofol should be decreased and the succinylcholine increased in the obese patient as compared to the alcoholic patient.
   D. On a mg/kg basis, the dosing of propofol should be decreased and the succinylcholine equivalent in the obese patient as compared to the alcoholic patient.
   E. On a mg/kg basis, the dosing of propofol should be equivalent and the succinylcholine decreased in the obese patient as compared to the alcoholic patient.

The correct answer is D. There are multiple concerns that must be considered in tailoring the dosing of drugs for each individual patient. Are there differences in the volumes of distribution and clearance? Are there differences in the protein binding of drugs? Are there differences in metabolism?

In this scenario, there are clear physiological differences that could affect the dosing of anesthetic agents. The obese patient has a larger volume of distribution for lipophilic drugs, whereas the alcoholic patient with ascites has a larger volume of distribution for hydrophilic drugs. The obese patient may have an overall higher metabolic rate, whereas the alcoholic patient may either have an induced rate of phase 1 and 2 biotransformation or enough liver damage to decrease rates of metabolism, as well as decreased protein binding of drugs. Furthermore, all of these changes must be taken in context of the specific agent used.

In this case, the dosing of propofol would be best considered in terms of lean body weight (LBW), as the drug has its effect in the vessel-rich group, after which, secondary to it both being rapidly redistributed and undergoing a high extraction rate and clearance in the liver, it has a short distribution half-life of 2 to 8 min. For a single-bolus dose, there is little concern in regard to any deposition in adipose tissue. Because it is already in a lipid formulation, protein binding is not an important consideration. Furthermore, the pharmacokinetics of propofol do not appear to be affected by obesity or cirrhosis. However, in the chronic alcoholic patient, it has been demonstrated that induction doses of propofol are increased as compared to normal patients.

In regard to succinylcholine, studies have shown that dosing according to total body weight (TBW) is preferable. Because there may be a somewhat higher level of overall metabolism in the obese, and due to the very efficient metabolism by pseudocholinesterase, only a small fraction ever reaches the neuromuscular junction, and doses do not have to be adjusted according to LBW in the obese. Although pseudocholinesterase levels have been shown to be decreased in patients with cirrhosis and liver damage, pseudocholinesterase levels must be decreased by more than 75% before any significant prolongation of neuromuscular blockade by succinylcholine is demonstrated.

Therefore, although the dose of propofol should be decreased in the obese as compared to the alcoholic patient on a mg/kg basis, the dosing of succinylcholine should be equivalent. The best answer is option D.

2. After intubation, you decide to maintain relaxation of both patients with a rocuronium IV infusion. Which of the following would be the most appropriate dosing for maintenance of muscle relaxation?

A. Dose both patients according to LBW.
B. Dose both patients according to TBW.
C. Dose the obese patient by TBW and the cirrhotic patient by LBW.
D. Dose the obese patient by LBW and the cirrhotic patient by TBW.

The correct answer is A. Nondepolarizing muscle relaxants are hydrophilic drugs. Therefore, although their volumes of distribution and clearance would not be increased in obese patients, they would be in patients with ascites. Furthermore, liver disease, especially liver failure, will prolong the blockade produced by rocuronium. So although initial dosing may be increased in cirrhotic patients, maintenance dosing should be reduced. Although obese patients do not possess the same increase in volumes of distribution and clearance as do cirrhotic patients, it has been demonstrated that dosing obese patients by TBW as opposed to LBW produces a predictable prolongation of the blockade commensurate with the amount of dosing increased beyond LBW. Therefore, in both instances, the most appropriate dosing for rocuronium for maintenance relaxation should be by LBW.

3. The decision is made to use an inhaled, halogenated agent to maintain anesthesia. In order to ensure a prompt emergence from anesthesia at the end of the case, the best choice would be which of the following?

A. Use an agent with a low blood and tissue solubility, such as desflurane, for the obese patient.
B. Use an agent with a high blood and tissue solubility, such as halothane, for the cirrhotic patient.
C. Use an agent that is more rapidly metabolized, such as halothane, in the obese patient.
D. Use an agent that is more rapidly metabolized, such as halothane, in the cirrhotic patient.
E. Use an agent with both low blood and tissue solubility and rapid metabolism in both patients.

The correct answer is A. The anesthesia effect of the halogenated vapors is terminated not by redistribution and metabolism as is true for IV agents, but by exhalation. Therefore, although metabolic considerations are important for their potential side effects, such as halothane-induced hepatitis and decreased hepatic blood flow, metabolism of vapor anesthetics makes almost no contribution to emergence from anesthesia. Instead, emergence from anesthesia is dependent on the blood and tissue solubilities of the vapor anesthetics. In general, the more soluble the vapor, the longer it will persist in the patient. Therefore, a patient given a vapor with low solubility such as desflurane will more predictably awaken from anesthesia at a faster rate than the same patient given isoflurane in the same way. Wake-up times are approximately 50% shorter with desflurane than with isoflurane. Desflurane has been marketed as the most appropriate inhalation anesthetic for obese patients. However, with greater degrees of obesity, blood flow per gram of fat decreases, so partition coefficients of anesthetics have a complex relationship to compartmental distribution. Furthermore, both desflurane and the more soluble anesthetic isoflurane have long time constants to reach steady state with fat tissue. These two factors of extended time constants and decreasing perfusion to fatty tissue will tend to reduce the effect of high tissue solubility in routine cases.

DID YOU LEARN?

- Volume of distribution of hydrophilic and lipophilic drugs.
- Termination of inhalational anesthetics.
- Factors influencing volume of distribution of anesthetic drugs.
- Effects of blood and tissue solubility and metabolism on termination of volatile anesthesia.

Recommended Readings

Ansari J, Carvalho B, Shafer SL, Flood P. Pharmacokinetics and pharmacodynamics of drugs commonly used in pregnancy and parturition. *Anesth Analg.* 2016;122:786.

Bailey JM. Context-sensitive half-times: What are they and how valuable are they in anaesthesiology? *Clin Pharmacokinet.* 2002;41:793.

Brunton LL, Knollman BC, eds. *Goodman & Gilman's The Pharmacological Basis of Therapeutics.* 13th ed. New York, NY: McGraw-Hill; 2017: chap 2.

Butterworth IV JF, Mackey DC, Wasnick JD, eds. Pharmacological principles. In: *Morgan & Mikhail's Clinical Anesthesiology.* 6th ed. New York, NY: McGraw-Hill Education; 2018:139-148.

Shargel L, Yu ABC, eds. *Applied Biopharmaceutics & Pharmacokinetics.* 7th ed. New York, NY: McGraw-Hill; 2016.

CHAPTER 8
Inhalation Anesthetics

CASE 1 Child for Repair of Atrial Septal Defect

Katrina Von Kriegenbergh, MD, and Mukesh Wadhwa, DO

A 3-year-old boy is scheduled for repair of an atrial septal defect (ASD) with a left-to-right shunt. In the operating room, preinduction vital signs are within normal limits, and he undergoes a smooth and uneventful inhalation induction with sevoflurane and oxygen.

1. The dial on the sevoflurane vaporizer is set to 2%, but the inspired sevoflurane concentration is 0.5%. Which of the following *does not* explain the difference between the set concentration on the dial and the inspiratory concentration (F_I) of sevoflurane?

   A. Low fresh gas flow rate.
   B. Large volume of the breathing circuit.
   C. High absorptive capacity of the breathing circuit.
   D. Ventilation/perfusion (V/Q) mismatch.

The correct answer is D. The number on the dial of the vaporizer is the concentration of volatile anesthetic that leaves the vaporizer, but does not necessarily equal the concentration of anesthetic gas that reaches the patient during inspiration. The fresh gas leaving the anesthesia machine mixes with gases in the breathing circuit before being inspired by the patient. Factors affecting F_I of a volatile anesthetic are fresh gas flow rate, volume of the breathing system, and any anesthetic absorption by the machine or breathing circuit. Inspired volatile anesthetic concentration will approach fresh gas concentration with higher fresh gas flow rates, smaller circuit volumes, and lower circuit absorption. The arterial gas concentration (F_a), not the (F_I), is affected by V/Q mismatch. Effects upon F_I, F_a, and F_A are demonstrated in the following figure.

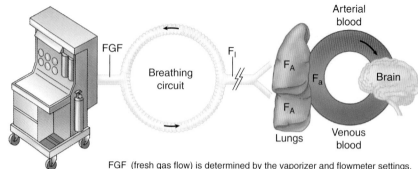

FGF (fresh gas flow) is determined by the vaporizer and flowmeter settings.

Anesthesia machine

F_I (inspired gas concentration) is determined by (1) FGF rate; (2) breathing-circuit volume; and (3) circuit absorption.

F_A (alveolar gas concentration) is determined by (1) uptake; (2) ventilation; (3) concentration effect; and (4) second gas effect (when nitrous oxide is present).

F_a (arterial gas concentration) is affected by ventilation/perfusion mismatching.

(Reproduced with permission from Butterworth JF, Mackey DC, Wasnick JD: *Morgan and Mikhail's Clinical Anesthesiology*, 6th ed. New York, NY: McGraw-Hill Education; 2018.)

2. Sevoflurane and halothane are compared in terms of inhalational induction. If the cardiac output is doubled from previous values, which agent will result in a greater increase in F_A/F_I and the rate of change of F_A/F_I?

   A. Sevoflurane will increase greater than halothane.
   B. Halothane will increase greater than sevoflurane.
   C. Both will increase the same.
   D. Cannot be determined.

The correct answer is A. The blood–gas solubilities of sevoflurane and halothane are 0.69 and 2.4, respectively. Factors affecting F_A (alveolar anesthetic concentration) are uptake of the anesthetic into the pulmonary circulation, alveolar ventilation, and inspired concentration. The amount of anesthetic uptake into the pulmonary circulation is directly proportional to anesthetic blood solubility, alveolar blood flow, and the difference in partial pressure of the volatile anesthetic in the alveolus and venous blood. If there were no uptake, F_A would rapidly approach F_I (inspiratory volatile anesthetic concentration), as is seen with insoluble agents, like desflurane. However, F_A lags behind F_I, so that the rate of rise (F_A/F_I) is <1 for soluble agents. Soluble agents such as halothane have greater uptake into the pulmonary circulation than less soluble agents, like sevoflurane. In the absence of pulmonary shunting, alveolar blood flow equals cardiac output. As cardiac output increases, anesthetic uptake increases, especially for soluble anesthetic agents. Tissue uptake causes a gradient between alveolar and venous blood partial pressures. The larger the uptake by tissue, the greater are the gradient and uptake into the pulmonary circulation. Increasing alveolar ventilation and inspired concentration serves to offset the effects of pulmonary circulation uptake, especially for relatively more soluble agents like halothane.

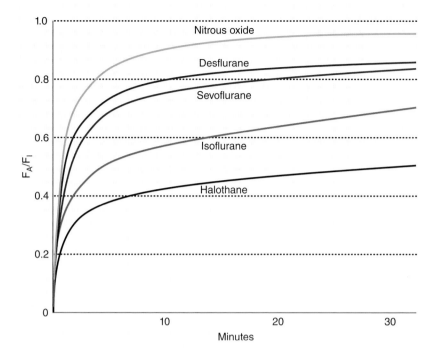

F_A rises toward F_I faster with nitrous oxide (an insoluble agent) than with halothane (a soluble agent). (Reproduced with permission frm Butterworth JF, Mackey DC, Wasnick JD: *Morgan and Mikhail's Clinical Anesthesiology*, 6th ed. New York, NY: McGraw-Hill Education; 2018.)

3. The presence of which type of shunt would *most* likely decrease the rate of rise in F_A/F_I for sevoflurane, thus slowing inhalational induction?

   A. 10% left-to-right shunt.
   B. 20% left-to-right shunt.
   C. 20% right-to-left shunt.
   D. 10% right-to-left shunt.

The correct answer is C. In the presence of a left-to-right intracardiac shunt, oxygenated blood is mixed with the systemic venous return. Having passed through the lungs, the blood also contains anesthetic gas. There is no anesthetic partial pressure difference with left-to-right shunts, as the blood entering the systemic circulation is at same partial pressure as it traverses the pulmonary circulation. In the presence of a right-to-left intracardiac shunt, there is a decrease in alveolar blood volume as a portion of deoxygenated blood flows from the right to the left heart instead of through the pulmonary circulation. The overall effect is an increase in the alveolar partial pressure for highly soluble agents, such as halothane, and a decrease in the arterial partial pressure for the more insoluble agents, such as sevoflurane. Clinically, this presents as slower rates of inhalation induction, which affects relatively insoluble agents more than highly soluble agents.

4. Factors that promote right-to-left shunting include all of the following *except*:

   A. Increased inspiratory oxygen concentration.
   B. Decreased ventilation.
   C. Elevated pulmonary artery pressures.
   D. Right endobronchial intubation.

The correct answer is A. Increasing inspiratory oxygen concentration results in decreasing pulmonary vascular resistance, promoting pulmonary blood flow. Factors that can increase pulmonary vascular resistance exacerbate right-to-left shunting and include hypoxemia, hypercarbia, acidosis, increased pulmonary artery pressures, high peak airway pressures, and endobronchial intubation. Hypercarbia associated with decreased ventilation causes pulmonary vasoconstriction and reductions in pulmonary blood flow, favoring shunt flow. Increased resistance to right-ventricular outflow likewise promotes right-to-left shunt flow, as seen in pulmonary hypertension. Finally, a right mainstem intubation results in increased hypoxic pulmonary vasoconstriction, increasing the likelihood of right-to-left blood flow through an anatomic shunt. Additionally, an endobronchial intubation results in a ventilation/perfusion mismatch, as the left lung is perfused but not ventilated.

5. If the patient has a right-to-left anatomic shunt, which invasive monitoring is needed to access blood samples to calculate the percentage of cardiac output that is shunted past the pulmonary circulation?

   A. Radial arterial line and internal jugular triple-lumen central venous line.
   B. Radial arterial line and subclavian triple-lumen central venous line.
   C. Femoral arterial line and pulmonary artery catheter.
   D. Ulnar arterial line and internal jugular catheter.

The correct answer is C. The pulmonary artery catheter allows calculation of the mixed venous oxygen saturation and content.

The shunt equation is:

$$\dot{Q}_s/\dot{Q}_T = \frac{C_c'O_2 - C_aO_2}{C_c'O_2 - C_{\bar{v}}O_2}$$

where

$\dot{Q}_s/\dot{Q}_T$ = percent shunt.
$C_c'O_2$ = ideal end-pulmonary capillary oxygen content.
C_aO_2 = arterial oxygen content.
$C_{\bar{v}}O_2$ = mixed venous oxygen content.

Oxygen content can be calculated with the following equation:

$$O_2 \text{ content } (C_xO_2) = (S_xO_2 \times Hb\ 1.31\ \text{mL/dL blood})$$
$$+ (P_xO_2 \times 0.003\ \text{mL/dL blood per mm Hg}).$$

The partial pressure of alveolar oxygen (P_AO_2) can be used in place of $P_c'O_2$ to approximate $C_c'O_2$, C_aO_2 can be calculated from values from the arterial blood gas (ABG), and $C_{\bar{v}}O_2$ can be calculated with $P_{\bar{v}}O_2$ and $S_{\bar{v}}O_2$ obtained via pulmonary catheter. Because pulmonary catheterization is not feasible in all patients, there are other means of estimating percent shunt. The alveolar-to-arterial difference can be used estimate venous admixture. As the shunt fraction increases, increasing inspired oxygen concentration fails to alter arterial oxygen tension. See the graph below.

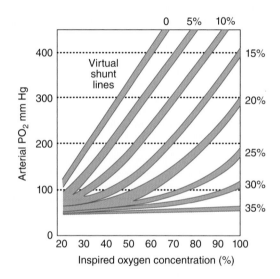

DID YOU LEARN?

- Factors affecting inspiratory concentration (F_I) of an anesthetic agent.
- Factors affecting alveolar concentration (F_A) of an anesthetic agent.
- Factors affecting arterial concentration (F_a) of an anesthetic agent.
- Effect of anesthetic uptake by the pulmonary circulation on anesthetic inhalation induction.
- Effect of cardiac output and ventilation on anesthetic inhalation induction.
- Difference between right-to-left and left-to-right shunting and its effect on inhalation induction.
- Components necessary to calculate percent shunt and the effect of shunt on arterial oxygen tension.

CASE 2 | Patient for Emergency Orthopedic Surgery

Katrina Von Kriegenbergh, MD, and Swapna Chaudhuri, MD, PhD

A 20-year-old, 108-kg, 5'9" man is scheduled for emergent fixation of bilateral femoral mid-shaft fractures following a motor vehicle accident that occurred 4 h earlier. During preanesthetic evaluation, the patient denies any major medical illnesses other than asthma, which is controlled with albuterol inhaler prn; an uneventful surgical history includes only a tonsillectomy at age 6 and a laparoscopic appendectomy 2 years ago. He is restless and complaining of pain; blood pressure is 94/68 mm Hg, heart rate is 112 beats/min, and respiratory rate is 20 breaths/min. Admission laboratory values reveal a hemoglobin of 11.2 mg/dL and blood alcohol of 0.2%. Fractures of right ribs 6 to 8 and a small right pneumothorax are visible on the chest radiograph.

1. Your choice of sevoflurane over desflurane for maintenance of general anesthesia in this patient is influenced by all of the following characteristics *except*:

   A. Sevoflurane usually produces less decline in blood pressure and less increase in heart rate compared to desflurane.
   B. Sevoflurane is less likely to induce bronchospasm than desflurane.
   C. Sevoflurane has greater blood solubility than desflurane.
   D. Sevoflurane undergoes more metabolism than desflurane.

The correct answer is D. Volatile anesthetics share similar effects on various organ systems, often making distinctions between the agents more theoretical than useful or practical. However, patient comorbidities and presentation may suggest which one is most suitable for a particular individual, at least in theory. Sevoflurane is metabolized 10 to 25 times more than desflurane by the cytochrome P-450 2E1 enzyme. This enzyme system can be induced if ethanol is present in the patient's circulation, resulting in a rise in potentially nephrotoxic inorganic fluoride. Nonetheless, kidney failure following sevoflurane anesthesia secondary to flouride ion toxicity is virtually nonexistent. Desflurane, and to a lesser extent sevoflurane, decrease systemic blood pressure via a reduction in systemic vascular resistance. However, cardiac output is not as well maintained with sevoflurane because it does not increase heart rate as greatly as does desflurane. All volatile anesthetics cause respiratory depression and blunt the normal ventilatory response to hypoxia and hypercarbia. Sevoflurane is less likely to produce bronchospasm compared to desflurane, making it a preferred agent for inhalational induction. Sevoflurane is minimally more soluble in blood than desflurane. The blood gas partition coefficients for desflurane and sevoflurane are 0.42 and 0.65, respectively. At steady state, this means that 1 mL of blood has only 0.42 times the amount of desflurane as air. As a consequence of limited solubility, alveolar partial pressure rises rapidly with either desflurane or sevoflurane, but more so with desflurane. In this patient with a potentially full stomach, it is unlikely that inhalation induction would be performed.

2. The sevoflurane vaporizer is empty, so you decide to use halothane; all of the following factors can enhance the rate of rise of F_A/F_I with halothane *except*:

A. High fresh gas flow.
B. Facilitation of rebreathing.
C. Low breathing circuit volume and absorption.
D. Increased ventilation.

The correct answer is B. Induction of anesthesia with volatile anesthetics is dependent on several factors that begin at the anesthesia machine and end in the target organ, the brain. High fresh gas flow rate, small breathing system volume, low breathing circuit absorption, and elimination of rebreathing contribute to increasing the concentration of volatile anesthetic delivered to the patient with each inspiration (F_I) and expediting induction. Within the patient's lungs, the volatile anesthetic reaches a certain concentration in the alveoli (F_A) that is affected by uptake, ventilation, and concentration. Anesthetic uptake into the pulmonary circulation decreases the rate at which F_A approaches F_I and results in prolonged induction times $(F_A/F_I < 1.0)$. Uptake is greater with more soluble anesthetics like halothane, during episodes of increased cardiac output, and when tissue uptake causes increased partial pressure differences in alveolar gas and venous blood. Increased ventilation and inspired concentration serve to offset the effect of uptake on F_A (increasing F_A/F_I) and induction of anesthesia, especially for soluble anesthetics like halothane.

3. Which of the following factors has been demonstrated to produce a decrease in minimal alveolar concentration (MAC)?

A. Hypernatremia.
B. Acute alcohol intoxication.
C. Hypothyroidism.
D. Acute amphetamine use.

The correct answer is B. MAC is defined as the concentration of an inhaled anesthetic that prevents movement to surgical stimulus in 50% of patients. There are several factors that have been shown to decrease MAC, including hyponatremia, acute alcohol intoxication, and chronic amphetamine use; conversely, hypernatremia, chronic alcohol abuse, and acute amphetamine use have been shown to increase MAC. Other drugs that increase MAC include cocaine and ephedrine. MAC declines with age, and volatile anesthetics are similar in their association with age. Except for in infants (where it can be lower), MAC decreases linearly with increasing age. Hypo- and hyperthryoidism, sex, and duration of anesthesia produce no change of MAC.

Factors Affecting Minimum Alveolar Concentration (MAC)[a]

Variable	Effect on MAC	Comments	Variable	Effect on MAC	Comments
Temperature			**Electrolytes**		
Hypothermia	→		Hypercalcemia	→	
Hyperthermia	→	↑ if >42°C	Hypernatremia	←	Caused by altered CSF[b]
Age			Hyponatremia	→	Caused by altered CSF
Young	←		Pregnancy	→	MAC decreased by one-third at 8 weeks' gestation; normal by 72 h postpartum
Elderly	→				
Alcohol			**Drugs**		
Acute intoxication	→		Local anesthetics	→	Except cocaine
Chronic abuse	←		Opioids	→	
Anemia			Ketamine	→	
Hematocrit <10%	→		Barbiturates	→	
PaO₂			Benzodiazepines	→	
<40 mm Hg	→		Verapamil	→	
PaCO₂			Lithium	→	
>95 mm Hg	→	Caused by < pH in CSF	Sympatholytics		
Thyroid			Methyldopa	→	
Hyperthyroid	No change		Clonidine	→	
Hypothyroid	No change		Dexmedetomidine	→	
Blood pressure			Sympathomimetics		
Mean arterial pressure	→		Amphetamine		
<40 mm Hg			Chronic	→	
			Acute	←	
			Cocaine	←	
			Ephedrine	→	

[a]These conclusions are based on human and animal studies.
[b]CSF, cerebrospinal fluid.

4. Seventy-two hours after uneventful surgery, the patient develops abnormal liver function tests: serum bilirubin 6.5 μmol/L, alanine aminotransferase (ALT) 1022 U/L, and prothrombin time (PT) 21.5 s. What is the most likely cause for the perioperative liver failure?

A. Viral hepatitis.
B. Shock liver.
C. Anesthetic-mediated hepatitis.
D. Cannot determine.

The correct answer is D. Regardless of etiology, acute hepatic failure has characteristic features, including increased serum aminotransferase levels, hyperbilirubinemia, prolongation of coagulation indices (PT/international normalized ratio [INR]), and encephalopathy. The timing of signs and the derangement in liver function tests can aid in identifying etiology. Volatile anesthetic-mediated hepatitis is rare, and signs related to hepatocyte injury appear within 2 weeks following volatile anesthetic exposure. These may include significantly increased serum ALT, jaundice secondary to elevated bilirubin, and encephalopathy. In viral hepatitis, there is a nonspecific viral prodromal phase that includes malaise and anorexia accompanied by nausea and vomiting. The icteric phase follows in 3 to 10 days, and jaundice peaks within 1 to 2 weeks. Intrahepatic cholestasis occasionally develops after major surgery, especially after abdominal or cardiovascular procedures. Increased levels of bile acids, γ-glutamyl transferase (GGT), and alkaline phosphatase are seen; however, increases in aminotransferase and bilirubin present as signs of hepatocellular damage. Both sepsis and hemolysis can contribute to multifactorial mixed hyperbilirubinemia, the most common cause of postoperative jaundice. Liver function tests reveal markedly elevated bilirubin with mild increases in aminotransferase and alkaline phosphatase levels. Shock states can also result in hepatic failure. This patient had a traumatic injury that could have resulted in a shock state. Additionally, the patient shows evidence of alcohol use, which might indicate previous alcohol-induced liver toxicity.

5. All of the following are characteristic features of halothane hepatitis *except*:

A. Necrosis of hepatocytes with a centrilobular pattern.
B. Immune-mediated injury.
C. Single exposure producing fulminant disease occurs most commonly.
D. Familial predisposition is considered an increased risk.

The correct answer is C. Two distinct types of hepatic injury have been described with clinical use of halothane. Mild injury is observed in about 20% of adults who have received halothane, with laboratory tests demonstrating mild elevations in ALT and aspartate aminotransferase (AST). The second type of injury is a fulminant form, commonly known as *halothane hepatitis*. Halothane hepatitis is extremely rare; nevertheless, patients with a history of multiple exposures to halothane at short intervals, middle-aged obese women, and those with a history of toxicity (either personally or within the family) are at increased risk. If exposed to halothane under hypoxic conditions, centrilobular necrosis of hepatocytes is seen in both humans and rats. This supports a reductive metabolite or hypoxic mechanism of action. However, there is also evidence for an immune-mediated allergic type of reaction. Circulating antibodies have been detected in patients with fulminant hepatic failure following halothane exposure that reacts specifically with the cell membrane of hepatocytes isolated from halothane-anesthetized rabbits.

DID YOU LEARN?

- The distinguishing cardiorespiratory effects of sevoflurane and desflurane.
- Factors that influence MAC.
- The differential diagnosis of perioperative liver failure.
- Key characteristics of halothane-induced hepatitis.

Recommended Readings

Butterworth IV JF, Mackey DC, Wasnick JD, eds. Inhalation anesthetics. In: *Morgan & Mikhail's Clinical Anesthesiology*. 6th ed. New York, NY: McGraw-Hill Education; 2018:149-170.

DeHert S, Preckel B, Schlack W. Update on inhaltional anaesthetics. *Curr Opin Anaesthesiol.* 2009;22:491.

Njoku D, Laster MJ, Gong DH. Biotransformation of halothane, enflurane, isoflurane and desflurane to trifluoroacetylated liver proteins: association between protein acylation and hepatic injury. *Anesth Analg.* 1997:84:173.

CHAPTER 9

Neuromuscular Blocking Agents

CASE 1 | Patient for Dilatation and Curettage

Bettina Schmitz, MD, and Spencer Thomas, MD

A 35-year-old woman with a past medical history that includes type 2 diabetes, hypertension, and hypothyroidism is scheduled for a dilation and curettage following a spontaneous abortion. The patient's past surgical history includes a cesarean delivery performed under spinal anesthesia. The patient does not know her family history, as she was adopted as an infant.

Prior to the start of the procedure, the patient is premedicated with 2 mg of IV midazolam. Standard American Society of Anesthesiologists (ASA) monitors are applied, and the patient is preoxygenated with 100% oxygen for 3 min. General anesthesia is induced with propofol and succinylcholine. The patient is successfully intubated, and anesthesia is maintained with 1 MAC of sevoflurane in a 1:1 air/O_2 mixture. Further muscle relaxation is not considered to be necessary, and no nondepolarizing muscle relaxant is used. The case proceeds uneventfully for 30 min. Ten minutes after the discontinuation of the volatile anesthetic, the expiratory sevoflurane concentration is less than 0.2%, but the patient makes no efforts to breathe spontaneously and does not respond to physical or verbal stimulation. The anesthetist obtains an arterial blood gas analysis, which shows a pH of 7.31, PCO_2 of 43, PO_2 of 109, HCO_3 of 19, and lactate of 2.0. The patient was transferred to the surgical intensive care unit with positive-pressure ventilation, where she was observed for signs of recovery from anesthesia.

1. A delay in recovery from anesthesia can be caused by which of the following?

   A. Preexisting medical conditions.
   B. Drug effects of the medication given during general anesthesia.
   C. Metabolic disturbances.
   D. All of the above.

The correct answer is D. Each of the above can contribute to delayed emergence from general anesthesia. Preexisting medical conditions (such as kidney or liver failure or hypothyroidism) can alter availability and metabolism of anesthetic agents, resulting in an unexpectedly prolonged emergence. Comorbidities such as sleep apnea and chronic obstructive pulmonary disease can result in increased CO_2 retention and somnolence.

Excessive doses of opioids, amnestics, and muscle relaxants can likewise result in delayed emergence. Individual variation in drug responses can contribute to an emergence delay despite apparently appropriate drug dosing.

Hypothermia, hypoglycemia, hyperglycemia, and hyponatremia can result in delayed recovery from anesthesia. Strokes, seizures, and other central nervous system events, while rare, must also be considered.

2. Without additional information, what action should *not* be performed at this moment?

    A. Review of patient's medical history.
    B. Physical examination of the patient.
    C. Review of patient's anesthesia record.
    D. Reversal with neostigmine and glycopyrrolate.

The correct answer is D. Whenever there is a delayed emergence from general anesthesia, the patient's medical record, medication history, and anesthetic record should be reviewed. It is also crucial to assess the patient's physical status for a possible explanation for her delayed emergence.

The patient's medical history was described previously. The intraoperative anesthesia course was uneventful. There were no periods of hypertension, hyponatremia, or hypoxemia. Opioids were given at appropriate doses. The patient did not receive a nondepolarizing muscle relaxant. So unless there is evidence for a resolving phase II block, reversal of neuromuscular nondepolarizing agents is not indicated. Adequacy of thyroid replacement therapy should be assessed preoperatively.

To identify residual muscle paralysis, a peripheral nerve stimulator is employed.

3. Which of the following is *not* correct?

    A. A phase II depolarizing block presents with a fading response to a tetanic stimulus.
    B. A nondepolarizing block presents a posttetanic potentiation.
    C. A phase I depolarizing block presents with constant but diminished double-burst stimulation.
    D. A nondepolarizing block presents with a fading train-of-four.
    E. A phase I depolarizing block presents with a fading response to a train-of-four.

The correct answer is E. A phase I depolarizing block shows a diminished but constant response to train-of-four, tetanic and double-burst stimulation, and no posttetanic potentiation. Both a phase II depolarizing block and a nondepolarizing block present with a fading response to train-of-four, tetanic, and double-burst stimulation, and a posttetanic potentiation.

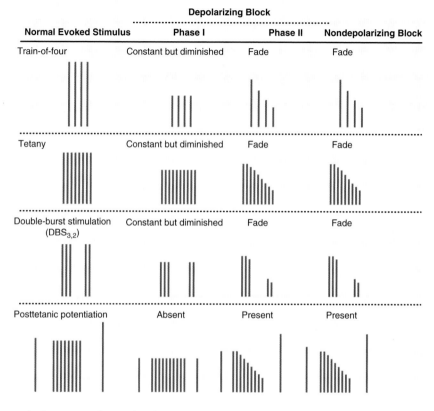

Evoked responses during depolarizing (phase I and phase II) and nondepolarizing block. (Reproduced with permission from Butterworth JF, Mackey DC, Wasnick JD: *Morgan and Mikhail's Clinical Anesthesiology*, 6th ed. New York, NY: McGraw-Hill Education; 2018.)

In this case, there was no response to train-of-four stimulation or tetanic stimulation. The clinical diagnosis of prolonged muscle relaxation caused by delayed succinylcholine metabolism is made and is thought likely to be secondary to homozygous pseudocholinesterase deficiency.

4. Treatment options include which of the following?

   A. Intravenous neostigmine/glycopyrrolate.
   B. Intravenous pyridostigmine/glycopyrrolate.
   C. Intravenous sugammadex.
   D. Sedation and continued ventilation until patient regains normal muscle function.

The correct answer is D. Cholinesterase antagonists (neostigmine and pyridostigmine) prolong the action of succinylcholine and are contraindicated in a patient with a pseudocholinesterase deficiency. Sugammadex selectively reverses the action of rocuronium or vecuronium.

Sedation and continuous mechanical ventilation until restoration of normal muscle function are the only options in a patient with prolonged muscle paralysis after succinylcholine. A recovery time of 4 to 8 h can be expected in patients with a homozygous pseudocholinesterase deficiency.

5. What dibucaine number is typical for a patient with homozygote pseudocholinesterase deficiency?

   A. 80%.
   B. 60%.
   C. 40%.
   D. 20%.

The correct answer is D. The dibucaine number is the percentage of pseudocholinesterase activity inhibited by dibucaine, a local anesthetic. Dibucaine inhibits normal pseudocholinesterase by 80%. Patients with a heterozygote gene for pseudocholinesterase will present with a dibucaine number between 40% and 60%, while dibucaine inhibits only 20% of the atypical pseudocholinesterase found in homozygote patients.

DID YOU LEARN?

- The differential diagnosis of delayed emergence from general anesthesia.
- Peripheral nerve stimulator responses indicative of phase I and phase II block.
- The meaning of the dibucaine number.

Recommended Readings

Brull SJ, Kopman AF. Current status of neuromuscular reversal and monitoring: Challenges and opportunities. *Anesthesiology.* 2017;126:173.

Butterworth IV JF, Mackey DC, Wasnick JD, eds. Neuromuscular blocking agents. In: *Morgan & Mikhail's Clinical Anesthesiology.* 6th ed. New York, NY: McGraw-Hill Education; 2018:199-220.

deBacker J, Hart N, Fan E. Neuromuscular blockade in the 21st century management of the critically ill patient. *Chest.* 2017;151:697.

Heerdt PM, Sunaga H, Savarese JJ. Novel neuromuscular blocking drugs and antagonists. *Curr Opin Anaesthesiol.* 2015;28:403.

Madsen MV, Staehr-Rye AK, Gätke MR, Claudius C. Neuromuscular blockade for optimising surgical conditions during abdominal and gynaecological surgery: A systematic review. *Acta Anaesthesiol Scand.* 2015;59:1.

Schreiber JU. Management of neuromuscular blockade in ambulatory patients. *Curr Opin Anaesthesiol.* 2014;27:583.

Tran DT, Newton EK, Mount VA, et al. Rocuronium versus succinylcholine for rapid sequence induction intubation. *Cochrane Database Syst Rev.* 2015;(10):CD002788.

CHAPTER 10

Cholinesterase Inhibitors & Other Pharmacological Antagonists to Neuromuscular Blocking Agents

| CASE 1 | Resuscitation of Patient Following Cardiac Arrest |

Spencer Thomas, MD, and Suzanne Northcutt, MD

You are called to assist in the resuscitation of a 5′ tall, 150-kg, 25-year-old woman who has suffered a cardiac arrest upon emergence from anesthesia following elective laparoscopic cholecystectomy. Anesthesia maintenance was with desflurane, fentanyl, and rocuronium. Reversal with glycopyrrolate (0.2 mg) and neostigmine (5 mg) had been administered 5 min prior to the arrest.

1. The ECG shows asystole. What is the most likely cause in your differential diagnosis?

   A. Prolonged QT syndrome.
   B. Inadequate glycopyrrolate administration.
   C. Autonomic neuropathy.
   D. Airway compromise and hypoxemia.

The correct answer is B. Prolonged QT syndrome could have been missed preoperatively leading to *torsades de pointes* arrhythmias. QT interval prolongation can be seen in the setting of congenital abnormalities and drug toxicity associated with antidepressants, phenothiazines, and antiarrythmic agents. Airway compromise on emergence with hypoxemia can lead to profound bradycardia and asystole. Such an occurrence would warrant immediate reestablishment of the airway by mask, intubation, or surgical/invasive airway management. This patient has a relatively high body mass index (BMI), and as such, airway difficulties upon emergence should always be expected. Although her obesity places her at risk for diabetes with autonomic dysfunction, this is not mentioned in the case history. Patients can arrest secondary to unknown cardiac disease perioperatively. Previously undetected cardiomyopathies, arrhythmias, and ischemic heart disease can unexpectedly lead to patient arrest during emergence. Although not impossible in a relatively young, albeit obese woman, such an event would be uncommon.

Routinely, 0.2 mg of glycopyrrolate is administered for every milligram of neostigmine administered. In this case, inadequate anticholinergic medication has been given to offset the effects of increased acetylcholine at the muscarinic receptors, resulting in bradycardia and asystole.

2. Appropriate actions at this point include all of the following *except*:

A. Calling for help.
B. Initiating cardiopulmonary resuscitation (CPR).
C. Administering atropine 2 mg IV.
D. Administering vasopressin 40 U IV.
E. Administering epinephrine 1 mg IV.

The correct answer is D. Calling for help and activating the operating room's emergency response is appropriate. CPR should commence immediately. Atropine is an anticholinergic with potent effects upon the heart and bronchial smooth muscle. Vasopressin has been removed from the advanced cardiac life support (ACLS) protocol in favor of the simplicity of epinephrine administration. This patient is asystolic secondary to drug effects. However, antagonism of acetylcholine at the muscarinic receptors of the heart is most likely to restore cardiac rhythm.

3. Following intubation and resuscitation, the arterial blood gas values obtained are pH 7.30, PaO_2 150 mm Hg, $PaCO_2$ 55 mm Hg, and HCO_3 27 mEq/L. These values reflect:

A. Respiratory alkalosis.
B. Respiratory acidosis without metabolic compensation
C. Respiratory acidosis with metabolic compensation.
D. Metabolic acidosis with respiratory compensation.

The correct answer is C. The patient has retained CO_2, producing a respiratory acidosis. Hypercarbia and respiratory acidosis can occur during laparoscopic surgery from absorption of peritoneal carbon dioxide. Inadequate ventilation following anesthesia is not uncommon. This patient also has a high BMI and may have elements of sleep apnea, leading to CO_2 retention following surgery. The patient's HCO_3 concentration is elevated perhaps secondary to chronic compensation from CO_2 retention secondary to sleep apnea. Of course, in this patient following an arrest situation, the possibility also exists that sodium bicarbonate was administered inappropriately during the arrest, resulting in an elevated bicarbonate concentration.

4. Which anticholinesterase agent crosses the blood–brain barrier?

The molecular structures of neostigmine, pyridostigmine, edrophonium, and physostigmine. (Reproduced with permission from Butterworth JF, Mackey DC, Wasnick JD: *Morgan and Mikhail's Clinical Anesthesiology*, 6th ed. New York, NY: McGraw-Hill Education; 2018.)

A. Neostigmine.
B. Pyridostigmine.
C. Edrophonium.
D. Physostigmine.

The correct answer is D. Neostigmine, pryidostigmine, and edrophonium have a charged quartenary amine group, limiting blood–brain barrier penetration. Physostigmine lacks a charged amine, facilitating lipid solubility. Physostigmine is useful in the treatment of central anticholinergic toxicity from atropine or scopolamine.

DID YOU LEARN?

- The differential diagnosis for cardiac arrest during emergence.
- Response to operating room cardiac arrest.
- Blood gas interpretation.
- The structural differences between neostigmine and physostigmine.

Recommended Readings

Baysal A, Dogukan M, Toman H, et al. The use of sugammadex for reversal of residual blockade after administration of neostigmine and atropine: 9AP1-9 *Eur J Anaesth*. 2013;30:142.

Brull SJ, Kopman AF. Current status of neuromuscular reversal and monitoring: Challenges and opportunities. *Anesthesiology.* 2017;126:173.

Butterworth IV JF, Mackey DC, Wasnick JD, eds. Cholinesterase inhibitors & other pharmacological antagonists to neuromuscular blocking agents. In: *Morgan & Mikhail's Clinical Anesthesiology.* 6th ed. New York, NY: McGraw-Hill Education; 2018:221-232.

Dirkman D, Britten M, Henning P, et al. Anticoagulant effect of sugammadex. *Anesthesiology.* 2016;124:1277.

Haeter F, Simons J, Foerster U, et al. Comparative effectiveness of calabadion and sugammadex to reverse nondepolarizing neuromuscular blocking agents. *Anesthesiology.* 2015;123:1337.

Heerdt P, Sunaga H, Savarese J. Novel neuromuscular blocking drugs and antagonists. *Curr Opin Anesthesiol.* 2015;28:403.

Hoffmann U, Grosse-Sundrup M, Eikermann-Haeter K, et al. Calabadion: A new agent to reverse the effects of benzylisoquinoline and steroidal neuromuscular blocking agents. *Anesthesiology.* 2013;119:317.

Kusha N, Singh D, Shetti A, et al. Sugammadex; a revolutionary drug in neuromuscular pharmacology. *Anesth Essays Res.* 2013;7:302.

Lien CA. Development and potential clinical impact of ultra-short acting neuromuscular blocking agents. *Br J Anaesth.* 2011;107(S1):160.

Meistelman C, Donati F. Do we really need sugammadex as an antagonist of muscle relaxants in anesthesia? *Curr Opin Anesthesiol.* 2016;29:462.

Naguib M. Sugammadex: Another milestone in clinical neuromuscular pharmacology. *Anesth Analg.* 2007;104:575.

Naguib M, Lien CA. Pharmacology of muscle relaxants and their antagonists. In: Miller RD, Eriksson LI, Fleisher L, Wiener-Kronish JP, Young WL, eds. *Miller's Anesthesia.* 8th ed. London: Churchill Livingstone; 2015.

Savarese JJ, McGilvra JD, Sunaga H, et al. Rapid chemical antagonism of neuromuscular blockade by L-cysteine adduction to and inactivation of the olefinic (double-bonded) isoquinoliniumdiester compounds gantacurium (AV430A), CW 002, and CW 011. *Anesthesiology.* 2010;113:58.

Taylor P. Anticholinesterase agents. In: Brunton LL, Knollmann BC, Hilal-Dandan R, eds. *Goodman and Gilman's Pharmacological Basis of Therapeutics.* 13th ed. New York, NY: McGraw-Hill; 2018.

References

Casati A, et al. Effects of pneumoperitoneum and reverse trendelenburg position on cardiopulmonary function in morbidly obese patients receiving laparoscopic gastric banding. *Eur J Anaesthesiol.* 2000;17:300-305.

Sprung J, et al. Perioperative cardiac arrests. *Signa Vitae.* 2008;3(2):8-12.

Usher S, Shaw A. Peri-operative asystole in a patient with diabetic autonomic neuropathy. *Anaesthesia.* 1999;54:1110-1129.

CHAPTER 11

Hypotensive Agents

CASE 1 | Patient Following Aortic Valve Replacement

Ron Banister, MD

1. An 83-year-old patient is returned to the cardiac surgery intensive care unit following aortic valve replacement. Vital signs on admission to the intensive care unit include blood pressure of 130/45 mm Hg and atrial-paced heart rhythm of 80 beats/min. The patient is receiving volume-controlled ventilation. The patient has a history of opioid use related to chronic back pain. As the patient emerges from anesthesia, blood pressure progressively increases to 185/100 mm Hg. Options to control the hypertension include:

   A. Propofol infusion.
   B. Dexmedetomidine infusion.
   C. Clevidipine infusion.
   D. Opioid administration.
   E. All of the above.
   F. None of the above.

The correct answer is E. Hypertension following surgery in general, and cardiac surgery in particular, may contribute to postoperative bleeding. Ideally, patients are normotensive during emergence from anesthesia following heart surgery. In this instance, administration of any combination of the above agents could be used to lower blood pressure. A patient with a history of opioid use can be particularly challenging perioperatively and would likely benefit from a multimodal approach to postoperative analgesia including nonopioid analgesics, lidocaine and/or ketamine infusions, and—as is true for all patients undergoing major surgery—enrollment in an enhanced recovery program. There is also the possibility that this patient may be physically opioid-dependent, and his hypertension may be secondary to opioid withdrawal.

2. Although the blood pressure is immediately controlled, chest tube drainage remains greater than 300 mL/h for the next 3 h. The cardiac index falls from 2.2 L/min/m^2 to 1.2 L/min/m^2, and the patient develops metabolic acidosis. Additionally, blood pressure has now fallen to 90/60 mm Hg. The best course of action at this time is:

A. Administer additional sodium bicarbonate.
B. Administer two units of packed red blood cells.
C. Begin an infusion of milrinone.
D. Notify the surgeon that the patient likely requires reexploration.
E. Perform an emergent echocardiographic examination.
F. Both D and E.

The correct answer is F. This patient likely has ongoing bleeding that requires surgical attention. An emergent echocardiographic examination could be additionally helpful in discerning why the patient's cardiac index has fallen. Possibilities include hypovolemia from ongoing blood loss in addition to pericardial tamponade. Although bicarbonate administration, packed red blood cells, and milrinone may be necessary, determining the cause of hemodynamic instability is of paramount importance. The differential diagnosis of low cardiac index following heart surgery includes hypovolemia, right ventricular failure, left ventricular failure, and pericardial tamponade. Transesophageal echocardiography typically can discern the etiology of hemodynamic decline.

DID YOU LEARN?

• Management of post–cardiac surgery hypertension.
• Differential diagnosis of post–cardiac surgery hemodynamic instability.

Recommended Readings

Ansari Barodka V, Joshi B, Berkowitz D, Hogue CW Jr, Nyhan D. Implications of vascular aging. *Anesth Analg.* 2011;112:1048.

Butterworth IV JF, Mackey DC, Wasnick JD, eds. Hypotensive agents. In: *Morgan & Mikhail's Clinical Anesthesiology.* 6th ed. New York, NY: McGraw-Hill Education; 2018:253-260.

Espinosa A, Ripollés-Melchor J, Casans-Francés R, et al; Evidence Anesthesia Review Group. Perioperative use of clevidipine: A systematic review and meta-analysis. *PLoS One.* 2016;11:e0150625.

Gillies MA, Kakar V, Parker RJ, Honoré PM, Ostermann M. Fenoldopam to prevent acute kidney injury after major surgery—a systematic review and meta-analysis. *Crit Care.* 2015;19:449.

Hottinger DG, Beebe DS, Kozhimannil T, Prielipp RC, Belani KG. Sodium nitroprusside in 2014: A clinical concepts review. *J Anaesthesiol Clin Pharmacol.* 2014;30:462.

Jain A, Elgendy IY, Al-Ani M, Agarwal N, Pepine CJ. Advancements in pharmacotherapy for angina. *Expert Opin Pharmacother.* 2017;18:457.

Moerman AT, De Hert SG, Jacobs TF, et al. Cerebral oxygen desaturation during beach chair position. *Eur J Anaesthesiol.* 2012;29:82.

Pilkington SA, Taboada D, Martinez G. Pulmonary hypertension and its management in patients undergoing non-cardiac surgery. *Anaesthesia.* 2015;70:56.

Oren O, Goldberg S. Heart failure with preserved ejection fraction: Diagnosis and management. *Am J Med.* 2017;130:510.

Williams-Russo P, Sharrock NE, Mattis S. Randomized trial of hypotensive epidural anesthesia in older adults. *Anesthesiology.* 1999;91:926.

Zhao N, Xu J, Singh B, et al. Nitrates for the prevention of cardiac morbidity and mortality in patients undergoing non cardiac surgery. *Cochrane Database Syst Rev.* 2016;(8):CD010726.

CHAPTER 12

Local Anesthetics

CASE 1 — Regional Anesthesia for Dialysis Access

John F. Butterworth IV, MD

1. You are asked by a colleague to place a peripheral nerve block in a patient scheduled for revision of an arteriovenous fistula for dialysis access. The medical history is notable for hypertension, insulin-dependent diabetes, and, of course, end-stage renal disease (ESRD). The patient was last dialyzed yesterday. As you prepare to place a single-shot supraclavicular block with 20 mL of mepivacaine 1.5%, a colleague asks about the possibility of a prolonged duration of blockade when using mepivacaine given the patient's renal disease. The best response is:

   A. Duration of mepivacaine anesthesia would be prolonged and blood levels increased in a patient with pseudocholinesterase deficiency.
   B. Duration of mepivacaine anesthesia would not be prolonged and blood levels would not be increased in ESRD.
   C. Mepivacaine duration will be prolonged due to increased blood levels of active metabolites in a patient with hepatic failure.
   D. Mepivacaine block duration will not be prolonged; however, this patient is at increased risk of methemoglobinemia from accumulation of local anesthetic metabolites.

The correct answer is B. In general, regional anesthesia is terminated by redistribution of local anesthetics, not by metabolism. There is no evidence that regional anesthesia has a longer duration in patients with ESRD, and indeed, some experts believe that regional anesthesia has a shorter duration in patients with ESRD. Mepivacaine and all other amide local anesthetics are metabolized by hepatic microsomal P-450 enzymes, specifically undergoing N-dealkylation and hydroxylation. Although decreases in hepatic blood flow or hepatic function may result in patients having increased concentrations of local anesthetic in blood, decreases in renal function have little effect on amide local anesthetic metabolism. Very little unmetabolized local anesthetic is excreted in urine. Only ester local anesthetics are dependent on pseudocholinesterase for metabolism via ester hydrolysis, and in any case, resolution of regional anesthesia with ester local anesthetics is almost exclusively due to redistribution, not metabolism. Methemoglobinemia is of greatest concern when using prilocaine or benzocaine, not mepivacaine.

2. If this same patient were presenting for open reduction and internal fixation of a forearm fracture instead of arteriovenous fistula revision, the goals of the block may change to include postoperative analgesia as well as intraoperative anesthesia. Your consulting colleague now suggests that you use a 1:1 mixture of mepivacaine 1.5% and bupivacaine 0.5% for fast onset and a prolonged duration of action. Which of the following statements is true?

A. In general, the highly lipid-soluble local anesthetics have a shorter duration of action than less lipid-soluble agents.
B. In general, the highly lipid-soluble local anesthetics have a more rapid onset than less lipid-soluble agents.
C. When mepivacaine is combined with bupivacaine in a 1:1 ratio, the duration of analgesia will be just as long as an equal volume of bupivacaine given alone.
D. The site of injection influences the duration of the nerve block.
E. The lower the pH, the more rapid is the speed of onset.

The correct answer is D. The onset of action of local anesthetics is generally slower for those agents with greater potency and lipid solubility, with the sole exception of the rarely-used etidocaine (which is potent, highly lipid soluble, and has a relatively rapid onset). The pK_a of a drug is the pH at which the percentage of ionized and neutral forms is equal, and the speed of onset of clinical anesthesia is *generally* faster when the pH is greater (and the fraction of the local anesthetic in the protonated versus free base form is smaller). In order to most readily permeate the neuronal plasma membrane, the drug must be in a neutral (ie, uncharged, more lipid soluble) form. This is why some clinicians routinely add small amounts of $NaHCO_3$ to local anesthetic solutions.

The duration of action of a local anesthetic associates with its lipid solubility and its potency. Those agents with increased potency and lipid solubility tend to be longer acting (for example, bupivacaine, ropivacaine, and tetracaine). The site of injection of the local anesthetic plays an important role both in its uptake and duration. The duration of bupivacaine spinal anesthesia is only a few hours, whereas bupivacaine provides brachial plexus blocks lasting 10 to 16 h. The rate of absorption is increased with increasing vascularity of the site, with intravenous > tracheal > intercostal > paracervical > epidural > brachial plexus > sciatic > subcutaneous. The addition of vasoconstrictors to local anesthetics prolongs the duration, decreases systemic absorption, and enhances the quality of analgesia, particularly of relatively shorter-acting agents such as lidocaine. Local anesthetics combinations of 1:1 produce blocks with onset times and durations of analgesia intermediate between the two agents.

DID YOU LEARN?

- The different mechanisms of metabolism of local anesthetics based on their chemical structure.
- Factors that affect the onset and duration of nerve blockade.
- The relationship of pH and pK_a to membrane permeation
- The relative rates of absorption for various sites of injection of local anesthetics

CASE 2   Lidocaine Infusion for Analgesia

John F. Butterworth IV, MD

1. A 65-year-old, 68-kg man has undergone colon resection for cancer under general anesthesia. In an attempt to minimize his postoperative analgesic requirements, an IV infusion of lidocaine 2 mg/min was administered intraoperatively and continued in the postanesthesia care unit. You are called by his nurse to evaluate him for hypoxemia and somnolence. When you arrive at the bedside, you note a reading of 94% on the pulse oximeter while the patient is receiving 6 L/min O_2 via nasal cannula. An arterial blood gas reveals the following values: pH 7.26, PCO_2 56 mm Hg, pO_2 82 mm Hg, and HCO_3 26 mEq/L. Which of the following is true regarding local anesthetic toxicity?

   A. For a given dose, the likelihood of local anesthetic toxicity is independent of site of injection.
   B. Hypercarbia may exacerbate local anesthetic systemic toxicity.
   C. Lidocaine inhibits cardiac Na channels in a more prolonged way than bupivacaine due to lidocaine's slower unbinding from the channel.
   D. Hypoxemia has little effect on local anesthetic systemic toxicity.
   E. Signs of cardiovascular local anesthetic toxicity are unlikely to precede central nervous system signs.

The correct answer is B. Systemic toxicity of local anesthetics is enhanced by hypercarbia, hypoxemia, and acidosis. After gaining entry into the cell, it is the protonated form of the drug that more potently exerts its action at the Na channel and thus exerts a toxic effect. Bupivacaine has a high affinity for cardiac Na channels, and it unbinds from this channel more slowly than does lidocaine. Lidocaine is a less potent local anesthetic, and while it may cause cardiotoxicity, its cardiac depressant effects are seen at much higher plasma concentrations than with bupivacaine or ropivacaine. Whereas bupivacaine is more likely to cause ventricular arrhythmias and sudden cardiovascular collapse, lidocaine toxicity is more often associated with progressive hypotension and bradycardia from left-ventricular depression. Arrhythmias are rarely the presenting sign of cardiac toxicity from lidocaine. Classic descriptions of local anesthetic systemic toxicity include a progression from mild central nervous system signs, such as tinnitus, perioral numbness, and dizziness, to excitatory signs, such as agitation and restlessness with progression to muscle twitching and seizure activity. In "classic" descriptions, signs of cardiac toxicity including cardiac depression and arrhythmias most often occurred *after* these neurologic "warning signs." In recent years, it has become clear that cardiovascular toxicity, particularly with bupivacaine and other potent local anesthetics, may occur before or concurrently with central nervous system signs or symptoms. The site of local anesthetic injection is important given the variability of degree and rate of uptake from various sites (eg, intercostal blocks versus local infiltration).

2. While you are reviewing the patient's laboratory values and his medical history, he becomes restless, shows myoclonic jerks, and then has a generalized seizure. His heart rate rises from 80 to 95 beats/min, and SpO_2 remains at 94% with a respiratory rate of 12 breaths/min. The blood pressure is 122/70 mm Hg. Of the following five options, what is the most appropriate next step?

   A. Administer an immediate bolus of 20% intralipid.
   B. Administer propofol 100 mg.
   C. Intubation with manual ventilation.
   D. Administer midazolam in 1-mg increments to terminate the seizure.
   E. Maintain an open airway.

The correct answer is D. This patient is demonstrating signs and symptoms consistent with local anesthetic toxicity. He became restless and was then noted to exhibit muscular twitching, which preceded convulsions. While oxygenation is of paramount importance, this patient may not require intubation. Cessation of seizure activity decreases the metabolic requirement for oxygen and prevents excessive CO_2 production and acidosis; therefore, appropriate anticonvulsant therapy should be promptly initiated. Benzodiazepines are the first-line choice in this case. Propofol may be administered as it also increases the seizure threshold; however, a dose of 100 mg may cause apnea and could exacerbate toxicity. Patients with suspected local anesthetic toxicity who begin to exhibit signs of cardiovascular toxicity should be treated with an intralipid bolus, particularly when ropivacaine or bupivacaine is the "offending" local anesthetic. This patient received lidocaine and has not shown signs of progression to more serious toxicity; thus, intralipid is not indicated. Should this patient's toxicity progress, a modified advanced cardiac life support (ACLS) protocol may be initiated.

3. You administer midazolam, 2 mg IV push. The patient's vital signs remain stable, and the convulsions appear to cease. About 2 min later, the nurse draws

your attention to the monitor. You see that the patient's blood pressure is now 92/50 mm Hg, with a heart rate of 64 beats/min. The SpO_2 is now 90%. You realize the lidocaine infusion continues to run and fear impending cardiovascular depression. You immediately discontinue the infusion. Which of the following interventions is the most appropriate for treatment of cardiovascular compromise in the setting of suspected local anesthetic toxicity?

A. Vasopressin bolus, 40 units, to replace the first dose of epinephrine.
B. Diltiazam for supraventricular arrhythmias.
C. Lidocaine bolus for refractory ventricular tachycardia.
D. Epinephrine, 70 mcg IV push every 3 to 5 min.
E. Metoprolol bolus for narrow-complex tachycardia.

The correct answer is D. The treatment of cardiovascular compromise/arrest in the setting of suspected local anesthetic toxicity requires modification of ACLS protocols. Calcium channel blockers, β-blockers, and local anesthetics should all be avoided in this setting, as they may worsen the clinical condition. Epinephrine is an acceptable drug choice; however, the dose should be reduced from the usual 1 mg IV push to less than 1 mcg/kg/dose. Animal studies suggest that vasopressin administered after bupivacaine-induced cardiac arrest may increase the incidence of pulmonary edema. Whether humans would respond similarly remains unknown. In this patient population, the trachea should be intubated and ventilation should commence with 100% oxygen. Propofol should be avoided in patients with signs of cardiovascular instability. The lipid content is not great enough to replace lipid emulsion, and the cardiac depression that follows is likely to hinder resuscitation. Twenty percent lipid emulsion therapy is the treatment of choice for cardiac toxicity with bupicaine or ropivacaine, and it should be administered initially as a bolus, 1.5 mL/kg of lean body mass over 1 min, or roughly 100 mL in an average adult. An infusion of 0.25 mL/kg/min, approximately 20 mL/min, should follow. For persistent collapse, the bolus may be repeated and the infusion increased to 0.5 mL/kg/min. Once the patient is stable, the infusion should be continued for at least another 10 min. It is unclear whether treatment with lipid emulsions is as effective for the less lipid-soluble agents (eg, lidocaine or mepivacaine) as it is for bupivacaine and ropivacaine.

DID YOU LEARN?

- The effects of hypercarbia, hypoxemia, and acidosis on local anesthetic toxicity.
- Differences in toxicity profiles between commonly used local anesthetics.
- Signs and symptoms of systemic local anesthetic toxicity.
- Modifications of resuscitation protocols for patients with cardiovascular compromise in the setting of local anesthetic toxicity.

Recommended Readings

Brunton LL, Knollmann BC, Hilal-Dandan R, eds. *Goodman and Gilman's The Pharmacological Basis of Therapeutics*. 13th ed. New York, NY: McGraw-Hill; 2018.

Butterworth IV JF, Mackey DC, Wasnick JD, eds. Local anesthetics. In: *Morgan & Mikhail's Clinical Anesthesiology*. 6th ed. New York, NY: McGraw-Hill Education; 2018:261-274.

Cousins MJ, Carr DB, Horlocker TT, Bridenbaugh PO, eds. *Cousins & Bridenbaugh's Neural Blockade in Clinical Anesthesia and Pain Medicine*. 4th ed. Philadelphia, PA: Lippincott, Williams & Wilkins; 2009.

El-Boghdadly K, Chin KJ. Local anesthetic systemic toxicity: Continuing professional development. *Can J Anaesth*. 2016;63:330.

Hadzic A, ed. *Textbook of Regional Anesthesia and Acute Pain Management*. New York, NY: McGraw-Hill; 2016. Includes discussions of the selection of local anesthetic agents.

Kirksey MA, Haskins SC, Cheng J, Liu SS. Local anesthetic peripheral nerve block adjuvants for prolongation of analgesia: A systematic qualitative review. *PLoS One*. 2015;10:e0137312.

Liu SS, Ortolan S, Sandoval MV, et al. Cardiac arrest and seizures caused by local anesthetic systemic toxicity after peripheral nerve blocks: Should we still fear the reaper? *Reg Anesth Pain Med*. 2016;41:5.

Matsen FA 3rd, Papadonikolakis A. Published evidence demonstrating the causation of glenohumeral chondrolysis by postoperative infusion of local anesthetic via a pain pump. *J Bone Joint Surg Am*. 2013;95:1126.

Neal JM, Bernards CM, Butterworth JF 4th, et al. ASRA practice advisory on local anesthetic systemic toxicity. *Reg Anesth Pain Med*. 2010;35:152.

Neal JM, Woodward CM, Harrison TK. The American Society of Regional Anesthesia and Pain Medicine Checklist for managing local anesthetic systemic toxicity: 2017 version. *Reg Anesth Pain Med*. 2018;43:150-153.

Vasques F, Behr AU, Weinberg G, Ori C, Di Gregorio G. A review of local anesthetic systemic toxicity cases since publication of the American Society of Regional Anesthesia recommendations: To whom it may concern. *Reg Anesth Pain Med*. 2015;40:698.

CHAPTER 13

Adjuncts to Anesthesia

CASE 1   Patient with Full Stomach

Kallol Chaudhuri, MD, PhD

1. A 22-year-old, 70-kg woman presents with ectopic pregnancy for emergency laparoscopic surgery. She ate a fast-food hamburger with fries 2 h prior to the onset of abdominal pain. In the holding area, she has abdominal pain and is actively vomiting. Her past history is significant for depression. To lower the gastric pH, the patient is given a combination of antacids, antihistamines, and metoclopramide. H_1 histamine receptor stimulation has which of the following effects?

    A. Increases myocardial contractility.
    B. Increases capillary permeability.
    C. Dilates bronchiolar smooth muscle.
    D. Activates suppressor T-lymphocytes.

The correct answer is B. Histamine is found in the central nervous system, in the gastric mucosa, and in other peripheral tissues. Histamine plays a major role in promoting the secretion of hydrochloric acid by the parietal cells in the stomach. Multiple receptors mediate the effects of histamine. The H_1 receptor activates phopholipase C and produces increased capillary permeability, enhanced ventricular irritability, bronchiolar constriction, and intestinal smooth muscle contraction, and attracts leukocytes, inducing the synthesis of prostaglandin. H_2-receptor stimulation increases heart rate and ventricular contractility, induces mild bronchodilatation, increases pulmonary vasoconstriction, increases gastric acid, and activates suppressor T-cells.

2. The patient is given 30 mL of 0.3 M sodium citrate prior to rapid-sequence induction. Of the following conditions, which is the one that is not an independent risk factor for postoperative nausea and vomiting?

A. Obesity.
B. Female gender.
C. History of motion sickness.
D. Use of opioids.

The correct answer is A. Obesity is not an independent risk factor for the development of postoperative nausea and vomiting (PONV). Anxiety and reversal of neuromuscular blockade are similarly not found to be independently associated with PONV. Risks of PONV are summarized below.

Risk Factors for Postoperative Nausea and Vomiting (PONV)[1]

Patient-specific risk factors:
  Female gender
  Nonsmoking status
  History of PONV/motion sickness
Anesthetic risk factors:
  Use of volatile anesthetics
  Use of nitrous oxide
  Use of intraoperative and postoperative opioids
Surgical risk factors:
  Duration of surgery (each 30-min increase in duration increases PONV risk by 60%, so that a baseline risk of 10% is increased by 16% after 30 min)
  Type of surgery

[1]Risk factors are assigned points and an increasing number of points increases the likelihood of PONV. Refer to the Society of Ambulatory Anesthesia (SAMBA) guidelines. Modified with permission from Gan TJ, Meyer TA, Apfel CC, et al: Society for Ambulatory Anesthesia guidelines for the management of postoperative nausea and vomiting, *Anesth Analg.* 2007 Dec;105(6):1615-1628.

3. The patient is given ondansetron. Of the cardiac conditions listed, with which should 5-HT$_3$ receptor antagonists such as ondansetron be used with caution?

A. Atrial fibrillation.
B. Prolonged QT interval.
C. Ventricular ectopy.
D. Wolf–Parkinson–White syndrome.

The correct answer is B. All of the 5-HT$_3$ antagonists can cause an increase in the QT interval, most commonly seen with dolasetron. The butyrophenone droperidol (0.625–1.25 mg) was previously used routinely for PONV prophylaxis; however, the U.S. Food and Drug Administration (FDA) has placed a warning indicating that it can produce QT prolongation, leading to the development of torsades des pointes arrythmia. This has been reported only at doses much larger than those used for PONV treatment.

4. An anticholinergic, scopolamine, is administered transdermally to further augment PONV prophylaxis. Of the anticholinergics below, which is incapable of crossing the blood–brain barrier?

(Reproduced with permission from Butterworth JF, Mackey DC, Wasnick JD: *Morgan and Mikhail's Clinical Anesthesiology*, 6th ed. New York, NY: McGraw-Hill Education; 2018.)

The correct answer is C. Glycopyrrolate has a quartenary structure, hindering its ability to cross the blood–brain barrier. Atropine (option A) and scopolamine (option B) cross the blood–brain barrier.

5. The patient has been treated with various antidepressants and antipsychotics with antimuscarinic properties. In the postanesthesia care unit, the patient becomes agitated with impaired vision, dry mouth, and tachycardia. It is concluded that the patient most likely demonstrates central anticholinergic syndrome. Which is the most effective cholinesterase inhibitor to administer?

(Reproduced with permission from Butterworth JF, Mackey DC, Wasnick JD: *Morgan and Mikhail's Clinical Anesthesiology*, 6th ed. New York, NY: McGraw-Hill Education; 2018.)

The correct answer is D. The three other chemical structures are of neostigmine (option A), pyridostigmine (option B), and endrophonium (option C). Physostigmine, being a tertiary as opposed to a quarternary amine, has the ability to cross the blood–brain barrier, making it an effective treatment for central anticholinergic syndrome.

6. The patient successfully recovers from her ectopic pregnancy; however, her depression worsens and she undergoes electroconvulsive therapy (ECT). Anesthesia by mask is induced with propofol and succinylcholine. Following induction of anesthesia, the patient develops masseter muscle rigidity, tachycardia, and hypercarbia. Twenty mg of dantrolene are found in the ECT suite and are administered to the patient. Which of the following statements is true?

A. This amount of dantrolene exceeds the recommended dose for the initial treatment of this patient.
B. This amount of dantrolene is the recommended dose of the initial treatment of this patient.
C. This amount of dantrolene does not meet the recommended initial dose of this patient.
D. Dantrolene administration is not warranted at this time.

The correct answer is C. The initial dose of dantrolene for a suspected episode of malignant hyperthermia (MH) is 2.5 mg/kg every 5 min until the episode is terminated, with an upper limit of roughly 10 mg/kg. The ECT facility with only 20 mg of dantrolene available is grossly undersupplied to treat an episode of MH in this 70-g patient. Dantrolene is relatively safe and should be employed immediately in the treatment of suspected MH.

7. The patient returns 2 years later for elective cholecystectomy. She is a non-smoker and reports previous PONV. Which of the following is true about her risk of PONV?

A. Her risk of PONV is low.
B. Her risk of PONV is medium, and thus one or two interventions to prevent PONV are indicated.
C. Her risk of PONV is high, and more than two interventions are indicated to prevent PONV.
D. Nonsmokers are less likely to experience PONV.

The correct answer is C. The patient presents with a number of risk factors for PONV. The algorithm below can be helpful in mitigating PONV risk.

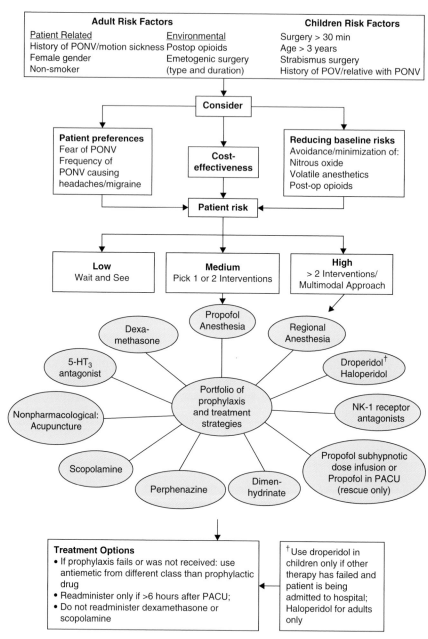

Adult Risk Factors		Children Risk Factors
Patient Related	Environmental	Surgery > 30 min
History of PONV/motion sickness	Postop opioids	Age > 3 years
Female gender	Emetogenic surgery	Strabismus surgery
Non-smoker	(type and duration)	History of POV/relative with PONV

Consider

Patient preferences
Fear of PONV
Frequency of PONV causing headaches/migraine

Cost-effectiveness

Reducing baseline risks
Avoidance/minimization of:
Nitrous oxide
Volatile anesthetics
Post-op opioids

Patient risk

Low
Wait and See

Medium
Pick 1 or 2 Interventions

High
> 2 Interventions/
Multimodal Approach

Portfolio of prophylaxis and treatment strategies

Propofol Anesthesia
Dexa-methasone
5-HT₃ antagonist
Nonpharmacological: Acupuncture
Scopolamine
Perphenazine
Dimen-hydrinate
Propofol subhypnotic dose infusion or Propofol in PACU (rescue only)
NK-1 receptor antagonists
Droperidol† Haloperidol
Regional Anesthesia

Treatment Options
- If prophylaxis fails or was not received: use antiemetic from different class than prophylactic drug
- Readminister only if >6 hours after PACU;
- Do not readminister dexamethasone or scopolamine

†Use droperidol in children only if other therapy has failed and patient is being admitted to hospital; Haloperidol for adults only

Algorithm for management of postoperative nausea and vomiting. PACU, postanesthesia care unit; PONV, postoperative nausea and vomiting; POV, postoperative vomiting. (Reproduced with permission from Gan TJ, Diemunsch P, Habib A, et al. Consensus guidelines for the management of postoperative nausea and vomiting. *Anesth Analg.* 2014 Jan;118(1):85-113.)

DID YOU LEARN?

- Properties of histamine receptors.
- Risk factors for PONV.
- Cardiac manifestations of 5-HT$_3$ antagonists.
- Manifestations and treatment for central anticholinergic syndrome.
- Proper dosing of dantrolene for the treatment of MH.

CHAPTER 13

Adjuncts to Anesthesia

Recommended Readings

2Butterworth IV JF, Mackey DC, Wasnick JD, eds. Adjuncts to anesthesia. In: *Morgan & Mikhail's Clinical Anesthesiology*. 6th ed. New York, NY: McGraw-Hill Education; 2018:275-294.

Dahl J, Nielsen V, Wetterslev L, et al. Postoperative effects of paracetamol, NSAIDs, glucocorticoids, gabapentinoids and their combinations: A topical review. *Acta Anaesthesiol Scand*. 2014;58:1165.

De Souza D, Doar L, Mehta S, et al. Aspiration prophylaxis and rapid sequence induction for elective cesarean delivery; time to reassess old dogma. *Anesth Analg*. 2010;110:1503.

Doleman B, Read D, Lund JN, Williams JP. Preventive acetaminophen reduces postoperative opioid consumption, vomiting, and pain scores after surgery: Systematic review and meta-analysis. *Reg Anesth Pain Med*. 2015;40:706.

Fabritius M, Geisler A, Petersen P, et al. Gabapentin for postoperative pain management—a systemic review with meta-analyses and trial sequential analyses. *Acta Anaesthesiol Scand*. 2016;60:1188.

George E, Hornuss C, Apfel C. Neurokinin 1 and novel serotonin antagonists for postoperative and postdischarge nausea and vomiting. *Curr Opin Anesth*. 2010;23:714.

Glass P, White P. Practice guidelines for the management of postoperative nausea and vomiting: Past, present and future. *Anesth Analg*. 2007;105:1528.

Kaye A, Ali S, Urman R. Perioperative analgesia: Ever changing technology and pharmacology. *Best Pract Res Clin Anaesthesiol*. 2014;28:3.

Kelly CJ, Walker RW. Perioperative pulmonary aspiration is infrequent and low risk in pediatric anesthetic practice. *Paediatr Anaesth*. 2015;25:36.

Lipp A, Kaliappan A. Focus on quality: Managing pain and PONV in day surgery. *Curr Anaesth Crit Care*. 2007;18:200.

Priebe HJ. Evidence no longer supports use of cricoid pressure. *Br J Anaesth*. 2016;117:537.

Sanchez Munoz MC, De Kock M, Forget P. What is the place of clonidine in anesthesia? Systematic review and meta-analyses of randomized controlled trials. *J Clin Anesth*. 2017;38:140.

Young A, Buvanendran A. Multimodal systemic and intra articular analgesics. *Int Anesth Clin*. 2011;49:117.

2222222

SECTION III

Anesthetic Management

CHAPTER 14

Preoperative Assessment, Premedication, & Perioperative Documentation

| CASE 1 | Informed Consent: The Discussion versus The Form |

Monica Rice Murphy, MD

You work providing obstetrical anesthesia in a high-volume delivery center. At 7 A.M. one morning you relieve a colleague and assume responsibility of a 28-year-old G2P1 having a repeat cesarean delivery under epidural anesthesia. The case is proceeding smoothly. When you review the patient's information in your hospital information system, you find that one of the anesthesiologists wrote a note during a preoperative visit the previous week, but you find no documentation of a preanesthetic evaluation during the current hospitalization.

1. Regarding the requirements for the documentation of the preanesthetic evaluation, which of the following is the most accurate statement?

   A. A preoperative note completed 1 week before the scheduled cesarean delivery would satisfy most insurers' requirements for a preanesthetic assessment.

   B. The Center for Medicare and Medicaid Services states that the preanesthetic evaluation must already be documented when the patient enters the operating room.

   C. All components of the preanesthetic evaluation must be performed within 48 h prior to the anesthetic.

   D. Lack of documentation of a preanesthetic evaluation before an anesthetic is submitted for payment may lead to audits and fines.

The correct answer is D. The U.S. Centers for Medicare and Medicaid Services (CMS) has extensive standards and regulations for billing. Most large insurers in the United States follow CMS regulations. CMS bundles preanesthetic evaluations, intraoperative care, and postanesthesia care into one service. In the United States, failure to comply with the CMS Conditions and Standards may subject an institution to fines, further audits, and charges of fraud. The *2011 CMS Revised Interpretive Guidelines* provide detailed guidance for those who wish to avoid such unpleasantness. The guidelines specify components of the preanesthesia assessment that must be performed within the 48 h preceding induction of anesthesia, and other components that may be performed within 30 days before the 48-h window. These must be reviewed and updated within the 48-h window. All preanesthesia documentation must take place before the first induction drug is administered.

Must Be Performed Within 48 h Before Induction	May Be Performed up to 30 Days Before Induction (but must be reviewed/ updated within 48 h before induction)
Review of medical history, anesthesia history, medications, allergies	Assignment of ASA class
	Attainment of labs/studies
Patient interview (if possible)	Identification of potential challenges
Physical examination	Development of anesthetic plan

2. On the following day, you relieve a colleague providing anesthesia for another cesarean delivery. The patient is a 21-year-old G1P0 who experienced arrest of the active phase of labor. The patient is stable and doing well, and the baby has been delivered. As you scroll through the chart to place postoperative orders, you cannot locate a signed anesthesia consent form. Which of the following statements is correct about informed consent?

A. Data from the American Society of Anesthesiologists (ASA) Closed Claims Database point to informed consent issues in more than 10% of claims.

B. An anesthesia-specific consent form, signed by the patient and witnessed by a nurse, proves that the patient gave informed consent.

C. Most jurisdictions apply the "reasonable patient standard" or the "reasonable practitioner standard" when assessing the adequacy of disclosure.

D. Lack of documentation of informed consent violates Medicare standards for the provision of anesthesia services.

The correct answer is C. Informed consent is a legal term that reflects societal support for the individual's right to accept or refuse treatment. The elements required for informed consent usually include: *disclosure* of risks, benefits, and alternatives; *capacity* of the patient or surrogate to understand and use the information to make a judgement; *comprehension* and *acceptance* of the information by the patient; and the *absence of coercion or manipulation* in the making of the decision.

In most jurisdictions in the United States, the standard for determining the adequacy of the *disclosure* element in a given circumstance is either the "reasonable patient standard" or the "reasonable practitioner standard," which ask the respective questions "What amount of information would satisfy a reasonable person?"

and "What amount of information would a reasonable practitioner disclose?" A less common but emerging standard advocates the tailoring of the disclosure to suit a particular patient's wants and needs ("the subjective patient standard").

What will be expected for documentation of consent for anesthesia varies across institutions in the United States. Medicare does not have an informed consent requirement for anesthesia services. The Joint Commission requires written documentation of informed consent but does not mandate its form. The ASA Closed Claims Database lists informed consent issues in only 1% of claims, making it difficult to provide evidence about the legal protection offered by a separate form. However, the implementation of a separate anesthesia consent form is becoming widespread as a growing number of anesthesiologists and their malpractice insurance carriers perceive this practice to have medical and legal benefits. Importantly, it is the meaningful discussion with the patient, not the signed document, that constitutes the informed consent; furthermore, a witness's signature on a consent form attests to the authenticity of the signature, not the content of the discussion.

DID YOU LEARN?

- Billing-imposed requirements for documenting a preanesthetic assessment.
- Components of the preanesthesia assessment that may be performed outside the 48-h preceding induction, provided they are reviewed/updated within the 48 h.
- Commonly invoked standards for the "disclosure" component of informed consent.
- "Subjective patient standard" for informed consent.

Recommended Reading

Tait AR, Teig MK, Voepel-Lewis T. Informed consent for anesthesia: A review of practice and strategies for optimizing the consent process. *Can J Anaesth*. 2014;61(9):832-842.

CASE 2   Fasting Before Sedation and Anesthesia

Monica Rice Murphy, MD

You are assigned by your chief of anesthesiology to a task force on "conscious sedation" for your hospital. A task force colleague proposes a 4-h period of NPO (nil per os) prior to all elective procedures requiring moderate or deep sedation. The example case is a 16-year-old with a closed fracture requiring sedation-analgesia prior to closed reduction. The chief of the emergency medicine department objects to any NPO requirement prior to sedation in her department.

1. Regarding NPO evidence and guidelines, which of the following is the most accurate?

A. For solid foods, a 6-h fast is superior to a 4-h fast for reducing emesis and pulmonary aspiration.
B. ASA and European Society of Anaesthesiologists guidelines agree that patients should fast from solids for at least 6 h and clear liquids for at least 2 h prior to an elective procedure requiring anesthesia.
C. The ASA guidelines specify a 4-h NPO time for patients requiring sedation in emergency room situations.
D. The ASA guidelines suggest cancelling elective procedures when the patient has not followed the fasting recommendations.

The correct answer is B. The European Society of Anaesthesiolgists (ESA) and the ASA have published preoperative fasting guidelines for elective procedures. Both guidelines recommend a 6-h fasting period for solid food, a 4-h fasting period for human milk, and a 2-h fasting period for clear liquids. In contrast to the ESA, the ASA further recommends an 8-h NPO period for fried or fatty food. Nevertheless, evidence is lacking as to how the timing of ingestion of solid food, infant formula, human milk, or clear liquids impacts the incidence of perioperative pulmonary aspiration. When fasting recommendations are not followed, the anesthesiologist should determine the amount and type of the ingested substance prior to estimating the risks and benefits of proceeding. ASA guidelines do not specify NPO periods for emergent or urgent situations, whether for monitored anesthesia care, regional anesthesia, or general anesthesia. The sedation practitioner must consider the possibility of pulmonary aspiration when choosing the timing of the procedure and the target level of sedation. In some cases, the risk of aspiration with deep sedation may be sufficiently great that general anesthesia with tracheal intubation may be a safer alternative. Of note, the American College of Emergency Physicians discourages delaying procedural sedation based on fasting times.

2. Your task force asks you to present published guidelines for granting privileges for administration of moderate sedation by practitioners who are not qualified anesthesia professionals. Based on your reading of the relevant guidelines, choose the best statement.

A. "Conscious sedation" is synonymous with minimal sedation/anxiolysis.
B. Patients under moderate sedation may require repeated or painful stimulation to elicit a purposeful response, and spontaneous ventilation may be inadequate.
C. Nonanesthesiologist practitioners who supervise moderate sedation are not required to have advanced airway skills sufficient to place a laryngeal mask airway or tracheal tube.
D. The ASA produces education materials to assist in the education and training of providers of moderate sedation who lack clinical privileges in anesthesia.

The correct answer is D. Statements for describing both requirements for Moderate Sedation privileges and materials for training sedation providers are available at asahq.org. Providers of moderate sedation must be able to recognize the various levels of sedation and general anesthesia (see table below). They must have a familiarity with the pharmacology of drugs used in sedation and the corresponding antagonists. Because intervention may be required to maintain a patent airway, providers of moderate sedation must be able to provide positive-pressure bag-mask ventilation. Supervisory practitioners should be trained in advanced life support measures appropriate to the ages of their patients. The term "conscious sedation" persists despite ongoing ridicule and attempts to expunge it, but it refers to moderate, not mild sedation.

	Minimal Sedation Anxiolysis	Moderate Sedation/ Analgesia ("Conscious Sedation")	Deep Sedation/ Analgesia	General Anesthesia
Responsiveness	Normal response to verbal stimulation	Purposeful response to verbal or tactile stimulation	Purposeful response following repeated or painful stimulation	Unarousable even with painful stimulus
Airway	Unaffected	No intervention required	Intervention may be required	Intervention often required
Spontaneous Ventilation	Unaffected	Adequate	May be inadequate	Frequently inadequate
Cardiovascular Function	Unaffected	Usually maintained	Usually maintained	May be impaired

Reproduced with permission from Practice Guidelines for Moderate Procedural Sedation and Analgesia 2018: A Report by the American Society of Anesthesiologists Task Force on Moderate Procedural Sedation and Analgesia, the American Association of Oral and Maxillofacial Surgeons, American College of Radiology, American Dental Association, American Society of Dentist Anesthesiologists, and Society of Interventional Radiology: *Anesthesiology.* 2018 Mar;128(3):437-479.

3. After your meeting, you return to the operating room to finish the day's cases. You interview a healthy 16-year-old scheduled for open reduction and internal fixation of a forearm fracture. He drank 400 mL of a clear liquid 2 h ago. Select the two statements below that have the support of both randomized controlled trials *and* meta-analysis.

A. Children given clear liquids 2 to 4 h before a procedure have increased (more favorable) gastric pH when compared to children who fast from clear liquids for more than 4 h.

B. Adults given clear liquids 2 to 4 h before a procedure have smaller gastric volume when compared to adults who fast from clear liquids for more than 4 h.

C. Infants given clear formula 4 h before surgery have higher gastric volumes than those who fast from infant formula for more than 6 h.

D. Adults given a light breakfast (eg, tea and toast) approximately 4 h before surgery had smaller gastric residual volumes than those who fasted overnight.

The correct answers are A and B. Adults who ingest clear liquids up to 2 h before surgery have smaller gastric residual volumes than those who fast from clear liquids for 4 h or more. Some randomized clinical trials have shown the same for children, but meta-analysis of all available trials has not confirmed that conclusion. Adults and children who ingest clear liquids up to 2 h before surgery have increased gastric pH values as compared to those who remained NPO. Studies comparing fasting times for infant formula have been observational. A randomized controlled trial was performed in adults comparing the effect on gastric volume of a light breakfast versus overnight fasting. The findings showed similar gastric volumes in the light breakfast group, but the presence of solid food in the stomach could not be ruled out.

4. The orthopedic surgeon, who trained first in Sweden, arrives and asks the patient: "Did you drink all of your high-carbohydrate drink?" The surgeon is referring to the clear liquid consumed 2 h ago. Your orthopedic colleague tells you the benefits of prescribing preoperative carbohydrate-rich drinks. When consumed 2 h before surgery, the literature suggests all of the following effects of carbohydrate-rich drinks *except*:

A. They decrease insulin resistance in the postoperative period.
B. They decrease the need for inotropes in bypass surgery.
C. They decrease hunger and anxiety in the preoperative period.
D. They increase gastric residual volume.

The correct answer is D. A Swedish study of patients undergoing hip arthroplasty demonstrated that preoperative ingestion of carbohydrate-rich liquids decreases insulin resistance in the postoperative period. Some evidence suggests that preoperative carbohydrate loading decreases the requirements for inotropic support when weaning from bypass in cardiac surgery. Carbohydrate-rich liquids given preoperatively decrease hunger and anxiety when compared to flavored water. Carbohydrate-rich liquids did not produce an increase in gastric pH or gastric residual volume when compared with flavored water.

DID YOU LEARN?

- Basic ASA and ESA fasting period guidelines.
- Evidence that supports the ingestion of clear liquids before surgery.
- Differences between moderate sedation, deep sedation, and general anesthesia.
- Potential benefits of carbohydrate loading before surgery.

Recommended Readings

Ayoub K, Nairooz R, Almomani A, et al. Perioperative heparin bridging in atrial fibrillation patients requiring temporary interruption of anticoagulation: Evidence from meta-analysis. *J Stroke Cerebrovasc Dis*. 2016;pii:S1052.

Butterworth IV JF, Mackey DC, Wasnick JD, eds. Preoperative assessment, premedication, & perioperative documentation. In: *Morgan & Mikhail's Clinical Anesthesiology*. 6th ed. New York, NY: McGraw-Hill Education; 2018:295-306.

Centers for Medicare and Medicaid Services (CMS). CMS Manual System. Pub 100-07 State Operations Provider Certification. DHHS. Available at: http://www.kdheks.gov/bhfr/download/Appendix_L.pdf. Accessed December 16, 2017.

Egbert LD, Battit G, Turndorf H, Beecher HK. The value of the preoperative visit by an anesthetist. A study of doctor-patient rapport. *JAMA*. 1963;185:553.

Jeong BH, Shin B, Eom JS, et al. Development of a prediction rule for estimating postoperative pulmonary complications. *PLoS One*. 2014;9:e113656.

Mendelson CL. The aspiration of stomach contents into the lungs during obstetric anesthesia. *Am J Obstet Gynecol*. 1946;52:191.

References

Continuum of depth of sedation. Definition of general anesthesia and levels of sedation-analgesia. *Eur J Anaesthesiol*. 2011;28:556-569.

Godwin SA, Burton JH, Gerardo CJ, American College of Emergency Physicians, et al. Clinical policy: procedural sedation and analgesia in the emergency department *Ann Emerg Med*. 2014;63(2):247-258.

Practice Guidelines for Moderate Procedural Sedation and Analgesia 2018: A report by the American Society of Anesthesiologists Task Force on Moderate Procedural Sedation and Analgesia, the American Association of Oral and Maxillofacial Surgeons, American College of Radiology, American Dental Association, American Society of Dentist Anesthesiologists, and Society of Interventional Radiology. *Anesthesiology*. 2018;128(3):437-479.

Practice Guidelines for Preoperative Fasting and the Use of Pharmacologic Agents to Reduce the Risk of Pulmonary Aspiration: Application to Healthy Patients Undergoing Elective Procedures: An updated report by the American Society of Anesthesiologists Task Force on Preoperative Fasting and the Use of Pharmacologic Agents to Reduce the Risk of Pulmonary Aspiration. *Anesthesiology*. 2017;126(3):376-393.

Statement of Granting Privileges for Administration of Moderate Sedation to Practitioners. Available at: https://www.asahq.org/standards-and-guidelines/statement-of-granting-privileges-for-administration-of-moderate-sedation-to-practitioners. Accessed September 29, 2019.

Statement on Granting Privileges to Non-Anesthesiologist Physicians for Personally Administering or Supervising Deep Sedation. Available at: https://www.asahq.org/standards-and-guidelines/statement-on-granting-privileges-to-nonanesthesiologist-physicians-for-personally-administering-or-supervising-deep-sedation. Accessed September 29, 2019.

CHAPTER 15
Airway Management

CASE 1 Patient with Angioedema

Christiane Vogt Harenkamp, MD, PhD, and Charlotte Walter, MD

1. You are called to the emergency center to evaluate a patient for intubation. When you arrive in the emergency center, you find a 30-year-old woman with extreme swelling of the face, tongue, lips, and neck. Her voice is muffled. Her oxygen saturation is 97%. Family members report she was recently started on the drug lisinopril. What is the most likely diagnosis?

   A. Epiglottitis.
   B. Angioedema.
   C. Ludwig angina.
   D. Facial trauma.

The correct answer is B. Angioedema is characterized by a transient swelling of the skin, mucosae, or both. Angioedema involves the dermis and subcutaneous and submucosal tissues, with swelling commonly involving the head, neck, and upper airway, as well as abdominal mucosae and genitals. Progression can be very rapid, and attacks that involve the mouth, tongue, or larynx constitute a medical emergency due to the potential for life-threatening airway obstruction.

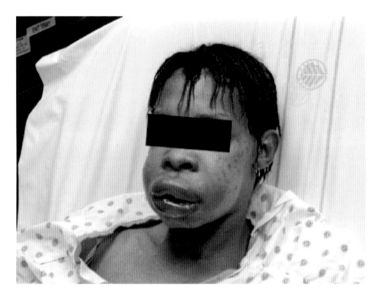

(Reproduced with permission from Hung OR, Murphy MF. *Hung's Difficult and Failed Airway Management*, 3rd ed. New York, NY: McGraw-Hill Education; 2018.)

The pathophysiology of angioedema involves vasodilatation and an increase in vascular permeability in the skin and submucosa, leading to local extravasation of plasma and consequent tissue swelling. Though similar in terms of clinical presentation, histamine-mediated angioedema and bradykinin-mediated angioedema respond to different treatments owing to their distinct pathophysiology.

The flow chart on page 103 summarizes the management of angioedema.

Angioedema can be classified as either hereditary angioedema (HAE) or non-hereditary angioedema. The majority of patients with HAE have the type 1 variety secondary to C1 inhibitor (C1-INH) deficiency, resulting in excessive bradykinin release. Angioedema can be caused by exposure to allergens, producing a characteristic histamine release from mast cells. C1-INH is a serine protease inhibitor protein and is the most important physiological inhibitor of plasma kallikrein and factors XIa and XIIa. C1-INH also inhibits proteinases of the fibrinolytic, clotting, and kinin pathways. Deficiency of C1-INH permits plasma kallikrein activation, which leads to the production of the vasoactive peptide bradykinin.

Though similar in terms of clinical presentation, histamine-mediated and bradykinin-mediated angioedema respond to different treatments owing to their distinct pathophysiology.

Inhibition of angiotensin-converting enzyme (ACE) prevents inactivation of a number of peptide mediators, including bradykinin.

The initial presentation of ACE inhibitor–induced angioedema can occur months or even years after the start of treatment. Irregular recurrences of angioedema during treatment with ACE inhibitors and late onset of angioedema weeks after treatment discontinuation have also been reported. Inhibition of ACE leads to an increase in bradykinin due to decreased degradation. This form of angioedema mostly affects the lips, face, and tongue, while abdominal involvement is

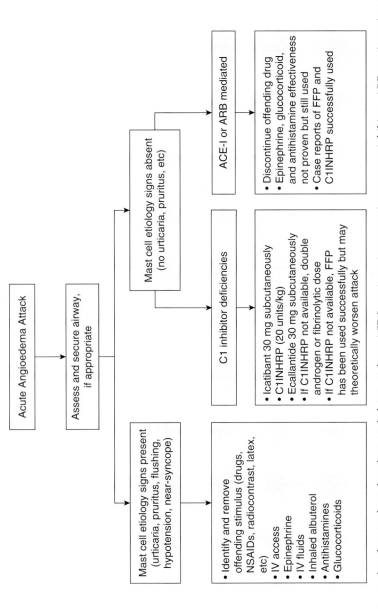

Treatment of acute attacks of angioedema based on underlying etiology. ACE-I, angiotensin-converting enzyme inhibitor; ARB, angiotensin receptor blocker; C1INHRP, C1 inhibitor replacement protein; FFP, fresh-frozen plasma; IV, intravenous; NSAIDs, nonsteroidal anti-inflammatory drugs. (Reproduced with permission from Barbara D, Ronan K, Maddox D, et al. Perioperative angioedema; background, diagnosis and management. *J Clin Anesth.* 2013 Jun;25(4):335-343.)

less common. Although ACE inhibitors are the only drugs for which there is clinical evidence in the literature, there are anecdotal reports of more than 200 agents involved in angioedema attacks.

Acute epiglottitis can be caused by bacteria (such as *Haemophilus influenzae* type B and *Streptococcus* B [adults]), viruses (such as herpes simplex), fungi (such as *Candida albicans*), and noninfectious insults (such as physical trauma, chemicals, and heat).

Acute epiglottitis may progress rapidly into life-threatening upper airway obstruction. Clinical features include stridor, dyspnea, odynophagia, drooling, and severe respiratory distress.

Ludwig angina is a rapidly progressive, potentially fulminant cellulitis or abscess involving the sublingual, submental, submandibular, and parapharyngeal spaces. Ludwig angina begins as a mild infection and progresses to induration of the upper neck with pain, trismus, and tongue elevation. The most serious complication is upper airway compromise. The bacterial agents commonly isolated include viridans streptococci, *Staphylococcus aureus*, and *Staphylococcus epidermidis*.

2. In preparing to intubate this patient, which of the following options should you consider?

   A. Tracheostomy.
   B. Cricothyrotomy.
   C. Awake fiberoptic nasal intubation.
   D. Video-assisted laryngoscopy with/without gum elastic bougie.
   E. All of the above.

The correct answer is E. All intubation options, including creation of a surgical airway, should be available.

Impending asphyxiation warrants an emergency cricothyrotomy. If there is severe swelling, but oxygenation and ventilation are maintained at tolerable levels, intubation using video-assisted laryngoscopy, awake nasal fiberoptic intubation, or a primary tracheostomy can be performed. Preparations should be made, and equipment and skilled personnel should be available at the bedside to perform all of the above procedures expeditiously and efficiently, as manipulation of the airway can rapidly result in deterioration of the patient's condition. Using heliox to improve gas flow across the obstructed airway may buy some time to prepare for intubation and/or creation of a surgical airway. Surgical airway access may be challenging in the patient with neck edema.

3. What nerve supplies the sensory innervations to the larynx above the vocal cords?
   A. The olfactory nerve.
   B. The trigeminal nerve.
   C. The glossopharyngeal nerve.
   D. The superior laryngeal nerve.

The correct answer is D. The sensory supply to the upper airway (mouth, pharynx, and larynx) is derived from the cranial nerves. The trigeminal nerve supplies the sensory innervations to the mucous membranes of the nose and hard and soft palate as well as the anterior two-thirds of the tongue. The glossopharyngeal nerve provides sensory innervation to the posterior one-third of the tongue. The glossopharyngeal nerve also innervates the roof of the pharynx, the tonsils, and the undersurface of the soft palate.

Divisions of the vagus nerve innervate the airway below the epiglottis. The internal branch of the superior laryngeal nerve provides sensory innervation to the mucosa above the vocal cords, while the recurrent laryngeal nerve provides motor and sensory innervation of and below the vocal cords and the trachea. See below.

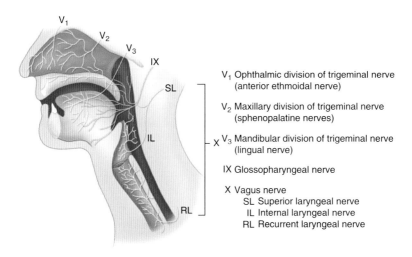

V_1 Ophthalmic division of trigeminal nerve (anterior ethmoidal nerve)

V_2 Maxillary division of trigeminal nerve (sphenopalatine nerves)

V_3 Mandibular division of trigeminal nerve (lingual nerve)

IX Glossopharyngeal nerve

X Vagus nerve
　SL Superior laryngeal nerve
　IL Internal laryngeal nerve
　RL Recurrent laryngeal nerve

(Reproduced with permission from Butterworth JF, Mackey DC, Wasnick JD: *Morgan and Mikhail's Clinical Anesthesiology*, 6th ed. New York, NY: McGraw-Hill Education; 2018.)

4. To anesthetize the airway, lidocaine is injected 1 cm below the greater cornu of the hyoid bone. What nerve is being anesthetized?

A. The recurrent laryngeal nerve.
B. The trigeminal nerve.
C. The glossopharyngeal nerve.
D. The superior laryngeal nerve.

The correct answer is D. The lingual nerve and glossopharyngeal nerve, which provide sensation to the posterior third of the tongue and oropharynx, are blocked by injecting local anesthetic into the base of the palatoglossal arch. See below.

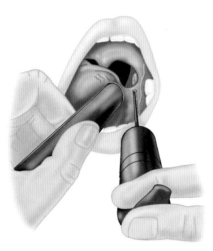

(Reproduced with permission from Butterworth JF, Mackey DC, Wasnick JD: *Morgan and Mikhail's Clinical Anesthesiology*, 6th ed. New York, NY: McGraw-Hill Education; 2018.)

The superior laryngeal nerve is blocked by injecting local anesthetics at the greater cornu of the hyoid.

The recurrent laryngeal nerve is blocked by injecting lidocaine through the cricothyroid membrane into the trachea, which induces coughing and spread of the local anesthetic along the surface. Atomized lidocaine provides a simpler alternative to airway anesthesia than various blocks. Topical benzocaine is also employed; however, it can produce methemeglobinemia.

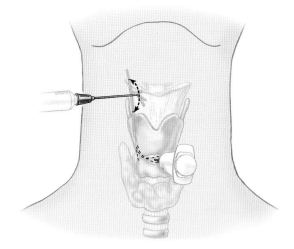

(Reproduced with permission from Butterworth JF, Mackey DC, Wasnick JD: *Morgan and Mikhail's Clinical Anesthesiology*, 6th ed. New York, NY: McGraw-Hill Education; 2018.)

In this emergent setting, local anesthesia delivery to the superior laryngeal nerve may not be possible or effective due to edema. Attempts at intubation can quickly result in loss of the airway, necessitating immediate creation of a surgical airway.

5. Upon return to the operating room, your next patient presents for emergent exploratory laparotomy. You anticipate a possibly difficult airway. The patient is Mallampati class III, the thyromental distance is less than three finger-breaths, and the patient's neck circumference is greater than 17 inches. You plan a rapid-sequence induction with video laryngoscopy. After three attempts, you are unable to intubate. Your next airway management action should be:

A. Insertion of a second-generation supraglottic airway device to restore ventilation.
B. Cricothyroidotomy.
C. Facemask ventilation.
D. None of the above.

The correct answer is A. Intubation has failed after numerous attempts; however, it may be possible to adequately ventilate the patient. Insertion of a second-generation supraglottic device will permit ventilation and gastric decompression. The Difficult Airway Society (DAS) provides intubation guidelines to assist in management. Both facemask ventilation and cricothryoidotomy are included in the algorithm but would not be the next step. Other options include intubating the patient through the supraglottic device and waking the patient up to proceed with an awake fiberoptic intubation. The DAS guidelines are summarized on the next page.

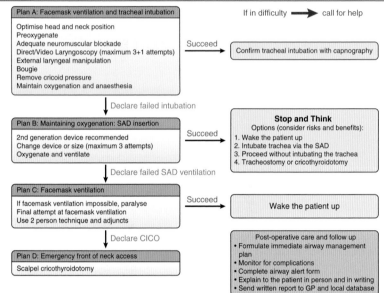

Management of unanticipated difficult tracheal intubation in adults
2015

Plan A: Facemask ventilation and tracheal intubation

Optimise head and neck position
Preoxygenate
Adequate neuromuscular blockade
Direct/Video Laryngoscopy (maximum 3+1 attempts)
External laryngeal manipulation
Bougie
Remove cricoid pressure
Maintain oxygenation and anaesthesia

If in difficulty ➔ call for help

Succeed ➔ Confirm tracheal intubation with capnography

Declare failed intubation

Plan B: Maintaining oxygenation: SAD insertion

2nd generation device recommended
Change device or size (maximum 3 attempts)
Oxygenate and ventilate

Succeed ➔

Stop and Think
Options (consider risks and benefits):
1. Wake the patient up
2. Intubate trachea via the SAD
3. Proceed without intubating the trachea
4. Tracheostomy or cricothyroidotomy

Declare failed SAD ventilation

Plan C: Facemask ventilation

If facemask ventilation impossible, paralyse
Final attempt at facemask ventilation
Use 2 person technique and adjuncts

Succeed ➔ Wake the patient up

Declare CICO

Plan D: Emergency front of neck access

Scalpel cricothyroidotomy

Post-operative care and follow up
• Formulate immediate airway management plan
• Monitor for complications
• Complete airway alert form
• Explain to the patient in person and in writing
• Send written report to GP and local database

This flowchart forms part of the DAS Guidelines for unanticipated difficult intubation in adults 2015 and should be used in conjunction with the text.

(Reproduced with permission from Frerk C, Mitchell V, McNarry A, et al. Difficult Airway Society 2015 guidelines for management of unanticipated difficult intubation in adults. *Br J Anaesth*. 2015 Dec;115(6):827-848.)

DID YOU LEARN?

- Management of angioedema.
- Innervation of the airway.
- Difficult airway algorithm.

Recommended Readings

Butterworth IV JF, Mackey DC, Wasnick JD, eds. Airway management. In: *Morgan & Mikhail's Clinical Anesthesiology*. 6th ed. New York, NY: McGraw-Hill Education; 2018: 307-342.

Cook TM. A new practical classification of laryngeal view. *Anaesthesia*. 2000;55:274.

El-Orbany M, Woehlck H, Ramez Salem M. Head and neck position for direct laryngoscopy. *Anesth Analg*. 2011;113:103.

Hurford WE. Orotracheal intubation outside the operating room: Anatomic considerations and techniques. *Respir Care*. 1999;44:615.

Kaplan M, Ward D, Hagberg C, et al. Seeing is believing: The importance of video laryngoscopy in teaching and in managing the difficult airway. *Surg Endosc*. 2006;20:S479.

Osman A, Sum KM. Role of upper airway ultrasound in airway management. *J Intensive Care*. 2016;4:52.

CHAPTER 16

Cardiovascular Physiology & Anesthesia

CASE 1 Patient with Ischemic Cardiomyopathy for Coronary Artery Bypass

Charlotte Walter, MD, Katrina Von Kriegenbergh, MD, Spencer Thomas, MD, and John Welker, MD

An 85-year-old patient with a history of ischemic cardiomyopathy presents for coronary artery bypass grafting. The patient has a left-ventricular ejection fraction of 20%. Preoperatively, the patient was managed in the intensive care unit with milrinone and furosemide infusions to improve cardiac function and to reduce pulmonary congestion.

1. Milrinone is a:

    A. Phosphodiesterase inhibitor.
    B. β_1-receptor agonist.
    C. β_1-receptor antagonist.
    D. Myofilament calcium sensitizer.

The correct answer is A. Milrinone is a phosphodiesterase inhibitor that increases the intracellular concentration of cyclic adenosine monophosphate (cAMP), resulting in increased myocyte calcium ion concentrations. Adrenergic agonists such as norepinephrine and epinephrine stimulate β-receptors and increase cAMP through stimulation of adenylyl cyclase. β-Blockers function as antagonists. Levosimendan, available outside of the United States, functions as a myofilament calcium sensitizer that enhances myocyte contractility.

2. An older colleague insists that prior to taking the patient to surgery, a pulmonary artery catheter is required to measure cardiac output and stroke volume. You remind the colleague that pulmonary artery catheters carry risks and may not improve perioperative outcomes. You suggest using perioperative transesophageal echocardiography (TEE) as a method to estimate the patient's cardiac output. Of the following, which measurement is *not* required to use TEE to estimate cardiac output?

A. Central venous pressure.
B. Heart rate.
C. Left-ventricular outflow tract (LVOT) diameter.
D. LVOT velocity time integral.

The correct answer is A. Central venous pressure is not necessary to estimate cardiac output using TEE. Cardiac output (CO) is the product of the heart rate (HR) multiplied by the stroke volume (SV).

$$CO = SV \times HR$$

Stroke volume = Left-ventricular end-diastolic volume
– Left-ventricular end-systolic volume

During each beat of the heart, the blood passes through the LVOT. The area of the LVOT can be approximated by the following formula:

$$Area = \pi Radius^2$$
$$Radius^2 = Diameter^2/4$$

or

$$Area = \pi\ Diameter^2/4$$

or

$$Area = 0.785 \times Diameter^2$$

Measuring the diameter of the LVOT can be done echocardiographically as demonstrated in the figure on the next page.

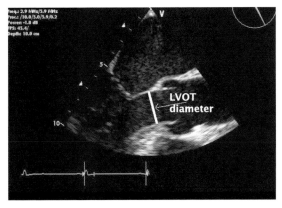

The midesophageal long-axis view is employed in this image to measure the diameter of the left-ventricular outflow tract (LVOT). Knowing the diameter of the LVOT permits calculation of the LVOT area. (Reproduced with permission from Wasnick J, Hillel Z, Kramer D, et al. *Cardiac Anesthesia & Transesophageal Echocardiography.* New York, NY: McGraw-Hill Education; 2011.)

Next, the distance that blood travels during a single stroke volume can be obtained from the time velocity integral (TVI). Knowing the area through which the blood travels in the LVOT and the distance the blood travels (the TVI), it is possible to discern the volume of blood passing through the LVOT during each heartbeat.

$$\text{Volume} = \text{Area} \times \text{Distance}$$

Therefore,

$$\text{Stroke volume} = \text{Area (LVOT)} \times \text{TVI (LVOT)}$$

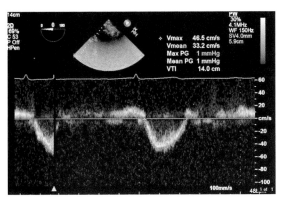

Pulsed wave Doppler is employed in this deep transgastric view interrogation of the left-ventricular outflow tract (LVOT). Blood is flowing in the LVOT away from the esophagus. Therefore, the flow velocities appear below the baseline. Flow velocity through the LVOT is 46.5 cm/s. This is as expected when there is no pathology noted as blood is ejected along the LVOT. Tracing the flow envelope (dotted lines) identifies the time-velocity interval (TVI). In this example the TVI is 14 cm. (Reproduced with permission from Wasnick J, Hillel Z, Kramer D, et al. *Cardiac Anesthesia & Transesophageal Echocardiography.* New York, NY: McGraw-Hill Education; 2011.)

For example, if the LVOT TVI is 14 cm and the LVOT diameter is 1.6 cm, the stroke volume would be:

$$SV = \text{Area (LVOT)} \times \text{TVI (LVOT)}$$
$$SV = (0.785 \times 1.6 \text{ cm}^2) \times 14 \text{ cm}$$
$$SV = 28 \text{ cm}^3 \text{ or } 28 \text{ mL}$$

If the heart rate is 60 beats/min, the patient's CO is:

$$CO = SV \times HR$$
$$CO = 28 \text{ mL} \times 60 \text{ beats/min}$$
$$CO = 1.68 \text{ L/min}$$

For an average-sized adult, a CO of approximately 1.7 L/min would be inadequate to meet metabolic requirements.

3. Compensatory mechanisms associated with systolic heart failure include all of the following *except*:

A. Decreased activation of the renin-angiotensin-aldosterone system.
B. Increased release of arginine vasopressin.
C. Activation of the sympathetic nervous system.
D. Ventricular dilatation.

The correct answer is A. The patient with systolic heart failure attempts to compensate by increasing sympathetic outflow, fluid retention, and activation of the renin-angiotensin-aldosterone system. Over time, the heart hypertrophies eccentrically, increasing the left-ventricular end-diastolic volume.

4. Which Starling curve (depicted in the figure below) is most likely to be found in a patient with cardiogenic shock?
   A. Curve A.
   B. Curve B.
   C. Curve C.
   D. Curve D.

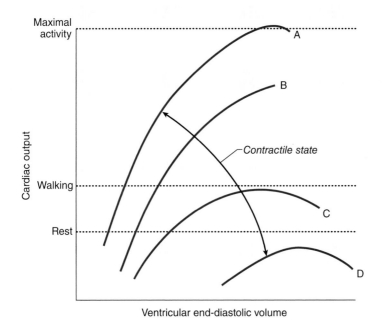

(Reproduced with permission from Braunwald E, Ross J, Sonnenblick EH. Mechanisms of contraction of the normal and failing heart. *N Engl J Med*. 1967 Oct 12;277(15):794-800.)

The correct answer is D. Curve D reflects the patient with cardiogenic shock. As the heart fails, higher filling volumes are required to produce ever-decreasing cardiac output. The healthy heart at rest and at exercise (curves B and A, respectively) generates increased cardiac output with relatively low end-diastolic volumes. As the heart fails, end-diastolic volume increases as a result of compensatory mechanisms. In shock states, the heart cannot pump sufficient blood to meet the body's metabolic needs, resulting in tissue ischemia, metabolic acidosis, and increased lactate concentration.

5. Line E-A on the pressure–volume loop depicted in the below figure represents:

A. An isovolumetric contraction.
B. Isovolumetric relaxation.
C. Ventricular systolic ejection.
D. Diastolic filling.

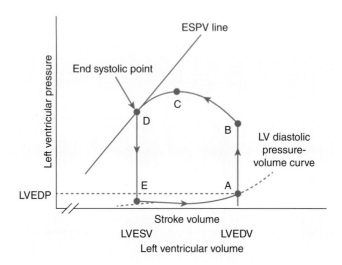

(Reproduced with permission from Hoffman WJ, Wasnick JD. *Postoperative Critical Care of the Massachusetts General Hospital*. 2nd ed. Boston, MA: Little, Brown and Company; 1992.)

The correct answer is D. The pressure–volume loop provides a schematic of hemodynamic changes in the left ventricle during a single stroke volume. Line A-B reflects isovolumetric contraction, B-D reflects systolic ejection of blood, and D-E reflects isovolumetric relaxation. Patients with systolic heart failure require increased left-ventricular end-diastolic volume as a compensatory mechanism to maintain the stroke volume. In patients with diastolic dysfunction, impaired ventricular relaxation results in higher left-ventricular pressure with the same volume compared with a normal ventricle (see below).

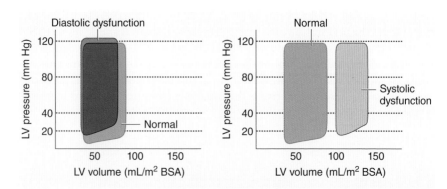

Ventricular pressure–volume relationships in isolated systolic and diastolic dysfunction. (Reproduced with permission from Butterworth JF, Mackey DC, Wasnick JD: *Morgan and Mikhail's Clinical Anesthesiology*, 6th ed. New York, NY: McGraw-Hill Education; 2018.)

6. Diastolic dysfunction can be identified with tissue Doppler imaging. Which of the following statements regarding the Doppler image shown below is false?

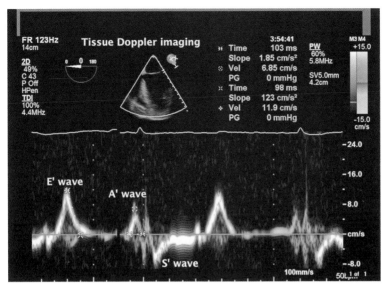

(Reproduced with permission from Wasnick JD, Nicoara A: *Cardiac Anesthesia and Transesophageal Echocardiography*, 2nd ed. New York, NY: McGraw-Hill Education; 2019.)

A. An E′ wave <8 cm/s is associated with diastolic dysfunction.

B. The E′ wave is associated with late diastolic filling.

C. The A′ wave reflects the atrial contribution to ventricular diastolic filling.

D. The S′ wave reflects the movement of the lateral mitral annulus away from the TEE probe during systole.

The correct answer is B. The E′ wave is associated with early diastolic filling. Patients with impaired diastolic function may generate increased left-ventricular diastolic pressure for a given left-ventricular diastolic volume as compared to patients with preserved diastolic function. Such patients can develop pulmonary vascular congestion when challenged with perioperative fluid administration.

7. The surgeon has placed three bypass grafts. When attempting to wean the patient from cardiopulmonary bypass, the anesthesiologist reports that there are new ventricular wall motion abnormalities on TEE examination in the area shaded blue.

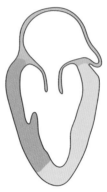

(Modifed with permission from Shanewise JS, Cheung AT, Aronson S, et al. ASE/SCA guidelines for performing a comprehensive intraoperative multiplane transesophageal echocardiography examination; recommendations of the American Society of Echocardiography Council for Intraoperative Echocardiography and the Society for Cardiovascular Anesthesiologists Task Force for Certification in Perioperative Transesophageal Echocardiography. *Anesth Analg.* 1999 Oct;89(4):870-884.)

The area shaded blue is the:

A. Inferior wall.
B. Anterior wall.
C. Anterolateral wall.
D. Septal wall.

The correct answer is B. The two-chamber view shown demonstrates the anterior wall (blue) and the inferior wall (green). When new wall motion abnormalities are seen upon separation from bypass, the surgeon should inspect the grafts placed supplying blood to that ventricular wall to ensure the graft remains patent.

8. The patient is returned to the cardiac intensive care unit following surgery, and the intensive care unit physician would like to estimate the pulmonary artery systolic pressure (PASP) using echocardiography. Of the following, which value is *not* required to perform that estimate?

A. Central venous pressure (CVP).
B. Peak velocity of the jet of tricuspid regurgitation.
C. Peak velocity of the jet of mitral regurgitation.
D. Absence of any pulmonary valvular disease.

The correct answer is C. It is not necessary to know the peak velocity of the jet of mitral regurgitation to estimate the PASP. If there is no pulmonary valve pathology, then the right-ventricular systolic pressure should equal the PASP. The pressure gradient between the right atrium and the right ventricle can be estimated using the Bernoulli equation for the peak velocity of the jet of tricuspid regurgitation. Thus,

RV systolic pressure (RVSP) = Pulmonary artery systolic pressure (PASP)

Pressure gradient = RVSP − CVP

Pressure gradient = $4V^2$, where V is the velocity in m/s of the peak velocity jet of tricuspid regurgitation

$$4V^2 = RVSP - CVP$$
$$4V^2 + CVP = RVSP = PASP$$

DID YOU LEARN?

- Mechanism of inotropes.
- TEE estimates of stroke volume.
- Compensatory responses to heart failure.
- Interpretation of pressure–volume loops.
- Echocardiographic diagnosis of diastolic dysfunction.
- Estimation of PASP by TEE.

Recommended Readings

Bollinger D, Seeberger M, Kasper J, et al. Different effects of sevoflurane, desflurane, and isoflurane on early and late left ventricular diastolic function in young healthy adults. *Br J Anaesth.* 2010;104:547.

Butterworth IV JF, Mackey DC, Wasnick JD, eds. Cardiovascular physiology & anesthesia. In: *Morgan & Mikhail's Clinical Anesthesiology.* 6th ed. New York, NY: McGraw-Hill Education; 2018:343-380.

Colson P, Ryckwaert F, Coriat P. Renin angiotensin system antagonists and anesthesia. *Anesth Analg.* 1999;89:1143.

de Baaij JH, Hoenderop JG, Bindels RJ. Magnesium in man: Implications for health and disease. *Physiol Rev.* 2015;95:1.

De Hert S. Physiology of hemodynamic homeostasis. *Best Pract Res Clin Anesthesiol.* 2012;26:409.

Duncan A, Alfirevic A, Sessler D, Popovic Z, Thomas J. Perioperative assessment of myocardial deformation. *Anesth Analg.* 2014;118:525.

Epstein AE, Olshansky B, Naccarelli GV, et al. Practical management guide for clinicians who treat patients with amiodarone. *Am J Med.* 2016;129:468.

Forrest P. Anaesthesia and right ventricular failure. *Anaesth Intensive Care.* 2009;37:370.

Francis G, Barots J, Adatya S. Inotropes. *J Am Coll Cardiol.* 2014;63:2069.

Groban L, Butterworth J. Perioperative management of chronic heart failure. *Anesth Analg.* 2006;103:557.

Harjola VP, Mebazaa A, Čelutkienė J, et al. Contemporary management of acute right ventricular failure: A statement from the heart failure association and the Working Group on Pulmonary Circulation and Right Ventricular Function of the European Society of Cardiology. *Eur J Heart Fail.* 2016;18:226.

Jacobsohn E, Chorn R, O'Connor M. The role of the vasculature in regulating venous return and cardiac output: Historical and graphical approach. *Can J Anaesth.* 1997;44:849.

Ross S, Foex P. Protective effects of anaesthetics in reversible and irreversible ischemia-reperfusion injury. *Br J Anaesth.* 1999;82:622.

Shi WY, Li S, Collins N, et al. Peri-operative levosimendan in patients undergoing cardiac surgery: An overview of the evidence. *Heart Lung Circ.* 2015;24:667.

Van Gelder IC, Tuinenburg AE, Schoonderwoerd BS, et al. Pharmacologic versus direct-current electrical cardioversion of atrial flutter and fibrillation. *Am J Cardiol.* 1999;84:147R.

Woods J, Monteiro P, Rhodes A. Right ventricular dysfunction. *Curr Opin Crit Care.* 2007;13:535.

Yost CS. Potassium channels. Basic aspects, functional roles and medical significance. *Anesthesiology.* 1999;90:1186.

CHAPTER 17

Anesthesia for Patients with Cardiovascular Disease

CASE 1   Preoperative Assessment Before
          Carotid Endarterectomy

Sarah Armour, MD

1. A 57-year-old woman with a past medical history of hypertension and hyperlipidemia presents for evaluation of transient ischemic attacks (TIAs). She has never had a stroke. She denies a history of myocardial infarction or coronary artery disease, but is known to have an abdominal aortic aneurysm (AAA) measuring 4.5 cm. Her social history is significant for smoking one pack of cigarettes per day for 20 years. After undergoing an imaging study, she is scheduled for carotid endarterectomy.

   According to the 2014 American College of Cardiology (ACC)/American Heart Association (AHA) guidelines on preoperative cardiovascular assessment, which of the following options is the next best step for this patient?

   A. Obtain a 12-lead ECG to evaluate the active cardiac disease.
   B. Obtain a vascular surgery consult given the presence of a 4.5-cm AAA.
   C. Assess the functional capacity of the patient.
   D. This is an emergent surgery, so proceed directly to the operating room.
   E. Cancel the surgery. This patient is not a surgical candidate based on the information given.

The correct answer is C. According to the ACC/AHA guidelines, carotid endarterectomy (CEA) has a risk of 1% to 5% of adverse cardiac outcomes. CEA is not an emergent surgery (option D), and the patient has no active cardiac conditions (eg, unstable coronary syndromes, significant arrhythmias, severe valvular disease, or congestive heart failure—option A). Vascular surgery does not need to be consulted given that the AAA is less than 5 cm (option B), and there is nothing in the information given to suggest the patient is not a surgical candidate at this time (option E). Option C is correct because this is the only information that might potentially change the management of the patient.

CASE 2 — Emergency Surgery with an Unclear Cardiac History

Sarah Armour, MD

1. A 25-year-old man presents with worsening right lower quadrant pain associated with nausea and vomiting over the past 24 h. Preoperative assessment for laparoscopic appendectomy reveals that the patient has a history of dyspnea and chest pain with exertion and has a family history of early cardiac death. Based on the information provided, appropriate anesthetic management of this patient might include all of the following *except*:

A. Transesophageal echocardiography (TEE).
B. Phenylephrine.
C. Fluid bolus.
D. Ephedrine.
E. β-Blocker.

The correct answer is D. This patient's history is concerning for the presence of hypertrophic cardiomyopathy, among other possibilities because of his family history of early cardiac death. Appropriate treatment of patients with hypertrophic cardiomyopathy is aimed at minimizing left-ventricular outflow tract (LVOT) obstruction by maintaining an adequate intravascular volume and afterload and reducing myocardial contractility (with β-blockers). Ephedrine might result in worsening LVOT obstruction by increasing contractility, and ephedrine (and other positive inotropic drugs) should be avoided in patients with hypertrophic cardiomyopathy. TEE can be helpful in establishing the diagnosis and monitoring for outflow obstruction.

CASE 3 — Recent Revascularization Before Mastectomy

Sarah Armour, MD

1. A 65-year-old woman is diagnosed with infiltrating ductal carcinoma of the breast. She is scheduled for right mastectomy and presents to you for a preanesthetic evaluation. One month prior to discovery of her breast cancer, she had a cardiac catheterization demonstrating a 70% mid-LAD lesion, and a drug-eluting stent was placed. She was started on dual antiplatelet therapy (aspirin

and clopidogrel). Which of the following is the best way to safely manage this patient's several medical problems?

A. Consult with the surgeon and cardiologist to compare the risk of surgical bleeding if dual antiplatelet therapy is continued versus the risk of a serious cardiac event if it is discontinued.
B. Discontinue aspirin 7 days before surgery but continue clopidogrel.
C. The patient should continue aspirin and clopidogrel up to the day of surgery because she is at high risk of catastrophic stent thrombosis if discontinued.
D. Continue aspirin through surgery, but discontinue clopidogrel 3 days before surgery.
E. Discontinue the clopidogrel and initiate a glycoprotein IIb/IIIa agent 5 days in advance of surgery.

The correct answer is A. This patient with breast adenocarcinoma must undergo surgery, and her recently placed drug-eluting stent presents a challenging management problem. Current guidelines state that dual antiplatelet therapy (ie, aspirin and a thienopyridine) should be continued uninterrupted for 12 months after placement of a drug-eluting stent and 4 to 6 weeks after placement of a bare-metal stent. This patient, however, requires nonelective surgery, and therefore, interruption of her anticoagulation may be necessary. A discussion with the surgeon and cardiologist should take place, and the risk of stopping antiplatelet therapy should be weighed against the benefit of reduction in bleeding complications from the planned surgery. Fortunately, breast surgery is unlikely to result in catastrophic bleeding. If thienopyridines must be discontinued before major surgery, aspirin should be continued and the thienopyridine restarted as soon as possible. There is no evidence that warfarin, antithrombotics, or glycoprotein IIb/IIIa agents will reduce the risk of stent thrombosis after discontinuation of oral antiplatelet agents.

CASE 4 — Pathophysiology of the Transplanted Heart

Sarah Armour, MD

1. A 39-year-old man presents for repair of a pelvic fracture. He underwent cardiac transplant 5 years earlier. Which of the following statements is *false* regarding the physiology and pharmacology of a typical transplanted heart?

A. Cardiac output is normal.
B. Cardiac conduction is normal.
C. Responses to circulating catecholamines are enhanced.
D. Transplanted hearts are notably preload dependent.
E. Coronary autoregulation is lost.

The correct answer is E. Each of the other alternatives is a true statement. Coronary autoregulation is preserved.

References

Fleisher LA. The value of preoperative assessment before noncardiac surgery in the era of value-based care. *Circulation.* 2017;136(19):1769-1771.

Fleisher LA, Fleischmann KE, Auerbach AD, et al. 2014 ACC/AHA guideline on perioperative cardiovascular evaluation and management of patients undergoing noncardiac surgery: a report of the American College of Cardiology/American Heart Association Task Force on Practice Guidelines. *Circulation.* 2014;130:e278-e333.

Rabin J, Kaczorowski DJ. Perioperative management of the cardiac transplant recipient. *Crit Care Clin.* 2019;35(1):45-60.

CASE 5   Cardiac Assessments in the Preoperative Clinic

Robert Johnston, MD, Thomas McHugh, MD, and Johannes DeRiese, MD

1. A 77-year-old patient with bladder cancer presents in the preoperative evaluation clinic for assessment prior to surgery. The patient reports good exercise tolerance, but has a past history of smoking and hyperlipidemia that has been treated with a statin. According to ACC/AHA guidelines, the next evaluative step for this patient preoperatively should be?

   A. Schedule for a cardiac catheterization.
   B. Schedule for an exercise stress test.
   C. Estimate perioperative risk of major adverse cardiac events (MACE).
   D. Estimate diastolic and systolic function using transthoracic echocardiography.

The correct answer is C. Current ACC/AHA guidelines suggest that if the risk of MACE is less than 1%, no further testing is required and the patient should proceed to surgery. Only if the risk of MACE is elevated in the setting of poor exercise tolerance (<4 METs) is additional cardiac evaluation recommended. The 2014 ACC/AHA guidelines for perioperative evaluation are summarized in the table below.

Summary of Recommendations for Supplemental Preoperative Evaluation

Recommendations	COR	LOE
The 12-lead ECG		
Preoperative resting 12-lead ECG is reasonable for patients with known coronary heart disease or other significant structural heart disease, except for low-risk surgery	IIa	B
Preoperative resting 12-lead ECG may be considered for asymptomatic patients, except for low-risk surgery	IIb	B
Routine preoperative resting 12-lead ECG is not useful for asymptomatic patients undergoing low-risk surgical procedures	III: No Benefit	B

(Continued)

Recommendations	COR	LOE
Assessment of LV function		
It is reasonable for patients with dyspnea of unknown origin to undergo preoperative evaluation of LV function	IIa	C
It is reasonable for patients with HF with worsening dyspnea or other charge in clinical status to undergo preoperative evaluation of LV function	IIa	C
Reassessment of LV function in clinically stable patients may be considered	IIb	C
Routine preoperative evaluation of LV function is not recomended	III: No Benefit	B
Exercise stress testing for myocardial ischemia and functional capacity		
For patients with elevated risk and excellent functional capacity, it is reasonable to forgo further exercise testing and preceed to surgery	IIa	B
For patients with elevated risk and unknown functional capacity it may be reasonable to perform exercise testing to assess for functional capacity if it will change management	IIb	B
For patients with elevated risk and moderate to good functional capacity, it may be reasonable to forgo further exercise testing and proceed to surgery	IIb	B
For patients with elevated risk and poor or unknown functional capacity, it may be reasonable to perform exercise testing with cardiac imaging to assess for myocardial ischemia	IIb	C
Routine screening with noninvasive stress testing is not useful for low-risk noncardiac surgery	III: No Benefit	B
Cardiopulmonary exercise testing		
Cardiopulmonary exercise testing may be considered for patients undergoing elevated risk procedures	IIb	B
Noninvasive pharmacological stress testing before noncardiac surgery		
It is reasonable for patients at elevated risk for noncardiac surgery with poor functional capacity to undergo either DSE or MPI if it will change management	IIa	B
Routine screening with noninvasive stress testing is not useful for low-risk noncardiac surgery	III: No Benefit	B
Preoperative coronary angiography		
Routine preoperative coronary angiography is not recommended	III: No Benefit	C

COR, class of recommendation; DSE, dobutamine stress echocardiogram; ECG, electrocardiogram, HF, heart failure; LOE, level of evidence; LV, left ventricular; MPI, myocardial perfusion imaging.
Reproduced with permission from Fleisher LA, Fleischman KE, Auerbach AD, et al. 2014 ACC/AHA guideline on perioperative cardiovascular evaluation and management of patients undergoing noncardiac surgery: A report of the American College of Cardiology/American Heart Association Task Force on practice guidelines. *J Am Coll Cardiol*. 2014 Dec 9;64(22):e77-e137.

2. A colleague informs you that she routinely orders stress testing for all patients over 75 years of age. According to ACC/AHA guidelines, this action would receive what class of recommendation?

A. Class I (benefit >>> risk).
B. Class IIa (benefit >> risk).
C. Class IIb (benefit >/= risk).
D. Class III (no benefit/harm).

The correct answer is D. Routine screening of patients at low risk is not indicated.

3. The next patient to be seen in the evaluation clinic is likewise scheduled for a cystoscopy. The patient has a history of heart failure with reduced ejection fraction (25%). Baseline medications include carvedilol and an angiotensin-converting enzyme inhibitor. The patient has known structural heart disease along with the signs and symptoms of heart failure. According to the American College of Cardiology Foundation (ACCF)/AHA guidelines, patients with structural heart disease and heart failure symptoms represent what stage of heart failure?

A. Stage A.
B. Stage B.
C. Stage C.
D. Stage D.

The correct answer is C. Patients with structural heart disease and symptoms of heart failure with either preserved or reduced ejection fraction are stage C. See the next figure.

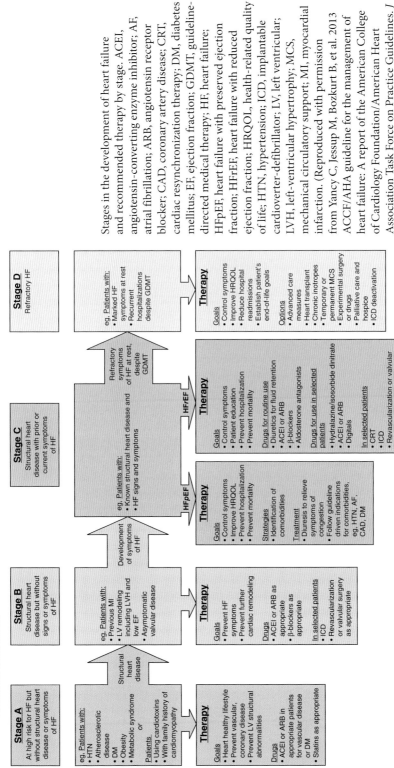

Heart failure

Stages in the development of heart failure and recommended therapy by stage. ACEI, angiotensin-converting enzyme inhibitor; AF, atrial fibrillation; ARB, angiotensin receptor blocker; CAD, coronary artery disease; CRT, cardiac resynchronization therapy; DM, diabetes mellitus; EF, ejection fraction; GDMT, guideline-directed medical therapy; HF, heart failure; HFpEF, heart failure with preserved ejection fraction; HFrEF, heart failure with reduced ejection fraction; HRQOL, health-related quality of life; HTN, hypertension; ICD, implantable cardioverter-defibrillator; LV, left ventricular; LVH, left-ventricular hypertrophy; MCS, mechanical circulatory support; MI, myocardial infarction. (Reproduced with permission from Yancy C, Jessup M, Bozkurt B, et al. 2013 ACCF/AHA guideline for the management of heart failure: A report of the American College of Cardiology Foundation/American Heart Association Task Force on Practice Guidelines. *J Am Coll Cardiol.* 2013 Oct 15;62(l6):e147–e239.)

4. The next patient for evaluation presents with a history of mitral stenosis from rheumatic heart disease. Of the following, which pressure–volume loop is consistent with the patient with mitral stenosis if loop A reflects the patient with normal heart function?

   A. Loop A.
   B. Loop B.
   C. Loop C.
   D. Loop D.
   E. Loop E.

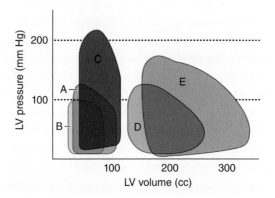

(Reproduced with permission from Jackson JM, Thomas SJ, Lowenstein E. Anesthetic management of patients with valvular heart disease. *Semin Anesth.* 1982;1:239.)

The correct answer is B. The patient with mitral stenosis underloads the left ventricle during diastole as diastolic inflow is restricted by the stenotic mitral valve. Diastolic filling worsens during periods of tachycardia, as the diastolic filling time is reduced. Atrial fibrillation likewise impedes diastolic filling secondary of loss of the atrial contraction to augment ventricular filling. Over time, patients with mitral stenosis develop pulmonary artery hypertension and right-ventricular failure, resulting in the potential for hemodynamic collapse at the time of induction of general anesthesia unless care is taken to maintain right ventricular preload.

5. Refer again to the figure above. Which pressure–volume loop reflects a patient with aortic stenosis?

   A. Loop A.
   B. Loop B.
   C. Loop C.
   D. Loop D.
   E. Loop E.

The correct answer is C. Patients with aortic stenosis (AS) develop high intra-ventricular pressures and left-ventricular hypertrophy to eject blood through the narrowed aortic valve orifice.

6. The anesthetic goals of the patient with severe AS include all of the following *except*:

    A. Maintain normal sinus rhythm.
    B. Reduce systemic vascular resistance.
    C. Maintain intravascular volume.
    D. Avoid tachycardia.

The correct answer is B. Lowering systemic vascular resistance will lead to hypo-tension in the AS patient. The narrowed aortic valve limits ejection from the left ventricle, leading to reduced blood pressure and reduced coronary artery per-fusion pressure in the settings of lower vascular tone. The AS patient generally requires normal sinus rhythm, a preserved heart rate, and maintained peripheral vascular resistance. Tachycardia reduces systolic ejection time, hampering the heart's ability to minimize end systolic volume and maintain cardiac output.

7. After being evaluated for anesthesia, a patient presents on the day of surgery with the following vital signs: heart rate 90 beats/min, blood pressure 190/100 mm Hg, and respiratory rate 20 breaths/min. The patient has taken his usual blood pres-sure medications, which consist of a thiazide diuretic and metoprolol. During the preoperative visit, the patient maintained a blood pressure of 150/80 mm Hg on the same medical regimen. The next best course of treatment is:

    A. Cancel the procedure.
    B. Agree to perform the procedure with neuraxial but not general anesthesia.
    C. Anesthetize the patient with general or neuraxial anesthesia.
    D. Anesthetize the patient and maintain blood pressure within 20% of the patient's baseline pressures as measured in the preoperative visit.

The correct answer is D. Transient increases in blood pressure often occur during the immediate preoperative period secondary to anxiety. This patient has taken his baseline medications and has previously been relatively well controlled on his current regimen. Hypertensive patients on diuretic and other antihypertensive therapy can experience wide swings in blood pressure perioperatively irrespec-tive of the anesthetic technique. In this instance, the patient should proceed to surgery. Despite controlling the blood pressure prior to induction, both hyper- and hypo-tension can readily occur. Anesthesia staff must be prepared to both augment and to reduce the blood pressure following anesthesia induction. Ideally the mean blood pressure should not be less than 65 mm Hg in normotensive patients and within 20% of the patient's baseline pressure. Hypertensive patients have altered autoregulation of cerebral blood, indicating that higher mean arterial pressures may be required to achieve adequate cerebral blood flow.

8. The color-flow jet in the image below is consistent with what valvular pathology?

A. Mitral stenosis.
B. Mitral regurgitation.
C. Aortic stenosis.
D. Tricuspid regurgitation.

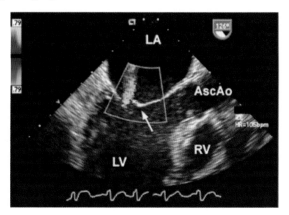

(Reproduced with permission from Mathew JP, Swaminathan M, Ayoub CM. *Clinical Manual and Review of Transesophageal Echocardiography*. 2nd ed. New York, NY: McGraw-Hill Education; 2010.)

The correct answer is B. This is a jet of mitral regurgitation. In this TEE image, one can see the left ventricle (LV), left atrium (LA), the anterior leaflet of the mitral valve (arrow), the right ventricle (RV), and the ascending aorta (AscAo).

9. A patient presents to the endoscopy unit for colonoscopy to evaluate intermittent gastrointestinal bleeding. The patient has advanced heart failure and is maintained with a continuous-flow left-ventricular assist device (LVAD). Inadequate loading of the LVAD can be secondary to all of the following *except*:

A. Hypovolemia.
B. Pulmonary hypertension.
C. Right heart failure.
D. Mitral stenosis.
E. Aortic regurgitation.

The correct answer is E. Answers A through D all result in reduced volume presented to the LVAD inflow located in the apex of the left ventricle. Aortic regurgitation does not affect LVAD inflow; however, blood leaking back into the left ventricle through the leaky aortic valve is not ejected into the system circulation, defeating the LVAD's ability to deliver blood to the tissues. Mitral stenosis and severe aortic regurgitation should be corrected surgically at the time of LVAD implantation. Likewise any patent foramen ovale or other connections between the right and left heart (eg, atrial septal defect) must be repaired to prevent the shunting of deoxygenated blood across the anatomic defect from right to left following initiation of LVAD flow.

DID YOU LEARN?

- Elements of preoperative cardiac evaluation.
- Stages of heart failure.
- Interpretation of pressure–volume loops.
- Possible causes of inadequate loading of a left-ventricular assist device.

Recommended Readings

Fleisher LA, Fleischmann KE, Auerbach AD, et al. 2014 ACC/AHA Guideline on Perioperative Cardiovascular Evaluation and Management of Patients Undergoing Noncardiac Surgery: A report of the American College of Cardiology/American Heart Association Task Force on Practice Guidelines. Available at: http://www.onlinejacc.org/content/64/22/e77. Accessed September 6, 2019.

Heart Failure Guidelines Toolkit. Available at: https://www.heart.org/en/health-topics/heart-failure/heart-failure-tools-resources/heart-failure-guidelines-toolkit. Accessed September 6, 2019.

CASE 6 — Patient with Fontan Circulation for Laparoscopic Cholecystectomy

Mukesh Wadhwa, DO, and Brian McClure, DO

A 32-year-old patient scheduled for a laparoscopic cholecystectomy presents with a total cavopulmonary Fontan physiology (see the figure on the following page). She has a history of congenital pulmonary and tricuspid atresia and has undergone several staged, single-ventricle procedures in the past. Additional history includes recurrent atrial flutter that was treated with radiofrequency ablation approximately 3 years ago. Her preoperative echocardiogram demonstrates good systemic ventricular function, patent Fontan pathways, no intraatrial shunting, and mild atrioventricular valve regurgitation. She has been followed closely by her cardiologist and has not needed further surgical intervention. The interview with the patient reveals good functional capacity without dyspnea with moderate exertion. A full preoperative evaluation is performed, options are discussed with the patient, and the decision is made to proceed with the laparoscopic cholecystectomy under general anesthesia.

1. The Fontan procedure involves which of the following?

   A. Replacement of an atretic tricuspid valve.
   B. Diversion of venous circulation from the right atrium directly to the pulmonary arteries.
   C. Creation of a shunt between the subclavian artery and pulmonary artery.
   D. Maintenance of a patent ductus arteriosus.

The correct answer is B. The Fontan procedure is usually the third stage of palliative surgery by which a patient's single ventricle (SV) is dedicated to the systemic circulation. Tricuspid atresia is one example of SV pathology. In patients with tricuspid atresia, pulmonary blood flow is inadequate, and initial survival is possible only via blood flow through an atrial septal defect and a patent ductus arteriosus.

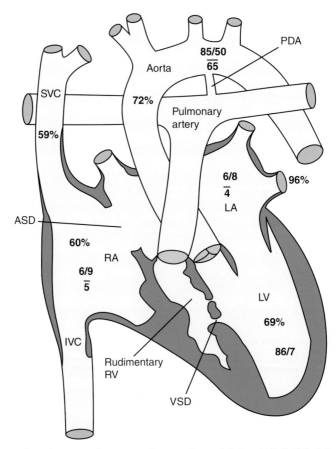

Single ventricle with tricuspid atresia and an atrial septal defect (ASD). (Modified with permission from Leyvi G, Wasnick JD: Single-ventricle patient: pathophysiology and anesthetic management, *J Cardiothorac Vasc Anesth.* 2010 Feb;24(1):121-130.)

Initial patient management is directed to improve pulmonary blood flow by maintenance of the patent ductus arteriosus. Prostaglandin infusions are employed to maintain ductal patency. To further augment pulmonary blood flow, a Blalock–Thomas–Taussig (BTT) shunt can be created, which will further relieve cyanosis. The BTT shunt is a systemic artery to pulmonary artery shunt. The schematic below demonstrates the new shunt and the change of expected oxygen saturation in the various chambers of the SV heart.

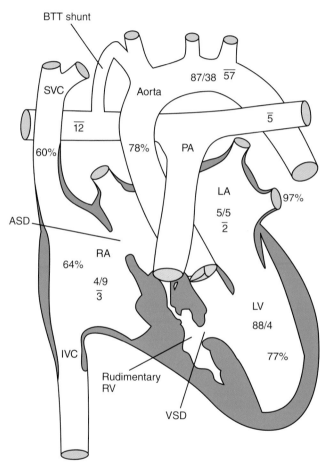

A BTT shunt has been placed to increase pulmonary blood flow in this cyanotic patient. (Modified with permission from Leyvi G, Wasnick JD: Single-ventricle patient: pathophysiology and anesthetic management, *J Cardiothorac Vasc Anesth*. 2010 Feb;24(1):121-130.)

The second stage of palliation includes creation of a Glenn shunt. In the Glenn procedure, venous blood from the superior vena cava (SVC) is directed into the pulmonary artery. Flow from the inferior vena cava (IVC) continues to return to the SV and enters the systemic circulation, contributing to ongoing cyanosis. See the figure on the following page.

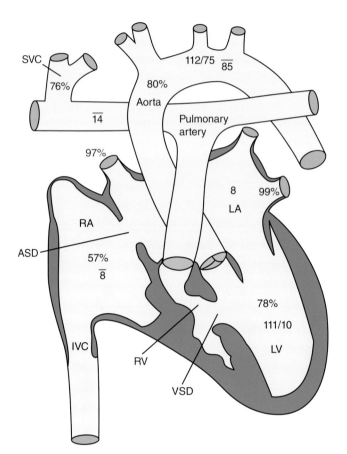

The Glenn procedure directs superior vena cava flow to the pulmonary artery. (Modified with permission from Leyvi G, Wasnick JD: Single-ventricle patient: pathophysiology and anesthetic management, *J Cardiothorac Vasc Anesth*. 2010 Feb;24(1):121-130.)

The Fontan procedure is the last stage of palliation for the tricuspid atresia patient. Flow from the IVC is directed to the pulmonary circulation, isolating the SV from systemic venous return, creating a total cavopulmonary connection. The main pulmonary artery is divided, and flow from the Glenn shunt (bidirectional Glenn [BDG]) is joined with IVC blood flow to direct venous flow directly to the pulmonary circulation, bypassing the heart. See the figure on page 133.

Option B is the correct answer because the Fontan procedure completes the redirection of venous blood flow to the pulmonary circulation. The atretic valve is not replaced. The right ventricle is underdeveloped in the tricuspid atresia patient. Options C and D are steps used to improve pulmonary blood flow in the tricuspid atresia patient but are performed before the final palliative surgery or Fontan procedure.

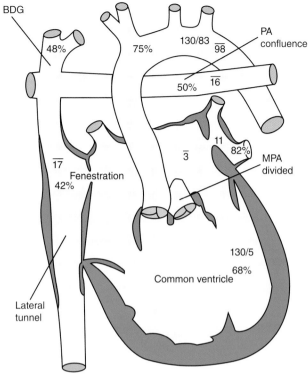

BDG

48%

75%

130/83 $\overline{98}$

PA confluence

50% $\overline{16}$

$\overline{17}$
Fenestration
42%

$\overline{3}$

11

82%

MPA divided

130/5

68%

Common ventricle

Lateral tunnel

Palliation of the single ventricle by the Fontan procedure using a lateral tunnel to direct venous flow to the pulmonary artery. (Modified with permission from Leyvi G, Wasnick JD: Single-ventricle patient: pathophysiology and anesthetic management, *J Cardiothorac Vasc Anesth.* 2010 Feb;24(1):121-130.)

2. The most common clinical finding in patients with tricuspid atresia is:

   A. Cyanosis.
   B. Pulmonary blood flow >> systemic blood flow.
   C. Pulmonary edema.
   D. SaO_2 >99%.

The correct answer is A. The patient with tricuspid atresia does not deliver sufficient blood flow through the atretic tricuspid valve to the right ventricle to be ejected into the pulmonary artery. Tricuspid atresia patients are cyanotic as blood shunts from the right to the left heart through atrial and ventricular septal defects. A patent ductus arteriosus is necessary to provide some pulmonary blood flow until a BTT shunt can be created.

Tricuspid atresia is associated with cyanosis. Increased pulmonary blood flow and pulmonary overload are associated primarily with increased pulmonary circulation, as is seen in patients with hypoplastic left heart syndrome.

In patients with hypoplastic heart syndrome (or aortic valve atresia), the left ventricle, as opposed to the right ventricle, is underdeveloped (see figure below). Pulmonary blood flow is excessive, leading to heart failure and pulmonary edema. In this condition, the systemic circulation, as opposed to the pulmonary circulation, is hypoperfused.

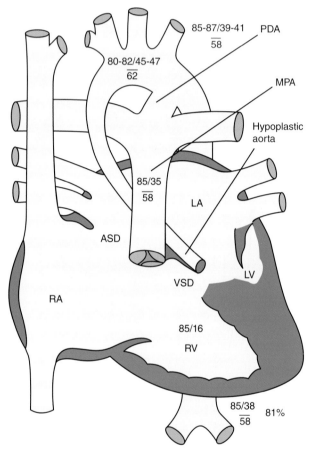

Hypoplastic left heart syndrome. (Reproduced with permission from Wasnick JD, Nicoara A: *Cardiac Anesthesia and Transesophageal Echocardiography*, 2nd ed. New York, NY: McGraw-Hill Education; 2019.)

3. The adult patient with Fontan circulation is now taken to the operating room for laparoscopic cholecystectomy, and routine monitors are placed with the addition of a preinduction arterial line for close blood pressure monitoring. General anesthesia is induced with propofol and rocuronium. The patient is intubated uneventfully. However, with institution of positive-pressure ventilation, the patient becomes hypotensive. The most appropriate next step is:

A. Place the patient on heliox.
B. Decrease the ventilator tidal volumes to decrease pulmonary vascular resistance.
C. Add positive end-expiratory pressure (PEEP).
D. None of the above.

The correct answer is B. Patients who have undergone the Fontan procedure depend on blood flow through the pulmonary circulation without the assistance of the right ventricle. The difference between central venous pressure and systemic ventricular end-diastolic pressure (termed the "transpulmonary gradient") is the primary force promoting pulmonary blood flow and, more importantly, cardiac output. Circulation in the Fontan patient is promoted by low pulmonary vascular resistance. Positive-pressure ventilation with increased tidal volumes, as described above, can result in excessive intrathoracic pressures, leading to decreased venous return to the heart and increased pulmonary vascular resistance. In periods of low oxygen saturation, 100% inspiratory oxygen, rather than a heliox mixture, is appropriate. The addition of PEEP will increase intrathoracic pressure, reducing venous return.

4. The schematic shown in the figure below reflects which congenital heart disease?

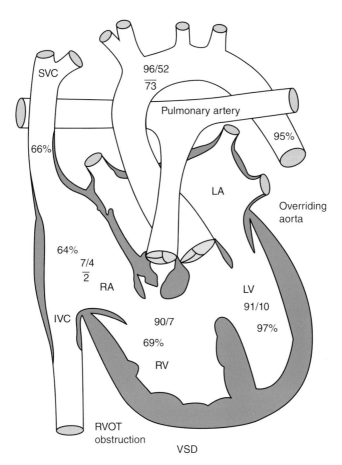

(Reproduced with permission from Wasnick JD, Nicoara A: *Cardiac Anesthesia and Transesophageal Echocardiography*, 2nd ed. New York, NY: McGraw-Hill Education; 2019.)

A. Secundum atrial septal defect.
B. Ventricular septal defect.
C. Complete atrioventricular canal.
D. Tetralogy of Fallot.

The correct answer is D. Tetralogy of Fallot is noted for right-ventricular hypertrophy, a ventricular septal defect, right-ventricular outflow obstruction, and an overriding aorta.

A secundum atrial septal defect is demonstrated in the figure below.

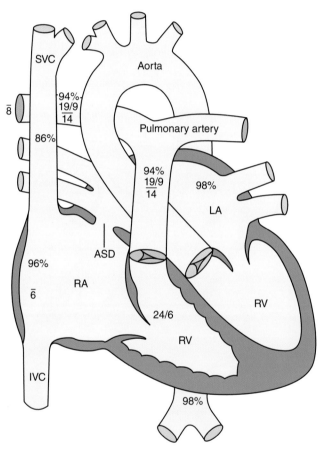

An ostium secundum atrial septal defect is seen in this schematic; pressures and oxygen saturations in the various parts of the heart are displayed. (Reproduced with permission from Wasnick JD, Nicoara A: *Cardiac Anesthesia and Transesophageal Echocardiography*, 2nd ed. New York, NY: McGraw-Hill Education; 2019.)

Blood flow is generally from left to right; however, as pulmonary hypertension develops, blood flow can shift to right to left, resulting in Eisenmenger syndrome.

There are many different types of ventricular septal defects (VSDs). Approximately 80% of VSDs are type II or perimembranous VSDs, as shown in the next figure.

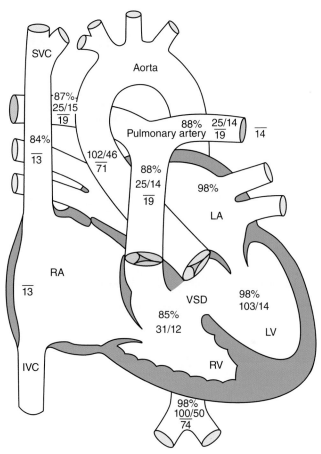

Type II VSD. (Reproduced with permission from Wasnick JD, Nicoara A: *Cardiac Anesthesia and Transesophageal Echocardiography*, 2nd ed. New York, NY: McGraw-Hill Education; 2019.)

Defects in formation of the atrioventricular canal or endocardial cushion can lead to development of a complete atrioventricular canal, including a primum atrial septal defect, a cleft mitral valve, and a VSD. This is shown in the following figure.

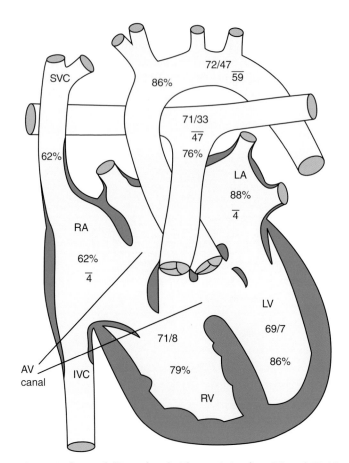

Complete atrioventricular canal. (Reproduced with permission from Wasnick JD, Nicoara A: *Cardiac Anesthesia and Transesophageal Echocardiography*, 2nd ed. New York, NY: McGraw-Hill Education; 2019.)

Management of the congenital heart disease patient is often focused on the correct balance of systemic and pulmonary blood flow. Ensuring equal pulmonary and systemic flow is critical to preventing cyanosis, avoiding pulmonary edema, and ensuring systemic perfusion.

DID YOU LEARN?

- The pathophysiology associated with congenital heart disease requiring the Fontan procedure.
- Symptoms associated with right-to-left shunts, with common presentations.
- Physiology of adults with the Fontan procedure.

Recommended Reading

Gewillig M, Brown SC. The Fontan circulation after 45 years: update in physiology. *Heart.* 2016;102(14):1081-1086.

CASE 7 Young Patient with Hemodynamic Instability

John Welker, MD, and Dennis Ho, DO

A 17-year-old patient presents emergently with a fractured femur following a football injury. Preoperative vital signs include temperature 37°C, heart rate 85 beats/min, blood pressure 100/60 mm Hg, and respiratory rate 18 breaths/min. Past medical history is unremarkable. Family anesthesia history is unremarkable; however, the patient's elder brother has occasional fainting episodes. The family attributes these episodes to opioid abuse. General anesthesia is preferred by the patient.

Following routine rapid-sequence induction, the patient's blood pressure falls to 50/30 mm Hg, SaO_2 decreases to 84%, and heart rate increases to 90 beats/min. Ephedrine 10 mg IV is administered, and the patient quickly develops ventricular fibrillation. Chest compressions are begun, and he is successfully defibrillated.

Auscultation of the heart reveals a systolic flow murmur, and the following TEE image is obtained.

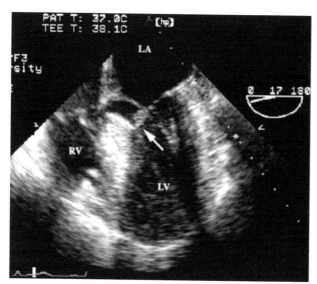

(Reproduced with permission from Mathew JP, Swaminathan M, Ayoub CM. Clinical Manual and Review of Transesophageal Echocardiography. 2nd ed. New York, NY: McGraw-Hill Education; 2010.)

1. What is the likely diagnosis?

    A. Coronary artery disease.
    B. Hypertrophic cardiomyopathy.
    C. Pneumothorax.
    D. Fat embolism.

The correct answer is B. The TEE image obtained demonstrates systolic anterior motion of the mitral valve abutting the hypertrophied septum (*arrow*) of this patient with hypertrophic cardiomyopathy (HCM). HCM is an autosomal dominant trait, with over one-half of patients affected having a relative with the disease. Both males and females are affected by HCM, with the risk in the general population being approximately 1:500. Many patients do not develop dynamic obstruction of the left-ventricular outflow tract, as seen here. However, sudden cardiac death can occur in the absence of dynamic obstruction and is often the first manifestation of the disease.

Symptoms include dyspnea, exercise intolerance, palpitations, chest pain, syncope, and sudden cardiac death. This patient has a family member with a history of syncope and thus may also present with HCM. Often patients with nonobstructive HCM develop diastolic dysfunction with concomitant increased left-ventricular end-diastolic pressure, resulting in dyspnea.

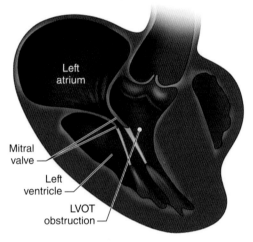

Left atrium

Mitral valve

Left ventricle

LVOT obstruction

(Reproduced with permission from Wasnick J, Hillel Z, Kramer D, et al. *Cardiac Anesthesia & Transesophageal Echocardiography*. New York, NY: McGraw-Hill Education; 2011.)

The image above demonstrates the area of dynamic obstruction that develops when the anterior leaflet of the mitral valve abuts the intraventricular septum. Pressure gradients develop within the left ventricle. Mitral regurgitation develops secondary to elevated left-ventricular cavity pressures.

2. Should the HCM patient become hypotensive perioperatively, appropriate therapies include all of the following *except*:

A. Milrinone.
B. β-Blockers.
C. Calcium antagonists.
D. Volume administration.
E. Phenylephrine.

The correct answer is A. Obstruction is decreased in patients with reduced myocardial contractility and increased left-ventricular volume. Likewise, drugs that increase vascular tone, such as vasopressin and phenylephrine, reduce the dynamic gradient generated during systole. Conversely, inotropic drugs such as dopamine, dobutamine, and milrinone increase contractility and may decrease vascular tone, further increasing the dynamic gradient and worsening hemodynamic performance.

Treatment for HCM includes surgical myectomy and mitral valve repair. Surgical therapies are designed to eliminate systolic anterior motion of the anterior leaflet of the mitral valve. Mitral valve repair is often included with surgical myectomy to move the coaptation point between the anterior and posterior leaflets of the mitral valve more posteriorly. Because of the risk of sudden cardiac death, HCM patients are often also managed with implantable cardioverter-defibrillator (ICD) devices.

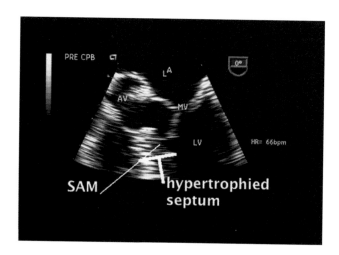

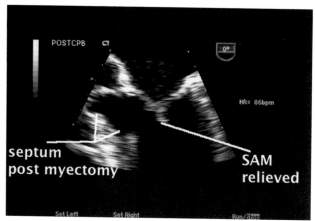

(Reproduced with permission from Wasnick J, Hillel Z, Kramer D, et al. *Cardiac Anesthesia & Transesophageal Echocardiography*. New York, NY: McGraw-Hill Education; 2011.)

Many patients are managed medically with β-blockers, calcium antagonists, and ICD placement.

DID YOU LEARN?

- Management of a patient with HCM.
- TEE imagery of a patient with HCM.

Recommended Reading

Veselka J, Anavekar NS, Charron P. Hypertrophic obstructive cardiomyopathy. *Lancet.* 2017;389(10075):1253-1267.

| CASE 8 | Heart Transplant Patient for Evaluation of a Lung Mass |

Gary Welch, MD, and Brian Hirsch, MD

A 60-year-old man with a history of heart transplantation presents for bronchoscopy and biopsy of a lung mass. The lung mass was discovered incidentally during an admission for endovascular abdominal aortic aneurysm repair. Surgical history includes orthotopic heart transplantation approximately 17 years previously secondary to severe cardiomyopathy. Current medications include antirejection medications, an angiotensin-converting enzyme inhibitor, a diuretic, and an adult low-dose aspirin.

1. Which of the following most commonly occurs over time in the heart transplant patient?

    A. Aortic stenosis.
    B. Posterior leaflet dysfunction of the mitral valve.
    C. Atrial fibrillation with rapid ventricular rate.
    D. Atrial thrombus formation.
    E. Coronary artery disease.

The correct answer is E. Coronary artery disease (CAD) is the most common of the above to occur in the heart transplant patient. CAD arises from a diffuse obliterative coronary arteriopathy that occurs in approximately 50% of heart transplant patients. This obliterative arteriopathy reflects a chronic rejection process in the vascular endothelium. An accumulation of lymphocytes promotes a chronic inflammatory state, leading to progressive scarring and occlusion. Tricuspid regurgitation, and not left heart valvulopathies, is most commonly seen in the posttransplant patient. Tricuspid regurgitation is often the result of residual pulmonary hypertension.

Irreversible pulmonary vascular disease with a pulmonary vascular resistance (PVR) of greater than 6 to 8 Wood units is generally a contraindication to ortho-topic heart transplantation. Such patients frequently require combined heart and lung transplants. Left heart failure can produce profound pulmonary hypertension with right-ventricular failure. The transplanted right heart, unaccustomed to these pressures, can frequently fail, requiring the use of inotropes, iloprost, and nitric oxide (NO) to lower PVR. The use of a right-ventricular assist device may also be necessary if the newly transplanted heart is unable to effectively load the left heart through an increased PVR.

2. Of the following agents, which would be least effective in augmenting cardiac output?

A. Ephedrine.
B. Epinephrine.
C. Isoproterenol.
D. Dobutamine.
E. Milrinone.

The correct answer is A. The grafted heart is denervated from the sympathetic and parasympathetic nervous system. Ephedrine is an indirect-acting agent work-ing primarily through the release of endogenous catecholamines. The other agents listed have a direct effect upon the heart, likely resulting in improved cardiac function.

3. Which answer best explains the following ECG tracing?

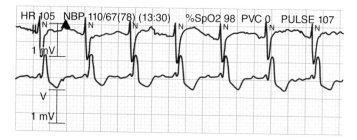

A. First-degree heart block.
B. Atrial fibrillation.
C. Nonconducted P wave.
D. Junctional rhythm.
E. Myocardial ischemia.

The correct answer is C. First-degree heart block can be eliminated because the P wave is followed by the QRS complex within 120 ms. The rhythm is regular, making atrial fibrillation unlikely. Junctional rhythm is excluded because the QRS follows the P wave. The conduction defect could make the diagnosis of myocardial ischemia difficult. The most likely answer is C. During transplantation, both donor and recipient atrial tissues are present, generating two separate P waves.

4. Match the immunosuppressive agent with its mechanism of action.

A. Calcineurin inhibition
B. Purine synthesis inhibition
C. Interleukin-2 receptor blockers
D. Steroid immune suppression

1. Azathioprine
2. Methylprednisolone
3. Basiliximab
4. Cyclosporine A

The correct matches are:

A → 4 (Cyclosporine A).
B → 1 (Azathioprine).
C → 3 (Basiliximab).
D → 2 (Methylprednisolone).

Management of immune suppression often involves a number of agents. Discussion with the transplant team as to their desired time for administration (prior to restoration of circulation to the transplanted heart) is essential. Immunosuppression, while essential for graft survival, can lead to long-term problems with malignancy and infection.

5. During performance of the bronchoscopy under general endotracheal anesthesia, copious amounts of blood appear in the endotracheal tube. The surgeon asks for placement of a left double-lumen endobronchial tube to facilitate lung isolation. Blood in the airway obscures the bronchoscopic view to guide double-lumen placement. You inflate the tracheal cuff and note bilateral breath sounds. You next inflate the bronchial cuff and clamp the tracheal lumen. You listen for isolated left breath sounds, but note the persistence of bilateral breath sounds. This indicates:

A. The bronchial lumen is still in the trachea.
B. The bronchial lumen is in the right bronchus.
C. The endobronchial tube is inserted too far into the left bronchus.
D. The endobronchial tube is not inserted far enough into the right lumen.

The correct answer is A. Persistence of bilateral breath sounds indicates that the bronchial lumen has not been advanced into the bronchus. If the bronchial lumen of a left-sided double-lumen tube is placed in the right bronchus with the tracheal lumen clamped, then there would only be right-sided breath sounds. An endobronchial tube inserted too far into the left bronchus will likewise generate only single-sided breath sounds. The bronchial lumen of a left-sided tube should be placed on the left so as to avoid inadvertent collapse of the right upper lobe.

DID YOU LEARN?

- Potential complications in the heart transplant patient.
- Identification by auscultation of double-lumen endotracheal tube placement.

CASE 9 Patient with Unexpected Hemodynamic Instability

Toni Manougian, MD

A 17-year-old male patient is scheduled for repair of a wrist fracture following a fall during basketball practice. There are no other injuries reported. There is no past anesthesia history, and the patient prefers general anesthesia. The patient is alert and oriented; blood pressure is 100/60 mm Hg, heart rate is 70 beats/min, respiratory rate is 16 breaths/min, and he is afebrile.

General anesthesia is induced with propofol and rocuronium. Anesthetic maintenance is with sevoflurane in 30% oxygen/air.

Following induction, blood pressure falls to 60/40 mm Hg and heart rate increases. Lactated Ringer's solution is given along with 10 mg ephedrine. However, the patient develops ventricular fibrillation.

1. Which of the following should be your next action?

   A. Administer 40 units of vasopressin.
   B. Synchronized cardioversion.
   C. Attempt defibrillation × 3.
   D. Attempt defibrillation × 1.

The correct answer is D. Defibrillation should be immediately attempted followed by cardiopulmonary resuscitation (CPR) and drug therapy. Epinephrine is useful in the treatment of ventricular fibrillation. Stacking shocks is no longer recommended. Instead, a single shock is to be delivered followed by resumption of cardiac compressions. Synchronized cardioversion is appropriate for correction of rapid supraventricular rhythms with hemodynamic compromise as opposed to ventricular fibrillation.

2. Defibrillation is not successful. CPR is begun. An end-tidal CO_2 less than ____ and an arterial diastolic pressure less than ____ have been shown to be indicators of inadequate compressions.

   A. 20 mm Hg; 20 mm Hg.
   B. 10 mm Hg; 10 mm Hg.
   C. 10 mm Hg; 20 mm Hg.
   D. 20 mm Hg; 10 mm Hg.

The correct answer is C. New protocols for CPR emphasize the importance of the adequacy of chest compressions. An end-tidal CO_2 greater than 10 mm Hg is considered a sign of efficient chest compressions. Likewise, an arterial diastolic pressure greater than 20 mm Hg is an indicator of appropriate chest compressions. The algorithm below outlines the steps for management of the ventricular fibrillation patient.

Adult Cardiac Arrest Algorithm—2015 Update

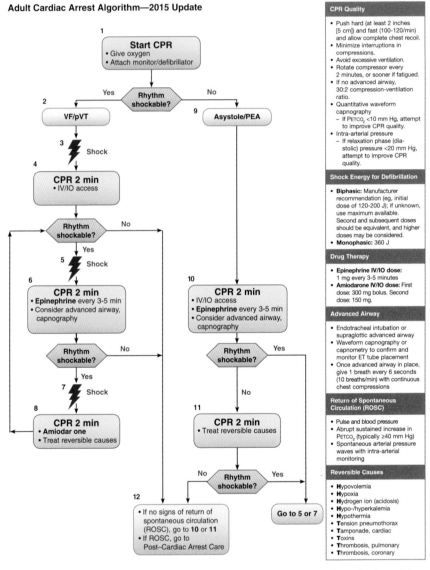

Algorithm for treating ventricular fibrillation and pulseless ventricular tachycardia (VF/VT). Pulseless ventricular tachycardia should be treated in the same way as ventricular fibrillation. Note: This figure emphasizes the concept that rescuers and health care providers must assume that all unmonitored adult cardiac arrests are due to VF/VT. In each figure, the flow of the algorithm assumes that the arrhythmia is continuing. CPR, cardiopulmonary resuscitation; IV/IO, intravenous or intraosseous; PEA, pulseless electrical activity. (Reproduced with permission from Link MS, Berkow LC, Kudenchuk PJ, et al: Part 7: Adult Advanced Cardiovascular Life Support: 2015 American Heart Association Guidelines Update for Cardiopulmonary Resuscitation and Emergency Cardiovascular Care, *Circulation*. 2015 Nov 3;132(18 Suppl 2):S444-S464.)

The patient has a return of spontaneous circulation. An emergent transthoracic echocardiogram (TTE) is performed.

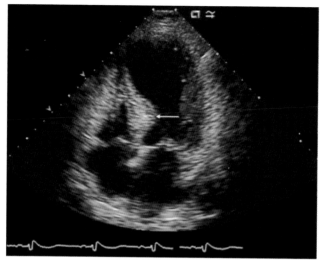

(Reproduced with permission from Levitov A, Mayo PH, Slonim AD: *Critical Care Ultrasonography,* 2nd ed. New York, NY: McGraw-Hill Education; 2014.)

3. The arrow is located in which cardiac chamber?

   A. Right atrium.
   B. Left atrium.
   C. Right ventricle.
   D. Left ventricle.

The correct answer is D. The following images demonstrate the cardiac chambers as identified by both TTE and TEE.

TTE:

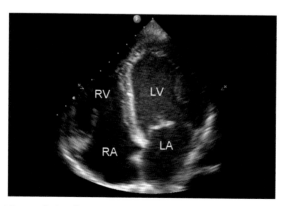

(Reproduced with permission from Carmody KA, Moore CL, *Feller-Kopman: Handbook of Critical Care and Emergency Ultrasound.* New York, NY: McGraw-Hill; 2011.)

TEE:

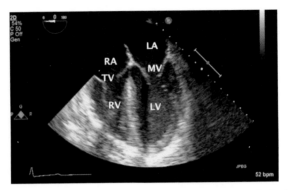

(Reproduced with permission from Wasnick J, Hillel Z, Kramer D, et al. *Cardiac Anesthesia & Transesophageal Echocardiography*. New York, NY: McGraw-Hill Education; 2011.)

4. The TTE image is likely to be associated with:

A. An early diastolic heart murmur.
B. An early systolic heart murmur.
C. A late systolic heart murmur.
D. A late diastolic heart murmur.

The correct answer is C. Hypertrophic cardiomyopathy (HCM) is an autosomal dominant trait that affects 1 in 500 adults. The arrow demonstrates the thick intraventricular septum associated with HCM. Many patients are unaware of the condition, and sudden cardiac death is often the initial manifestation. Symptoms include exercise intolerance, palpitations, and dyspnea. During periods of increased myocardial contractility, the anterior leaflet of the mitral valve can occlude the left-ventricular outflow tract (LVOT), producing elevated intraventricular pressure and mitral regurgitation. Treatment is directed to reduce myocardial contractility and to preserve ventricular volume. Adequate volume delivery is critical perioperatively. Hypotension is treated with agents such as phenylephrine or vasopressin, which primarily increase systemic vascular resistance.

A family medical history obtained after the arrest revealed the sudden cardiac death of the patient's 23-year-old brother 2 years earlier. The following figure demonstrates LVOT obstruction by the anterior mitral valve leaflet.

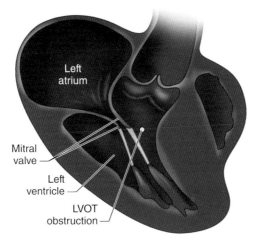

```
         Left
         atrium
```

Mitral
valve
Left
ventricle
LVOT
obstruction

(Reproduced with permission from Wasnick J, Hillel Z, Kramer D, et al. *Cardiac Anesthesia & Transesophageal Echocardiography*. New York, NY: McGraw-Hill Education; 2011.)

Medical therapy for HCM includes β-blockers and calcium antagonists. In patients with dynamic obstruction of the LVOT, surgical approaches can reduce the size of the intraventricular septum and relieve the surgical obstruction.

5. The patient is awakened and recovers uneventfully from his arrest and is started on medical therapy for HCM. He is returned to the operating room to repair his wrist fracture. A brachial plexus block is performed. The patient reports ringing in the ears followed by a seizure and cardiovascular collapse. The local anesthetic with the greatest cardiac toxicity is:

A. Lidocaine.
B. Levobupivacaine.
C. Bupivacaine.
D. Ropivacaine.

The correct answer is C. Bupivacaine has the greatest potential for cardiac toxicity of the agents mentioned. Both bupivacaine and ropivacaine have chiral carbons and thus can exist as two enantiomers or optical isomers. The R-isomer binds to Na channels with greater avidity than the S-isomer. Ropivacaine is formulated as an S-enantiomer. Levobupivacaine is likewise the S-enantiomer of bupivacaine. Bupivacaine is a racemic mixture. A 20% lipid emulsion should be started immediately, 1.5 mL/kg over the first minute, with infusion and repeated boluses as needed along with advanced cardiac life support (ACLS) until spontaneous circulation is restored.

DID YOU LEARN?

- Approach to defibrillation.
- TEE and TTE identification of cardiac chambers.

CHAPTER 17 Anesthesia for Patients with Cardiovascular Disease

CASE 10 Preoperative ECG Changes

Lydia Conlay, MD, PhD, MBA, and Clayton Adams, MD

A 92-kg, 67-year-old man presents to preoperative clinic for an elective incisional hernia repair. He has a history of hypertension, gout, and gastroesophageal reflux disease. He says he was prescribed medications but does not take them because he doesn't feel any better when he takes them. On interview, he reports no complications with prior surgeries. He reports having occasional palpitations, although he denies syncopal episodes. Regular work-up includes an ECG, shown in the following figure.

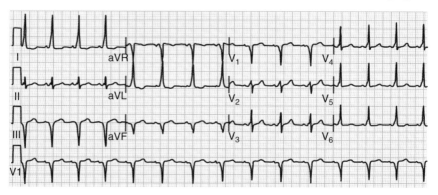

(Reproduced with permission from Knoop KJ, Stack LB, Storrow AB, et al: *The Atlas of Emergency Medicine*, 3rd ed. New York, NY: McGraw-Hill Education; 2016. ECG contributor: James V. Ritchie, MD.)

1. Upon reentering the exam room, you notice that the patient's heart rate has increased to 195 beats/min, blood pressure is 135/76 mm Hg, and oxygen saturation is 99%. The patient is breathing regularly at 14 breaths/min, and he is lethargic. The most appropriate next action is:

   A. Administer amiodarone.
   B. Administer metoprolol.
   C. Electrical cardioversion.
   D. Administer verapamil.

The correct answer is C. This patient has Wolff–Parkinson–White syndrome (WPW) demonstrated by the delta waves on the ECG. Patients with WPW who are experiencing severe symptoms such as mental status changes or blood pressure instability due to a tachyarrhythmia require electrical cardioversion. Medications that block the atrioventricular (AV) node should be avoided in patients with WPW, especially in the setting of acute tachyarrhytmias. By blocking the AV node, the WPW accessory pathways are favored, potentially leading to unstable ventricular rhythms. For this reason, β-blockers like metoprolol (option B) and calcium channel blockers like verapamil (option D) should be avoided. Intravenous amiodarone (option A) is also not recommended in this setting.

2. The patient returned to the previous rhythm following your management. As you are exiting the clinic room, he becomes tachycardic again, this time to a heart rate of 235 beats/min. His blood pressure remains stable at 130/75 mm Hg, but his oxygen saturation falls to 75% and he becomes lethargic again. The most appropriate next step in the management of this patient is:

A. Electrical cardioversion.
B. Administer amiodarone.
C. Intubate the patient.
D. Both A and C.

The correct answer is D. Patients who acutely decompensate must always be treated with appropriate stabilization. This patient's mental decline and poor oxygen saturation dictate that controlling the airway is a priority.

3. Several days later, you are covering the operating room when an emergent case is posted for a strangulated incisional hernia. You quickly realize this is the same patient you recently saw in the clinic. The patient is brought to the operating room and induced without incident. During the case, his heart rate increases to 165 beats/min, and on the monitor, it appears to be a narrow-complex tachycardia. The most appropriate next step is to:

A. Administer labetalol intravenously.
B. Perform cardioversion.
C. Deepen anesthetic with intravenous ketamine.
D. Begin esmolol infusion.

The correct answer is B. Reducing this patient's heart rate can be achieved in a variety of ways, but the most appropriate is by cardioversion. Labetalol administration will decrease the heart rate but is a poor choice in this patient due to the possibility of enhancing the aberrant conduction pathway, as discussed earlier. For this reason, an esmolol infusion is an incorrect answer. Administering ketamine may deepen the anesthetic, but this will not affect the arrhythmia due to the patient's underlying conduction abnormality. Cardioversion will allow the patient to regain intrinsic conduction function.

4. Following the procedure, the patient's son reflected on his own situation and worried about his father's risk of sudden cardiac death from his WPW. Which of the following factors most increases this patient's risk for sudden cardiac death?

A. Older age.
B. Male gender.
C. Single aberrant conduction pathway.
D. Long refractory period of conduction pathway.

The correct answer is B. Male gender is associated with an increased likelihood of sudden cardiac death with WPW. Other factors associated with an increased risk are younger age, multiple accessory pathways, and short refractory times of accessory pathways. The mechanism of sudden cardiac death in these patients usually involves rapid ventricular response to atrial fibrillation that degenerates into ventricular fibrillation. AV node blocking medications can increase the likelihood of this process. The patient's son should also be advised that around 4% of patients have a familial WPW that affects a first-degree relative.

DID YOU LEARN?

- Management techniques for symptomatic tachydysrhythmias in patients with WPW.
- Management of intraoperative tachydysrhythmias in the setting of WPW.
- Effects of various medications on aberrant conduction pathways.
- Risk factors for sudden cardiac death in WPW.

Recommended Readings

Amar D. Perioperative atrial tachyarrhythmias. *Anesthesiology.* 2002;97:1618.

Atlee JL, Bernstein AD. Cardiac rhythm management devices (part I). Indications, device selection, and function. *Anesthesiology.* 2001;95:1265.

Atlee JL, Bernstein AD. Cardiac rhythm management devices (part II). Perioperative management. *Anesthesiology.* 2001;95:1492.

Braunwald E, Zipes DP, Libby P. *Heart Disease.* 9th ed. Philadelphia, PA: W.B. Saunders; 2011.

Butterworth IV JF, Mackey DC, Wasnick JD, eds. Anesthesia for patients with cardiovascular disease. In: *Morgan & Mikhail's Clinical Anesthesiology.* 6th ed. New York, NY: McGraw-Hill Education; 2018:381-440.

Chassot PG, Delabays A, Spahn DR. Preoperative evaluation of patients with, or at risk of, CAD undergoing non-cardiac surgery. *Br J Anaesth.* 2002;89:747.

Etheridge SP, Escudero CA, Blaufox AD, et al. Life-threatening event risk in children with Wolff-Parkinson-White syndrome: A multicenter international study. *JACC Clin Electrophysiol.* 2018;4(4):433-444.

Howell SJ, Sear JW, Foex P. Hypertension, hypertensive heart disease and perioperative cardiac risk. *Br J Anaesth.* 2004;92:570.

James PA, Oparil S, Carter BL, et al. 2014 evidence based guidelines for the management of high blood pressure in adults: Report from the panel members appointed to the Eight Joint National Committee (JNC8). *JAMA.* 2014;311:507.

Lake CL. *Pediatric Cardiac Anesthesia.* 4th ed. Philadelphia, PA: Lippincott Williams and Wilkins; 2004.

Otto CM. *Valvular Heart Disease.* 3rd ed. Philadelphia, PA: W.B. Saunders; 2009.

Otto CM. *Textbook of Clinical Echocardiography.* 4th ed. Philadelphia, PA: W.B. Saunders; 2009.

Park KW. Preoperative cardiac evaluation. *Anesth Clin North Am.* 2004;22:199.

Wasnick J, Hillel Z, Kramer D, et al. *Cardiac Anesthesia & Transesophageal Echocardiography.* New York, NY: McGraw-Hill; 2011.

CHAPTER 18
Anesthesia for Cardiovascular Surgery

CASE 1 Patient for Cardiac Surgery

Elizabeth R. Rivas, MD

1. The cannula to deliver retrograde cardioplegia is placed in which structure of the heart below?

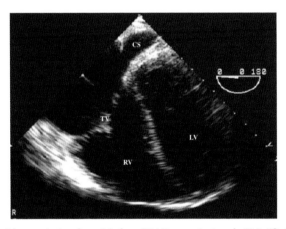

(Reproduced with permission from Mathew JP, Nicoara A, Ayoub CM. *Clinical Manual and Review of Transesophageal Echocardiography*, 3rd ed. New York, NY: McGraw-Hill Education; 2019.)

   A. Right ventricle (RV).
   B. Left ventricle (LV).
   C. Coronary sinus (CS).
   D. Tricuspid valve (TV).

The correct answer is C. Cardioplegia can be delivered to the heart in either or both anterograde and retrograde fashions. Anterograde cardioplegic solutions are delivered through a small cannula placed in the aorta by the surgeon. After aortic cross-clamping, cardioplegic solution is delivered via the native coronary arteries to the myocardium. Retrograde cardioplegia is delivered via a cannula placed in the coronary sinus (CS). The CS drains venous blood from the heart. With the CS cannula in place and the surrounding balloon inflated, cardioplegia solution is delivered in a retrograde fashion to the myocardium via the venous system. The other structures seen in this image are the tricuspid valve (TV), the right ventricle (RV), and the left ventricle (LV).

2. Upon the initiation of cardiopulmonary bypass (CPB), the serum concentration of which of the following drugs is likely to be reduced by a medically important amount?

A. Rocuronium.
B. Fentanyl.
C. Sufentanil.
D. All of the above.

The correct answer is A. Plasma and serum concentrations of most water-soluble drugs (eg, nondepolarizing muscle relaxants) acutely decrease at the onset of CPB, but the change is inconsequential for most lipid-soluble drugs (eg, fentanyl and sufentanil).

3. Initiation of CPB is associated with which of the following physiological changes?

A. Increased activation of the complement system.
B. Increased activation of the coagulation system.
C. Increased activation of the kallikrein system.
D. All of the above.

The correct answer is D. CPB activates all three systems and can produce a generalized inflammatory response leading to vasoplegia. Numerous studies have attempted to discern whether interventions (eg, steroid administration) that modulate the inflammatory response will improve patient outcomes. At the present time, no positive effects on outcomes have been established.

4. A 45-year-old patient has been cannulated, and the perfusionist is now attempting to initiate CPB. The perfusion reports increased pressure in the tubing leading to the aortic cannula. Your next intervention includes which of the following?

A. Administer antihypertensive medication.
B. Increase the depth of anesthesia.
C. Administer additional heparin.
D. Examine the aorta with transesophageal echocardiography (TEE) while the surgeon physically inspects the cannulation site.

The correct answer is D. Insertion of the aortic perfusion cannula can create a false lumen within the walls of the aorta, creating an aortic dissection. A high pressure in the cannula at the time of initiation of CPB alerts the perfusionist that the cannula may be misplaced or that the surgeon has failed to remove a tubing clamp. Aortic dissections can be seen on TEE examination, as demonstrated below, with both the true lumen (TL) and false lumen (FL) seen.

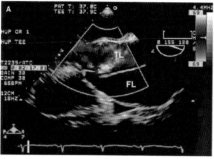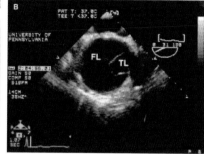

(Reproduced with permission from Longnecker DE, Mackey SC, Newman MF, et al: *Anesthesiology*, 3rd ed. New York, NY: McGraw-Hill Education; 2018.)

Aortic dissection associated with the initiation of CPB is a potentially lethal complication that necessitates aortic repair.

5. A 65-year-old patient is being weaned from CPB following replacement of the aortic valve and coronary artery bypass grafting. While administering protamine to reverse heparin anticoagulation, the patient becomes hypotensive and develops right-ventricular dysfunction as seen on TEE examination. Possible causes of acute right-ventricle failure include:

   A. Protamine reaction.
   B. Right coronary artery air embolism.
   C. Kinked right coronary artery bypass graft.
   D. A and B.
   E. A, B, and C.

The correct answer is E. A severe protamine reaction is often associated with increased pulmonary artery pressures and subsequent right-ventricular failure. Interference with the blood supply to the right ventricle either through a kinked bypass graft or air emboli could result in impaired right-ventricular function. The surgeon should inspect any coronary artery grafts while the anesthesiologist attempts to improve right ventricular function. Patients may require reheparinization and return to CPB to support hemodynamic function while the cause of right-ventricular dysfunction is evaluated.

6. It is concluded that the patient had a transient air embolism, and right-ventricular function has improved. The activated clotting times in the presence and absence of heparinase are identical and have returned to baseline values, but the patient has what appears to be persistent microvascular bleeding. What should your next management intervention be?

A. Administer 2 pheresis units of platelets.
B. Administer additional protamine.
C. Perform thromboelastography.
D. Discuss management with the surgeon.
E. C and D.

The correct answer is E. Ongoing hemorrhage following separation from CPB is a common occurrence. Surgeons must rule out any surgical bleeding sites. Thromboelastography permits targeted delivery of blood products based upon the diagnosis of various coagulopathic states such as factor deficiency, platelet dysfunction, and fibrinolysis. Nevertheless, empiric therapy could be indicated if diagnostic tests are not available or hemorrhage is rapidly progressing.

7. A 55-year-old patient with a severe left main coronary artery disease is taken to the operating room for coronary artery bypass grafting. Upon induction of anesthesia with ketamine, sufentanil, and midazolam, the patient's blood pressure falls to 60/30 mm Hg. ST-segment depression is noted on the ECG. Appropriate interventions at this time could include all of the following *except:*

A. Administer norepinephrine.
B. Administer vasopressin.
C. Administer nitroglycerin.
D. Prepare for emergent sternotomy and initiation of CPB.

The correct answer is C. The patient is hypotensive and ischemic following anesthesia induction. Efforts should be directed at increasing the blood pressure through administration of vasoconstrictor medications. Concurrently, the patient is at risk of further hemodynamic collapse, and emergent initiation of CPB may be required. Nitroglycerin administration at this time would likely worsen hypotension, leading to cardiac arrest.

8. The patient responds to administration of norepinephrine and the ST segments return to baseline. It is determined that emergent institution of CPB is not required; however, the anesthesiologist and surgeon decide that placement of an intraaortic balloon pump would be useful. All of the following statements regarding intraaortic balloon counter-pulsation are correct *except:*

A. The balloon inflates during systole.
B. The balloon should be positioned distal to the left subclavian artery.

C. Balloon counterpulsation should not be used in patients with aortic insufficiency.
D. The balloon inflates after the dicrotic notch on the aortic pressure tracing.

The correct answer is A. The balloon inflates during diastole, improving coronary artery perfusion pressure. Deflation of the balloon immediately prior to left-ventricular ejection decreases afterload, potentially augmenting ventricular ejection. To effectively increase coronary blood flow and cardiac output, the patient must not have aortic insufficiency.

9. The surgery proceeds uneventfully. Postoperatively, the patient becomes progressively acidotic with increasing vasopressor requirements. Cardiac index has fallen to 1.5 L/min/m^2, blood pressure is 90/60 mm Hg, and central venous pressure is 25 mm Hg. Which of the following is the most useful diagnostic action?

A. Place a pulmonary artery flotation catheter.
B. Determine stroke volume variation.
C. Administer a 500-mL bolus of normal saline.
D. Perform a diagnostic TEE examination.

The correct answer is D. The differential diagnosis for postcardiac surgery hemodynamic instability includes right- and left-ventricular failure, hypovolemia, drug reaction, and pericardial tamponade. Of the choices offered, none is as likely to identify the cause of perioperative hemodynamic instability as a rescue TEE examination. Elevated central venous pressure in the setting of a reduced cardiac index could be secondary to ventricular failure or pericardial tamponade. Tamponade necessitates a return to surgery to explore the chest. New ventricular failure can be secondary to bypass graft failure and might require a return to surgery or an emergency cardiac catheterization to assess graft patency.

DID YOU LEARN?

- Difference between anterograde and retrograde cardioplegia.
- Causes of perioperative right-ventricular failure.
- Inflation of an intraaortic balloon pump.

CASE 2   Problems with a Postoperative Cardiac Surgery Patient

John D. Wasnick, MD, MPH

1. You are called to the cardiac surgery intensive care unit to evaluate an intubated and ventilated 70-kg, 83-year-old patient who has been in the intensive care unit for 1 h following uneventful coronary artery bypass surgery. Vital signs include blood pressure 70/30 mm Hg, heart rate 100 beats/min (DDD paced), SaO_2 92%, central venous pressure 20 mm Hg, pulmonary artery pressure 40/20 mm Hg, and cardiac index 1.3 $L/min/m^2$. Nursing staff report that they have reached their protocol maximum for the amount of norepinephrine they can deliver without a supplemental physician order, which they would like you to now provide. Your next action is to:

   A. Increase the norepinephrine infusion.
   B. Begin an infusion of vasopressin.
   C. Place the CT surgery team on alert.
   D. Administer 1000 mL of colloid solution.

The correct answer is C. The postoperative period is potentially unstable for all patients following cardiac surgery. This patient appears to be developing cardiac tamponade, as indicated by increased filling pressures, decreased cardiac index, and reduced systemic pressures.

    The differential diagnosis includes bypass graft failure with subsequent ventricular failure, hypovolemia, and pericardial tamponade. Although additional vasoconstrictors and volume administration may improve hemodynamic performance, the surgery team should be put on notice that the patient may require surgical reexploration.

2. While contacting the surgeon, you administer intravenous fluid, start an epinephrine infusion, and order an arterial blood gas, which is reported as: pH 7.22, PaO_2 200 mm Hg, $PaCO_2$ 20 mm Hg, and HCO_3 12 mEq/L. This blood gas reflects which of the following?

   A. Metabolic alkalosis.
   B. Metabolic acidosis.
   C. Metabolic acidosis with respiratory alkalosis.
   D. Metabolic alkalosis with respiratory acidosis.

The correct answer is C. This patient is mechanically hyperventilated, resulting in a decrease in $PaCO_2$ to 20 mm Hg (normal, 35–45 mm Hg). The patient has metabolic acidosis with a decreased bicarbonate concentration of only 12 mEq/L. Hypoperfusion in shock states secondary to cardiogenic, hypovolemic, or redistributive shock can lead to metabolic acidosis. Treatment in such cases is directed at correcting the underlying cause of hypoperfusion.

3. Despite volume administration and increased vasopressor support, the patient continues to deteriorate with increasing pulmonary artery pressures and decreasing cardiac index. You place a TEE probe to facilitate the differential diagnosis (immediate postoperative TEE examination was normal). TEE demonstrates left-ventricular anterior wall hypokinesis. Based on the TEE diagnosis, your next course of action is to:

A. Perform bedside sternotomy.
B. Administer additional volume.
C. Place an intraaortic balloon pump.
D. Transport to the cardiac catheterization laboratory.

The correct answer is C. TEE demonstrates left-ventricular anterior wall akinesis. Immediate actions would include placement of an intraaortic balloon pump to improve myocardial perfusion and cardiac index and administration of inotropic agents. Possible causes of an acute wall motion abnormality include bypass graft kinking, bypass graft disruption, internal mammary artery bypass graft spasm, and/or air/particulate graft embolism. Close discussion with the surgeon is necessary to determine the next course of action to restore graft patency.

4. The surgeon elects to return the patient to the operating room to inspect the heart. The surgeon notes that the left internal mammary artery bypass graft to the left anterior descending artery has become kinked. Following heparin administration, the surgeon places the patient on full-flow cardiopulmonary bypass. The perfusionist reports that the patient has respiratory acidosis. Your next action is to:

A. Instruct the perfusionist to increase the sweep gas flow rate.
B. Obtain an arterial blood gas.
C. Increase respiratory rate.
D. Increase tidal volume and positive end-expiratory pressure.

The correct answer is A. During full cardiopulmonary bypass, increasing the sweep gas flow rate will increase removal of carbon dioxide (CO_2). Increased CO_2 tension in all patients is secondary to either increased CO_2 production or decreased CO_2 ventilation. Increased production can be secondary to thyroid disease, hyperalimentation, malignant hyperthermia, or generalized high metabolism. Decreased CO_2 ventilation during cardiopulmonary bypass is secondary to inadequate sweep gas flow. The pump oxygenator replaces the functions of the lungs during cardiopulmonary bypass. Hence, alterations in respiratory rate, tidal volume, or positive end-expiratory pressure will have little effect on gas exchange. An arterial blood gas should be checked to rule out metabolic acidosis and possible malignant hyperthermia.

DID YOU LEARN?

- The differential diagnosis of postcardiac surgery ventricular failure.
- The correct interpretation of a blood gas with mixed metabolic acidosis and respiratory alkalosis.
- TEE diagnosis of acute left-ventricular wall motion abnormalities.
- Management of hypercapnia on cardiopulmonary bypass.

Recommended Readings

Butterworth IV JF, Mackey DC, Wasnick JD, eds. Anesthesia for cardiovascular surgery. In: *Morgan & Mikhail's Clinical Anesthesiology*. 6th ed. New York, NY: McGraw-Hill Education; 2018:441-494.

Engelman R, Baker RA, Likosky DS, et al. The Society of Thoracic Surgeons, The Society of Cardiovascular Anesthesiologists, and The American Society of ExtraCorporeal Technology: Clinical Practice Guidelines for Cardiopulmonary Bypass—Temperature management during cardiopulmonary bypass. *J Extra Corpor Technol*. 2015;47:145.

Fedorow CA, Moon MC, Mutch WA, Grocott HP. Lumbar cerebrospinal fluid drainage for thoracoabdominal aortic surgery: Rationale and practical considerations for management. *Anesth Analg*. 2010;111:46.

Fudulu D, Benedetto U, Pecchinenda GG, et al. Current outcomes of off-pump versus on-pump coronary artery bypass grafting: Evidence from randomized controlled trials. *J Thorac Dis*. 2016;8(suppl 10):S758.

Hosseinian L, Weiner M, Levin MA, Fischer GW. Methylene blue: Magic bullet for vasoplegia? *Anesth Analg*. 2016;122:194.

Murphy GS, Hessel EA 2nd, Groom RC. Optimal perfusion during cardiopulmonary bypass: An evidence-based approach. *Anesth Analg*. 2009;108:1394.

Parissis H, Lau MC, Parissis M, et al. Current randomized control trials, observational studies and meta analysis in off-pump coronary surgery. *J Cardiothorac Surg*. 2015;10:185.

Ramakrishna H, Rehfeldt KH, Pajaro OE. Anesthetic pharmacology and perioperative considerations for heart transplantation. *Curr Clin Pharmacol*. 2015;10:3.

Scully M, Gates C, Neave L. How we manage patients with heparin induced thrombocytopenia. *Br J Haematol*. 2016;174:9.

Seco M, Edelman JJ, Van Boxtel B, et al. Neurologic injury and protection in adult cardiac and aortic surgery. *J Cardiothorac Vasc Anesth*. 2015;29:185.

Smilowitz NR, Berger JS. Perioperative management to reduce cardiovascular events. *Circulation*. 2016;133:1125.

van Veen JJ, Makris M. Management of peri-operative anti-thrombotic therapy. *Anaesthesia*. 2015;70(suppl 1):58.

Wilkey BJ, Weitzel NS. Anesthetic considerations for surgery on the aortic arch. *Semin Cardiothorac Vasc Anesth*. 2016;20:265.

Wong WT, Lai VK, Chee YE, Lee A. Fast-track cardiac care for adult cardiac surgical patients. *Cochrane Database Syst Rev*. 2016;(9):CD003587.

CHAPTER 19

Respiratory Physiology & Anesthesia

| CASE 1 | Interscalene Block for a Patient with a History of Smoking |

Bettina Schmitz, MD

A 52-year-old woman with a history of smoking and mild asthma is scheduled for left rotator cuff repair. The patient underwent preoperative pulmonary function tests (PFTs). An interscalene block of the brachial plexus is performed before the induction of general anesthesia for postoperative pain management.

1. Which of the following statements is correct?

    A. The tidal volume includes the expiratory reserve volume.
    B. The expiratory reserve volume is part of the inspiratory capacity.
    C. The vital capacity consists of the tidal volume and the expiratory reserve volume.
    D. The total lung capacity includes the vital capacity and the residual volume.

The correct answer is D. See the following figure.

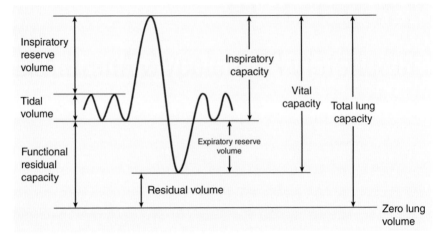

(Modified with permission from Lumb A. *Nunn's Applied Respiratory Physiology.* 8th ed. St. Louis, MO: Elsevier; 2017.)

2. What is usually the closing capacity of a 22-year-old woman who is not under any anesthesia?

A. Above the functional residual capacity (FRC) in upright position.
B. Below the FRC in supine and upright positions.
C. Above the FRC in supine position.
D. Above the FRC in supine and upright positions.

The correct answer is B. Closing capacity is defined as the lung volume where the airways close in the dependent areas of the lung while perfusion is preserved, thus resulting in an intrapulmonary shunt. In young persons, the closing capacity is below the FRC in upright and supine positions; however, it rises with age.

3. Of the following statements regarding pulmonary mechanics, which is *incorrect*?

A. FRC and closing volume are reduced to the same degree under general anesthesia.
B. The FRC is reduced by 0.8 to 2 L under general anesthesia.
C. The increase of the work of breathing under anesthesia is caused by an increase in airway resistance.
D. Stage III anesthesia with sevoflurane results in reduced tidal volumes with increased respiratory rate.

The correct answer is C. The FRC is reduced by 0.8 to 1 L in supine nonanesthetized patients. General anesthesia results in an additional reduction of the FRC by 0.4 to 0.5 L. Contributing factors are loss of inspiratory muscle tone, upward shift of the diaphragm, chest wall rigidity, and changes in the thoracic volume resulting in alveolar collapse and compression atelectasis. The dorsal part of the diaphragm moves upward under anesthesia. The FRC and closing capacity are usually equally reduced under anesthesia. Inhalational anesthetics have bronchodilating effects and prevent an increase of the airway resistance as a result of the decreased FRC. The increased work of breathing is caused by the reduced compliance of the lung and chest wall. Stage III general anesthesia with inhaled agents is usually associated with an increased respiratory rate and decreased tidal volume.

4. In the postanesthesia care unit, the patient complains about shortness of breath. What is the most common cause for this symptom in this patient?

   A. Pneumothorax.
   B. Hematothorax.
   C. High spinal anesthesia.
   D. Paralysis of the left hemidiaphragm.

The correct answer is D. The most likely cause for the shortness of breath in this patient is a paralysis of the left hemidiaphragm after an interscalene block of the brachial plexus. The phrenic nerve crosses the anterior scalene muscle in the interscalene groove, and the ipsilateral phrenic nerve is usually blocked with an interscalene brachial plexus block when the usual volumes of 15 to 25 mL of local anesthetic are injected (and the contralateral phrenic nerve may be blocked in up to 50% of cases). The reduction in vital capacity can cause dyspnea, hypoxemia, and hypercapnea. Patients with limited pulmonary reserve are not candidates for an interscalene block of the brachial plexus. Other neural structures inadvertently blocked with the interscalene approach are the recurrent laryngeal nerve with resulting hoarseness and the fibers of the cervicothoracic ganglion resulting in a Horner syndrome. Recent studies using reduced volumes of local anesthetics (5–7 mL) described a reduction of these side effects. Pneumothorax after interscalene brachial plexus block has been reported for both nerve stimulation-guided and ultrasound-guided block techniques.

Other, fortunately rare, complications of interscalene block include intravenous local anesthetic injection resulting in systemic local anesthetic toxicity; injection of local anesthetics into the vertebral artery resulting in seizures; intrathecal, subdural, and epidural spread of the local anesthetic causing a high spinal block; and injuries to the cervical spinal cord, nerve roots, or brachial plexus.

5. What would you expect when you review the preoperative PFTs?

   A. Forced vital capacity (FVC) normal, forced expiratory volume in 1 s (FEV_1)/ FVC of 60%.
   B. FVC reduced, FEV_1/FVC >80%.
   C. FVC normal , FEV_1/FVC of 75%.
   D. FVC significantly reduced, FEV_1/FVC >85%.

The correct answer is C. The FVC is the vital capacity measured with a fast and forceful expiration. The FEV_1 represents the volume exhaled in the first second of the forced expiration.

The FVC in patients with obstructive airway disease is usually normal; however, the FEV_1/FVC ratio is reduced proportional to the degree of airway obstruction. An FEV_1/FVC of 60% represents a significant obstruction; an FEV_1 of 75% is more likely to be present in a patient with mild asthma and a history of smoking. In restrictive lung disease, both FVC and FEV_1 are reduced.

DID YOU LEARN?

- Interpretation of PFTs.
- Complications of interscalene block.

CASE 2   A Trauma Patient Following Motor Vehicle Accident

Katrina von Kriegenbergh, MD, and Ashraf N. Farag, MD

A 55-year-old man is brought into the trauma bay following a motorcycle accident. The report from the ambulance crew states that the patient was ejected from his motorcycle and sustained an open left femoral fracture. There was no loss of consciousness. The patient's medical history includes obesity, hypertension, a six-pack of beer daily, and a 20-pack-year history of cigarette smoking. His complaints include left lower extremity pain, chest pain, and shortness of breath. Arterial blood gas (ABG) results are pH 7.42, $PaCO_2$ 42 mm Hg, PaO_2 55 mm Hg, bicarbonate 26 mEq/L, and S_aO_2 88%.

1. His hypoxemia is most likely due to which of the following?

   A. Bronchospasm.
   B. Hypovolemia.
   C. Pulmonary embolus.
   D. Pulmonary contusion and pneumothorax.

The correct answer is D. Lung injury and pneumothorax must always be considered in a patient following multiple trauma. Chest pain in this 55-year-old man could reflect both traumatic injury as well as myocardial ischemia. ECG, chest x-ray, and careful auscultation of the lungs would all be a part of the initial evaluation of this patient. Of the choices listed, pulmonary contusion and pneumothorax would be most likely in this setting. If myocardial ischemia were included, the information provided would not be sufficient to rule out that possibility. Had this patient lost consciousness, pulmonary aspiration would likewise need to be considered in the differential diagnosis of this patient's hypoxemia. Physiologically, hypoxemia often occurs secondary to inadequate matching of ventilation and perfusion. Lung collapse, as occurs with pneumothorax, and lung consolidation secondary to lung trauma reduce the ventilation/perfusion ratio, thereby leading to shunt. Shunt occurs when alveoli are perfused but not ventilated. Dead space ventilation is the opposite of shunt and implies ventilation without perfusion. Pulmonary embolism results in areas of the lung that are likely ventilated but not perfused.

2. 100% oxygen is administered to the patient, and a subsequent ABG shows that oxygenation has improved to PaO_2 90 mm Hg and SaO_2 to 95%. The patient's hemoglobin has been stable at 15 g/dL. How has the oxygen content of this patient's blood changed?

   A. It has increased by 24%.
   B. It has increased by 13%.
   C. It has increased by 9%.
   D. This cannot be determined without $PaCO_2$.

The correct answer is C. Oxygen content can be calculated with the following equation:

$$O_2 \text{ content } (CaO_2) = (SaO_2 \times Hb \times 1.31 \text{ mL/dL blood})$$
$$+ (PaO_2 \times 0.003 \text{ mL/dL blood/mm Hg})$$

Hb is hemoglobin concentration in g/dL blood.

SaO_2 is hemoglobin saturation at the given P_xO_2.

CaO_2 can be calculated with PaO_2 from the ABG:

$$CaO_2 = (SaO_2 \, Hb \times 1.31 \text{ mL/dL blood}) + (PaO_2 \times 0.003 \text{ mL/dL blood per mm Hg})$$
$$CaO_2 \text{ before } 100\% \, O_2 = (0.88 \times 15 \times 1.31) + (55 \times 0.003)$$
$$CaO_2 = 17.292 + 0.165$$
$$CaO_2 = 17.457 \text{ mL/dL blood}$$

$$CaO_2 \text{ after } 100\% \, O_2 = (0.95 \times 15 \times 1.31) + (90 \times 0.003)$$
$$CaO_2 = 18.6675 + 0.27$$
$$CaO_2 = 18.9375 \text{ mL/dL blood}$$
$$\frac{18.9375 - 17.457}{17.457} = 8.6\%$$

3. Chest x-ray and physical exam are consistent with pulmonary contusion, indicating an increased intrapulmonary shunt (normal is <5%). The most recent ABG shows PaO_2 200 mm Hg and SaO_2 100%. Assuming the patient is at sea level and his respiratory quotient is 0.8, what is the A–a gradient?

   A. 450 mm Hg.
   B. 550 mm Hg.
   C. 650 mm Hg.
   D. Cannot be determined without $PvCO_2$.

The correct answer is A.

A–a gradient = $PAO_2 - PaO_2$

PaO_2 is measured by taking an ABG.

PAO_2 is calculated by the alveolar gas equation:

$$PAO_2 = (P_{Atm} - P_{H_2O}) \times FiO_2 - (PaCO_2/R)$$

- PAO_2 is alveolar partial pressure.
- P_{Atm} is atmospheric pressure (760 mm Hg at sea level).
- P_{H_2O} is the water vapor pressure (47 mm Hg at room temperature).
- FiO_2 is the fraction of inspired oxygen.
- PaO_2 is the arterial partial pressure of oxygen measured by ABG.
- R is the respiratory quotient ($CO_{2\,eliminated}/O_{2\,consumed}$).

This equation shows how PAO_2 is affected by several variables. PAO_2 can change with elevation and temperature through P_{Atm} and P_{H2O}, respectively. R is dependent on the ongoing cellular metabolic processes that can change during the stress of infection and inflammation. Therefore, $PaCO_2$ is the only manipulable variable that would change PAO_2 significantly; $PaCO_2$ can be changed by modifying ventilation via rate or volume.

$$PAO_2 = (760 - 47) \times 1 - (44/0.8)$$
$$PAO_2 = 713 - 55$$
$$PAO_2 = 658 \text{ mm Hg}$$
$$658 - 200 = 458 \text{ mm Hg}$$

Normal A–a gradient is between 5 and 10 mm Hg in a young healthy patient and increases approximately 1 mm Hg per decade of increased age.

4. The patient is taken to surgery for repair of the femur fracture. During the procedure, systolic blood pressure suddenly declines to 40 mm Hg and end-tidal carbon dioxide (CO_2) to 15 mm Hg. Which of the following is the most likely cause of this decrease?

   A. Acute ST elevation myocardial infarction.
   B. Fat embolism.
   C. Sepsis.
   D. Acute hypovolemia.

The correct answer is B. Although all of the conditions above can result in hypotension, sepsis is not likely to produce a sudden decline in blood pressure or an acute fall in end-tidal CO_2 measurement. Ventricular failure, as might be seen with an acute myocardial infarction, can reduce both cardiac output and consequently increase dead space, resulting in reduced end-tidal CO_2 concentration, but this is not a likely presentation. Pulmonary embolism likewise will reduce alveolar perfusion while ventilation is maintained, thus increasing dead space and decreasing end-tidal CO_2. Acute hypovolemia will reduce cardiac output and increase dead space ventilation, but this would most likely be signaled by very evident and abundant blood loss.

5. The patient experiences significant blood loss intraoperatively and is rapidly given several units of packed red blood cells. All of the following should be expected *except*:

A. Leftward shift of the hemoglobin dissociation curve in packed red blood cells.
B. Increase in the PaO_2 where 50% of hemoglobin is saturated (P50) in packed red blood cells.
C. Rightward shift of the hemoglobin dissociation curve with acidosis.
D. Rightward shift of the hemoglobin dissociation curve with increased 2,3-diphosphogycerate (2,3-DPG).

The correct answer is B. The P50 shifts leftward in settings of decreased 2,3-DPG and in hypothermic conditions. Packed blood cells have decreased 2,3-DPG and are chilled, resulting in a lower P50. This implies that transfused cells have a greater avidity for oxygen—not releasing it to the tissues until lower than the normal oxygen tension (~27 mm Hg). In acidotic conditions, the curve shifts to the right, resulting in an increased release of oxygen to the tissues at higher oxygen tensions. See figure below.

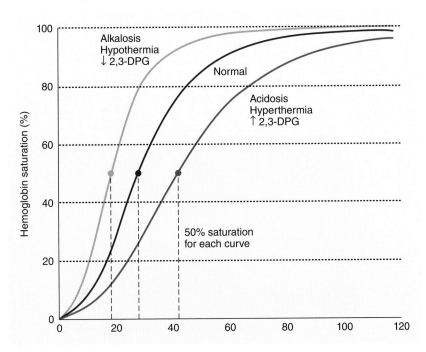

(Reproduced with permission from Butterworth JF, Mackey DC, Wasnick JD: *Morgan and Mikhail's Clinical Anesthesiology*, 6th ed. New York, NY: McGraw-Hill Education; 2018.)

6. The patient is taken to the intensive care unit. A transesophageal echocardiogram is performed during central line placement. The following image is obtained.

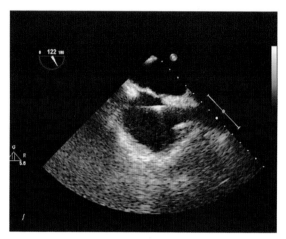

(Reproduced with permission from Butterworth JF, Mackey DC, Wasnick JD: *Morgan and Mikhail's Clinical Anesthesiology*, 6th ed. New York, NY: McGraw-Hill Education; 2018.)

The image demonstrates all of the following *except*:

A. The right atrium.
B. The left atrium.
C. A wire in the superior vena cava.
D. The left ventricle.
E. The intraatrial septum.

The correct answer is D. All of the above structures are seen with the exception of the left ventricle. This bicaval view is useful in the examination of the intraatrial septum and the superior and inferior vena cava. See image below.

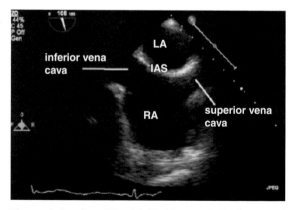

(Reproduced with permission from Wasnick JD, Nicoara A: *Cardiac Anesthesia and Transesophageal Echocardiography*, 2nd ed. New York, NY: McGraw-Hill Education; 2019.)

DID YOU LEARN?

- Calculation of oxygen content.
- The alveolar gas equation.
- The bicaval transesophageal echocardiography image structures.

Recommended Readings

Baumgardner JE, Hedenstierna G. Ventilation/perfusion distributions revisited. *Curr Opin Anaesthesiol.* 2016;29:2.

Butterworth IV JF, Mackey DC, Wasnick JD, eds. Respiratory physiology & anesthesia. In: *Morgan & Mikhail's Clinical Anesthesiology.* 6th ed. New York, NY: McGraw-Hill Education; 2018:495-534.

Campos J. Update on tracheobronchial anatomy and flexible fiberoptic bronchoscopy in thoracic anesthesia. *Curr Opin Anaesthesiol.* 2009;22:4.

Hedenstierna G, Edmark L. Effects of anesthesia on the respiratory system. *Best Pract Res Clin Anaesthesiol.* 2015;29:273.

Levitsky MG. *Pulmonary Physiology.* 8th ed. New York, NY: McGraw-Hill Education; 2013.

Lohser J. Evidence based management of one lung ventilation. *Anesthesiol Clin.* 2008;26:241.

Lumb AB, Slinger P. Hypoxic pulmonary vasoconstriction: Physiology and anesthetic implications. *Anesthesiology.* 2015;122:932.

Minnich D, Mathisen D. Anatomy of the trachea, carina, and bronchi. *Thorac Surg Clin.* 2007;17:571.

Warner DO. Diaphragm function during anesthesia: Still crazy after all these years. *Anesthesiology.* 2002;97:295.

CHAPTER 20

Anesthesia for Patients with Respiratory Disease

CASE 1   Perioperative Pulmonary Complications

Shady Adib, MD, and Lydia Conlay, MD, PhD, MBA

A 92-kg, 27-year-old man presents for an anterior cruciate ligament repair following a skiing injury. He has a history of asthma that is well controlled. He uses an albuterol inhaler three or four times a year, more often during allergy season, but also when he jogs during cold weather. He forgot to bring the inhaler with him. The patient denies dyspnea, wheezing, recent asthma attacks, or recent steroid therapy.

On examination the patient is not in distress. His lungs are clear, without audible wheezing or rhonchi, and there are no retractions noted in his respiratory effort.

1. The most critical time for asthmatic patients undergoing general anesthesia is:

    A. During intravenous induction of general anesthesia.
    B. During instrumentation of the airway.
    C. During initiation of surgical stimuli.
    D. After extubation.

The correct answer is B. This problem can be circumvented by deepening the anesthetic. Pain, emotional stress, or stimulation during light general anesthesia at either induction or emergence can precipitate bronchospasm.

A regional anesthetic eliminates the need to instrument the patient's airway, but it does not entirely eliminate the possibility of bronchospasm.

2. Reflex bronchospasm can be blunted before intubation by:

    A. Administering an additional dose of the intravenous induction agent.
    B. Ventilating the patient with 2 to 3 times the minimum alveolar concentration (MAC) of a volatile agent for 5 min.
    C. Administering intravenous or intratracheal lidocaine (1–2 mg/kg).
    D. All of the above.

The correct answer is D. Bronchospasm in response to instrumentation of the airway can be moderated or avoided entirely by first deepening the anesthetic with an additional dose of the induction agent, ventilating the patient with a 2 to 3 MAC of a volatile agent for 5 min, or administering intravenous or intratracheal lidocaine (1–2 mg/kg). Note that intratracheal lidocaine can in and of itself initiate bronchospasm if administered during an inadequately deep anesthetic.

3. Which of the following matches the capnograph of a patient with obstructive pulmonary disease?

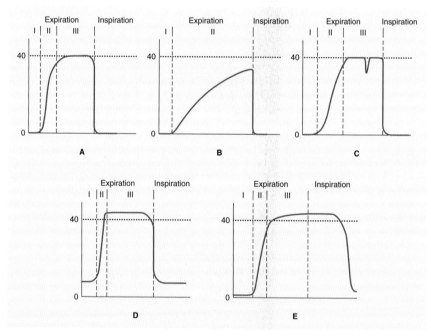

(Reproduced with permission from Butterworth JF, Mackey DC, Wasnick JD: *Morgan and Mikhail's Clinical Anesthesiology*, 6th ed. New York, NY: McGraw-Hill Education; 2018.)

    A. Graph A.
    B. Graph B.
    C. Graph C.
    D. Graph D.
    E. Graph E.

The correct answer is B. Graph A illustrates a normal capnograph demonstrating the three phases of expiration: phase I—dead space; phase II—mixture of dead space and alveolar gas; phase III—alveolar gas plateau.

Graph B illustrates the capnograph of a patient with severe chronic obstructive pulmonary disease. Severe bronchospasm is manifested by rising peak inspiratory pressures and incomplete exhalation, with no plateau before the next inspiration. The gradient between end-tidal CO_2 and arterial CO_2 is thus increased. The obstruction to airflow during expiration is demonstrated on capnography as a delayed rise of the end-tidal CO_2 value, and the severity of obstruction is inversely related to the rate of rise in end-tidal CO_2. Lower tidal volumes of 6 mL/kg or less with prolongation of the expiratory time may help avoid air trapping and barotrauma.

Graph C shows a downward deflection in the expiratory curve during phase III, indicating spontaneous respiratory effort.

Graph D shows a failure of the inspired CO_2 to return to zero. This may represent an incompetent expiratory valve or exhausted CO_2 absorbent.

Graph E demonstrates the persistence of exhaled gas during part of the inspiratory cycle and signals the presence of an incompetent inspiratory valve.

DID YOU LEARN?

- Risk factors for bronchospasm in anesthetized patients.
- Methods to reduce the risk of bronchospasm intraoperatively.
- Differential diagnoses of intraoperative bronchospasm.
- Capnographs display a waveform of CO_2 concentration that allows recognition of a variety of conditions.

CASE 2   Anesthesia for a Patient with Pulmonary Fibrosis

Robert Johnston, MD, and Thomas McHugh, MD

A 44-year-old woman presents emergently for laparoscopic appendectomy. Vital signs include heart rate 100 beats/min, respiratory rate 29 breaths/min, and blood pressure 90/60 mm Hg. Her past medical history is significant for primary pulmonary fibrosis. She has previously been treated with glucocorticoids and immunosuppressive therapy.

1. Upon review of the medical record, you expect the patient's pulmonary function tests to demonstrate all of the following *except*:

 A. Reduced forced expiratory volume in 1 s (FEV_1).
 B. Reduced forced vital capacity (FVC).
 C. Increased FEV_1/FVC ratio.
 D. Decreased pulmonary compliance.

The correct answer is C. Fibrotic lung disease is an example of restrictive lung disease. Although FEV_1 and FVC are both reduced in restrictive pulmonary diseases, the ratio of FEV_1/FVC is generally maintained. Restrictive pulmonary diseases are characterized by decreased lung compliance, and as a result, positive-pressure ventilation can often produce high inspiratory pressures with relatively small delivered tidal volumes. The work of breathing is often increased in patients with restrictive lung diseases, and they compensate by taking rapid, shallow breaths.

2. The medical record also indicates that the patient had previously been examined by transesophageal echocardiography to evaluate dyspnea. Echocardiographic findings associated with restrictive pulmonary disease include all of the following *except*:

   A. Mitral regurgitation.
   B. Dilated right ventricle.
   C. Flattening of the intraventricular septum.
   D. Tricuspid regurgitation.
   E. Right ventricular failure.

The correct answer is A. Patients with pulmonary fibrosis frequently develop pulmonary hypertension and right-ventricular failure. The right ventricle dilates and tricuspid regurgitation develops. The left ventricle may be underloaded secondary to right-ventricular failure. The interventricular septum flattens. Pulmonary hypertension generally leads to right heart abnormalities. The mitral valve is a left heart structure and therefore should not be directly impacted by changes in the right side of the heart. The echocardiographic image below demonstrates changes associated with right-ventricular dysfunction.

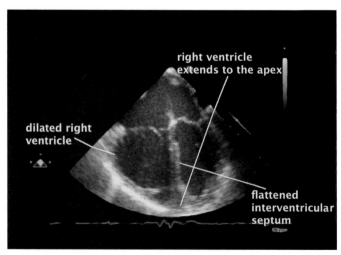

(Reproduced with permission from Wasnick JD, Nicoara A: *Cardiac Anesthesia and Transesophageal Echocardiography*, 2nd ed. New York, NY: McGraw-Hill Education; 2019.)

3. Following placement of an arterial line, general anesthesia is induced and the patient is successfully intubated. Tidal volumes 4 to 6 mL/kg are employed, and a peak inspiratory pressure of 30 mm Hg is noted. Surgery commences. The inspiratory pressure increases to 55 mm Hg and the patient becomes hypotensive to 60 mm Hg systolic. Immediate actions include all of the following *except*:

A. Have the surgeon release the pneumoperitoneum.
B. Auscultate the lungs.
C. Examine the endotracheal tube for kinks and occlusion.
D. Start inhaled nitric oxide.

The correct answer is D. Patients with right heart failure and restrictive lung disease may be unable to compensate for the increased intraabdominal pressure and increased intrathoracic pressure associated with positive-pressure ventilation and pneumoperitoneum. The result may be an abrupt fall in venous return and cardiac output. Release of the pneumoperitoneum at this time may lower the inspiratory pressure, improve venous return and cardiac output, and increase blood pressure. Nevertheless, any increased inspiratory pressure in any patient, either with or without lung disease, should prompt a thorough assessment of the patient's lungs and airway. Auscultation of the lungs and passage of a catheter down the endotracheal tube are indicated to rule out pneumothorax and any airway obstruction, respectively. Fiberoptic bronchoscopy may also be utilized, and a chest radiograph may be required for an uncertain diagnosis. Should the patient have right heart failure secondary to pulmonary hypertension, administration of nitric oxide (NO) may improve loading of the left ventricle and hemodynamic performance. NO therapy will never be an initial action when presented with an acute rise in inspiratory pressure.

4. A mucus plug is removed from the endotracheal tube, and the operation proceeds uneventfully. The patient is successfully extubated at the end of the procedure and delivered to the postanesthesia care unit. Two hours into her recovery, she acutely develops progressive hypotension (blood pressure 70/50 mm Hg). Appropriate initial actions include all of the following *except*:

A. Examine the abdomen for signs of distension.
B. Measure hemoglobin and hematocrit.
C. Perform a bedside transthoracic echocardiographic (TTE) examination.
D. Commence treatment with dopamine.
E. Obtain a chest x-ray.

The correct answer is D. While providing the patient with supplemental oxygen and administering intravenous volume, an immediate differential diagnosis should be generated to determine specific therapy. The abdomen is examined to determine if it is distended from bleeding. This patient was monitored with an arterial line, and a blood gas with electrolytes and hematocrit can be obtained. A pulse contour analysis monitor can be employed with the arterial waveform to estimate stroke volume to guide fluid and/or inotropic therapy. Bedside TTE examination can readily determine if the patient is hypovolemic, vasodilated, or in ventricular failure. Chest x-ray to rule out a previously undetected pneumothorax is also indicated. An inotrope such as dopamine may be employed should evaluation indicate ventricular failure. However, dopamine therapy would not be an initial action.

DID YOU LEARN?

- Pulmonary function tests and restrictive lung disease.
- Effects of pulmonary hypertension on right heart function.
- Management of sudden increase inspiratory pressure.

Recommended Readings

Butterworth IV JF, Mackey DC, Wasnick JD, eds. Anesthesia for patients with respiratory disease. In: *Morgan & Mikhail's Clinical Anesthesiology*. 6th ed. New York, NY: McGraw-Hill Education; 2018:535-552.

Canet J, Gallart L, Gomar C, et al. Prediction of postoperative pulmonary complications in a population based surgical cohort. *Anesthesiology*. 2010;113:1338.

Cox J, Jablons D. Operative and perioperative pulmonary emboli. *Thorac Surg Clin*. 2015;15:289.

Gallart L, Canet J. Post-operative pulmonary complications: Understanding definitions and risk assessment. *Best Pract Res Clin Anaesthesiol*. 2015;29:315.

Hedenstierna G, Edmark L. Effects of anesthesia on the respiratory system. *Best Pract Res Clin Anaesthesiol*. 2015;29:273.

Henzler T, Schoenberg S, Schoepf U, Fink C. Diagnosing acute pulmonary embolism: Systematic review of evidence base and cost effectiveness of imaging tests. *J Thorac Imaging*. 2012;27:304.

Hurford WE. The bronchospastic patient. *Int Anesthesiol Clin*. 2000;38:77.

Lakshminarasimhachar A, Smetana G. Preoperative evaluation: Estimation of pulmonary risk. *Anesthesiol Clin*. 2016;34:71.

Lee H, Kim J, Tagmazyan K. Treatment of stable chronic obstructive pulmonary disease: The GOLD guidelines. *Am Fam Physician*. 2013;88:655.

Radosevich M, Brown D. Anesthetic management of the adult patient with concomitant cardiac and pulmonary disease. *Anesthesiol Clin*. 2016;34:633.

Regli A, von Ungern-Sternberg B. Anesthesia and ventilation strategies in children with asthma: Part 1—preoperative assessment. *Curr Opin Anaesthesiol*. 2014;27:288.

Regli A, von Ungern-Sternberg B. Anesthesia and ventilation strategies in children with asthma: Part II—intraoperative management. *Curr Opin Anaesthesiol*. 2014;27:295.

Reilly JJ Jr. Evidence-based preoperative evaluation candidates for thoracotomy. *Chest*. 1999;116:474.

Salmasi V, Maheshwari K, Yang D, et al. Relationship between intraoperative hypotension, defined by either reduction from baseline or absolute thresholds, and acute kidney and myocardial injury after non cardiac surgery. *Anesthesiology*. 2017;126:47.

Smetana G. Postoperative pulmonary complications: An update on risk assessment and reduction. *Cleveland Clin J Med*. 2009;76(suppl 4):S60.

Sweitzer B, Smetana G. Identification and evaluation of the patient with lung disease. *Anesthesiol Clin*. 2009;27:673.

CHAPTER 21
Anesthesia for Thoracic Surgery

CASE 1	Patient for Tracheal Resection

Bettina Schmitz, MD, and Spencer Thomas, MD

A 64-year-old man is scheduled for a surgical repair of severe tracheal stenosis (lumen 5 mm). His past medical history is significant for type 2 diabetes mellitus controlled with oral agents and diet. He has a history of hypertension and coronary artery disease, the latter of which has been asymptomatic following stent placement 2 years previously. His past surgical history includes an appendectomy when he was 18 years old and a previous episode of severe urinary tract infection with sepsis and prolonged intensive care unit intubation. During your preoperative evaluation, you observe that the patient is experiencing respiratory distress despite supplemental oxygen through a nasal cannula. The patient presents with visual and auditory clues of stridor and labored breathing. He is using respiratory accessory muscles. He complains of severe dyspnea that prevents him from performing minimal tasks.

1. What interventions could you employ that might improve the patient's dyspnea prior to surgery?

   A. Administer 100% oxygen via a nonrebreather face mask.
   B. Administer a breathing treatment of albuterol nebulizer.
   C. Administer a helium–oxygen mixture of 79%/21% via face mask.
   D. All of the above.

The correct answer is D. The administration of a helium–oxygen mixture of 79%/21% is likely most efficacious. A helium–oxygen mixture is an effective treatment for patients who present with an airway obstruction pathology, including fixed tracheal obstructions. Helium decreases the density of the inspired gas, which results in a dramatic increase in flow through the obstruction, thus decreasing the work of breathing. Racemic epinephrine and/or albuterol may or may not have a beneficial effect depending upon the degree of airway edema present. The administration of 100% oxygen via a nonrebreather facemask may likewise be of benefit.

2. Prior to surgery, the patient underwent preoperative pulmonary test including flow–volume loops. What type of flow–volume loop would you expect to see due to the patient's large fixed obstruction?

A. Loop A.
B. Loop B.
C. Loop C.
D. Loop D.

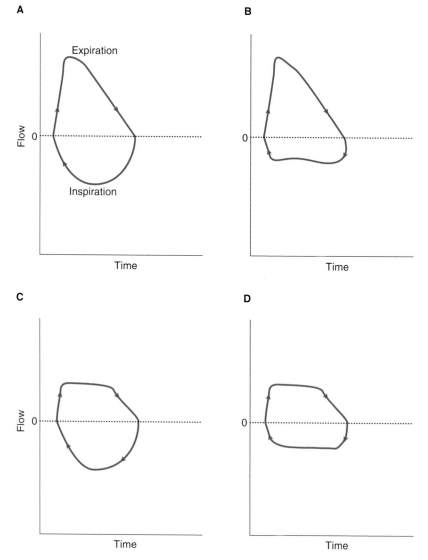

(Reproduced with permission from Butterworth JF, Mackey DC, Wasnick JD: *Morgan and Mikhail's Clinical Anesthesiology*, 6th ed. New York, NY: McGraw-Hill Education; 2018.)

The correct answer is D. Flow–volume loop A is typically observed in a patient without any obstruction. Loop B is observed in a patient with a variable extrathoracic obstruction, as the expiration is normal but inspiration is limited. Loop C is observed in a patient with a variable intrathoracic obstruction, with expiration now limited but inspiration preserved. Measurement of the flow–volume loops confirms the location of the obstruction and aids the clinician in evaluating the severity of the lesion.

3. What would be the most beneficial induction plan for a patient who presents with a large fixed-airway obstruction?

   A. Give the patient 2 mg midazolam preoperatively to relieve anxiety and dyspnea. Dry excessive secretions with an anticholinergic agent. Induce with intravenous (IV) propofol 2 mg/kg, fentanyl 2 μg/kg, lidocaine 1 mg/kg, and rocuronium 0.9 mg/kg.
   B. Give the patient 2 mg midazolam preoperatively to relieve the patient's anxiety and dyspnea. Induction with a rapid-sequence technique.
   C. Avoid preoperative sedation and induce with a rapid-sequence technique.
   D. Avoid preoperative sedation and perform an inhalation induction with sevoflurane and 100% oxygen, maintaining spontaneous ventilation while avoiding muscle relaxants.

The correct answer is D. Preservation of spontaneous ventilation is desirable in the airway stenosis patient. Ventilation with positive pressure may be inadequate. The use of anticholinergic agents to decrease airway secretions is controversial, as this may theoretically increase the risk of inspissation.

4. The case runs without any complications and you decide to leave the patient intubated and transport to the surgical intensive care unit (SICU), with the plan to extubate once the patient is stable. While giving a report to the SICU nurse, you get a page from the emergency department (ED) about a 6-year-old boy who is in severe respiratory distress. The patient has significant stridor, with a large amount of drooling. The ED nurse informs you that the patient received a lateral neck x-ray that was suspicious for a thumb-like epiglottic shadow. When you ask about the patient's condition, the nurse informs you that he is tachypneic with chest retractions, and that he is insisting that he remains in an upright position. What should be your main concern and the top of your differential?

   A. Rapid progression to airway obstruction resulting from infectious croup.
   B. Rapid progression to respiratory arrest due to fatigue resulting from a severe asthma attack.
   C. Rapid progression of airway obstruction resulting from epiglottitis.
   D. Rapid respiratory failure due to aspiration of a foreign object.

The correct answer is C. The patient presents with acute epiglottitis. He manifests classic signs including a neck x-ray showing a shadow epiglottis, respiratory distress, and the preference for upright positions. Recall that epiglottitis is a bacterial infection most commonly secondary to *Haemophilus influenzae* type B. Presentation is often in children age 2 to 6 years old. The patients can rapidly progress from a sore throat and dysphagia to complete airway obstruction. Because the inflammation includes all supraglottic structures, it has been termed supraglottitis as well.

5. What is the most appropriate management plan for the child?

   A. Manage conservatively with oxygen and humidified air. Give the patient racemic epinephrine and IV dexamethasone. Proceed with intubation if the patient progresses to severe intercostal retractions or respiratory fatigue or if central cyanosis is present.
   B. Proceed to the operating room (OR) for general anesthesia and elective tracheostomy.
   C. Proceed to the OR for general anesthesia and intubation and possible emergent tracheostomy.
   D. Perform immediate awake intubation in the ED.

The correct answer is C. The best plan for patients with epiglottitis is intubation and initiation of antibiotic therapy as these interventions can be lifesaving. The intubation should be performed in the OR, and adequate preparations for emergent tracheostomy must be made prior to induction of general anesthesia as total obstruction can occur at any moment. It is very important that laryngoscopy should not be performed before induction of general anesthesia because of the patient's increased risk for laryngospasm. Many experts recommend induction using inhaled sevoflurane (or halothane) with the patient in the upright position. The endotracheal tube should be ½ to 1 size smaller than the one that would be typically used for the patient.

Option A describes the treatment plan for croup, a consequence of an upper respiratory infection that involves the airway below the epiglottis. Intubation is rarely needed for this condition. The clinical description does not yet require tracheostomy as described in option B. Option D would be much less controlled and more dangerous than option C.

DID YOU LEARN?

- Management of the patient with tracheal stenosis.
- Differential diagnosis of acute epiglottitis.
- Management of childhood stridor.

Recommended Readings

Alam N. Lung resection in patients with marginal pulmonary function. *Thorac Surg Clin.* 2014;24:361.

Brunelli A, Kim A, Berger K, Addrizzo-Harris D. Physiologic evaluation of the patient with lung cancer being considered for resection surgery. *Chest.* 2013;143(suppl):e166S.

Butterworth IV JF, Mackey DC, Wasnick JD, eds. Anesthesia for thoracic surgery. In: *Morgan & Mikhail's Clinical Anesthesiology.* 6th ed. New York, NY: McGraw-Hill Education; 2018:553-582.

Campos J. An update on bronchial blockers during lung separation techniques in adults. *Anesth Analg.* 2003;97:1266.

Carney A, Dickinson M. Anesthesia for esophagectomy. *Anesthesiol Clin.* 2015;33:143.

Clayton-Smith A, Alston R, Adams G, et al. A comparison of the efficacy and adverse effects of double lumen endobronchial tubes and bronchial blockers in thoracic surgery: A systematic review and meta-analysis of randomized controlled trials. *J Cardiothorac Vasc Anesth.* 2015;29:955.

Della Rocca G, Coccia C. Acute lung injury in thoracic surgery. *Curr Opin Anesthesiol.* 2013;26:40.

Doan L, Augustus J, Androphy R, et al. Mitigating the impact of acute and chronic post thoracotomy pain. *J Cardiothorac Vasc Anesth.* 2014;28:1048.

Ehrenfeld JM, Walsh JL, Sandberg WS. Right- and left-sided Mallinckrodt double-lumen tubes have identical clinical performance. *Anesth Analg.* 2008;106:1847.

Falzon D, Alston RP, Coley E, Montgomery K. Lung isolation for thoracic surgery: From inception to evidence-based. *J Cardiothorac Vasc Anesth.* 2017;31:678.

Gemmill EH, Humes DJ, Catton JA. Systematic review of enhanced recovery after gastro-oesophageal cancer surgery. *Ann R Coll Surg Engl.* 2015;97:173.

Gimenez-Mila M, Klein A, Martinez G. Design and implementation of an enhanced recovery program in thoracic surgery. *J Thorac Dis.* 2016;8(suppl 1):S37.

Gothard J. Anesthetic considerations for patients with anterior mediastinal masses. *Anesthesiol Clin.* 2008;26:305.

Guldner A, Pelosi P, Abreu M. Nonventilatory strategies to prevent post operative pulmonary complications. *Curr Opin Anesthesiol.* 2013;26:141.

Hoechter D, von Dossow V. Lung transplantation: From the procedure to managing patients with lung transplantation. *Curr Opin Anesthesiol.* 2016;29:8.

Lohser J, Slinger P. Lung injury after one-lung ventilation; a review of the pathophysiologic mechanisms affecting the ventilated and collapsed lung. *Anesth Analg.* 2015;121:302.

Marseu K, Slinger P. Perioperative pulmonary dysfunction and protection. *Anaesthesia.* 2016;71(suppl 1):46.

Módolo NS, Módolo MP, Marton MA, et al. Intravenous versus inhalation anaesthesia for one-lung ventilation. *Cochrane Database Syst Rev.* 2013;(7):CD006313.

Neto A, Schultz M, Gama de Abreu M. Intraoperative ventilation strategies to prevent postoperative pulmonary complications: Systematic review, meta-analysis, and trial sequential analysis. *Best Pract Res Clin Anaesthesiol.* 2015;29:331.

Rodriguez-Aldrete D, Candiotti K, Janakiraman R, et al. Trends and new evidence in the management of acute and chronic post-thoracotomy pain—an overview of the literature from 2005–2015. *J Cardiothorac Vasc Anesth.* 2016;30:762.

Slinger P. Update on anesthetic management for pneumonectomy. *Curr Opin Anaesthesiol.* 2009;22:31.

Slinger P, Johnston M. Preoperative assessment: An anesthesiologist's perspective. *Thorac Surg Clin.* 2005;15:11.

Sylvester JT, Shimoda LA, Aaronson PI, Ward JP. Hypoxic pulmonary vasoconstriction. *Physiol Rev.* 2012;92:367.

CHAPTER 22
Anesthesia for Neurosurgery

CASE 1 | Posterior Fossa Craniotomy in the Sitting Position

Swapna Chaudhuri, MD, PhD, and John Welker, MD

A 22-year-old (73 kg, 5′7″) man is scheduled for a posterior fossa craniotomy. He was admitted to the hospital with a 5-week history of episodic headaches, vertigo, and ataxia. During preanesthetic evaluation in the holding area, the patient gave a history of new-onset hypertension. His surgical history is significant for fixation of a distal radius fracture at 8 years of age without any anesthetic complications. Current medications include levetiracetam, dexamethasone, and ondansetron. He is drowsy but otherwise oriented and appropriate; blood pressure is 156/82 mm Hg, heart rate is 80 beats/min, and respiratory rate is 16 breaths/min. Laboratory values reveal a normal hemoglobin concentration, normal electrolytes, and glucose of 160 mg/dL; magnetic resonance images (MRIs) show a 3-cm cystic lesion with mass effect in the left cerebellar tonsillar area. There is less surrounding edema in the latest images (obtained after initiation of dexamethasone).

1. The surgeon posts the patient for possible surgery in the sitting position. All of the following are possible contraindications of this position *except*:

    A. Hemodynamic instability.
    B. Persistent foramen ovale.
    C. Severe cervical stenosis.
    D. Morbid obesity.

The correct answer is D. With some explorations of the posterior fossa, the sitting (semi-recumbent) position is preferred by surgeons. However, this position uniquely increases certain risks, the most important being venous air embolism (VAE). In the upright position, and whenever the wound is above the level of the heart, a subatmospheric pressure can be created in the venous system. This can predispose patients to air entrainment in open veins or venous sinuses. A patent foramen ovale can permit passage of entrained air directly into the arterial circulation (paradoxical air embolism). After VAE, the upright position can worsen the subsequent hypotension and reduced cardiac output from venous pooling below the level of the right atrium. In patients with severe cervical stenosis, the neck flexion that occurs in the upright position can cause spinal cord compression and put the patient at risk for nerve injury or quadriplegia. Morbid obesity makes positioning in the sitting position technically difficult but is not a contraindication. Indeed, ventilation may be improved in the sitting position relative to supine in morbidly obese patients.

2. Complications associated with the sitting position relative to the supine position include all of the following *except*:

    A. Macroglossia and facial edema.
    B. Pneumocephalus.
    C. Increased blood loss.
    D. Quadriplegia.

The correct answer is C. In the sitting position, excessive neck flexion can predispose the patient to swelling of the face and upper airway due to venous congestion and concomitant facial edema. Because of decreased cerebrospinal fluid (CSF) volume and open subarachnoid space in the upright position, the patient is at increased risk for developing pneumocephalus. Following closure of the dura, this can cause compression of the brain, with potential delayed awakening and neurological impairment. As noted earlier, spinal cord compression from neck flexion in the sitting position can put the patient at risk for quadriplegia. The sitting position is not associated with increased blood loss. In fact, this type of positioning facilitates venous drainage, potentially decreases blood loss, and provides better surgical visualization.

3. Following intravenous induction and intubation, a peripheral arterial line and a central venous catheter are inserted uneventfully. Which of the following monitors is the *most* sensitive indicator for detection of VAE?

    A. Expiratory gas analysis for detection of nitrogen.
    B. Precordial Doppler sonography.
    C. Transesophageal echocardiography.
    D. Expired carbon dioxide (CO_2) monitoring.

The correct answer is C. There are several monitors available for detection of an intraoperative air embolism; however, transesophageal echocardiography (TEE) is considered the most sensitive. TEE can detect air bubbles as small as 0.25 mL. In addition, it allows visualization of a patent foramen ovale, as well as any change in cardiac function resulting from the VAE. Mass spectrometry for detection of nitrogen is specific for VAE, but it is less sensitive than TEE. Intraoperative capnography in the setting of VAE would be expected to show a sudden decrease in end-tidal CO_2 ($EtCO_2$); however, there are multiple other conditions that can lower $EtCO_2$ concentration, including decreased cardiac output, increased pulmonary dead space, and hyperventilation. For precordial Doppler sonography, the probe is placed over the right atrium (to the right of the sternum, between the third and sixth ribs) and taped in place. In the setting of VAE, the regular swishing of the Doppler signal is interrupted by a characteristic "mill-wheel" sound as air emboli enter the cardiac circulation. Intraoperative Doppler sonography is not as sensitive as TEE in detecting a small VAE.

4. A multiorifice catheter is chosen for central venous access. Optimal positioning of the catheter tip can be confirmed by each of the following *except*:

A. Intravascular electrocardiography demonstrating a "biphasic" P wave.
B. Fluoroscopy with radiocontrast injection ensuring that the tip is at the cavoatrial junction.
C. TEE.
D. Pullback from the right ventricle while monitoring intravascular pressure.

The correct answer is D. For optimal recovery of air following a VAE, the multiorifice central venous catheter should be positioned at the junction of the superior vena cava and the right atrium. Confirmation of correct positioning by intravascular electrocardiography is achieved by using a saline-filled catheter as a "V" lead. As the catheter is advanced toward the right atrium, a biphasic P wave appears; this characteristic changes to unidirectional deflection once the catheter tip enters farther into the heart. Fluoroscopy with radiocontrast injection could be used if one has this competency. Pulling back from the right ventricle while monitoring intravascular pressure can distinguish the right atrial pressure from the right ventricular pressure but cannot reliably identify the cavoatrial junction. Finally, visualization of the central venous catheter via TEE can be utilized for confirmation of correct catheter positioning, and it is the easiest and most convenient technique in most operating rooms.

5. Maintenance of anesthesia is accomplished with IV infusions of propofol, remifentanil, and minimal concentrations of isoflurane (0.3 MAC). However, the patient is observed to be very somnolent at the conclusion of a 5-h operative procedure. Common causes of delayed emergence in this patient include all of the following *except*:

A. Tension pneumocephalus.
B. Brain edema as a result of prolonged surgical retraction.
C. Propofol infusion syndrome.
D. Intraoperative cerebellar infarction.

The correct answer is C. Propofol infusion syndrome (PRIS) is quite rare and can occur with prolonged infusion (>48 h) in adult and pediatric patients. It is usually associated with metabolic acidosis, hypotension, elevated lactate, myoglobinuria, rhabdomyolysis, and triglyceridemia. PRIS is unlikely in the above setting. This clinical scenario could represent a patient with elevated intracranial pressure (ICP); in addition, entrapped air following closure of the dura can cause tension pneumocephalus. This is a neurosurgical emergency and requires prompt decompression. Brain edema can result from prolonged surgical manipulation and excessive tension; it can also result in elevated ICP. This, however, is not usually a surgical emergency; cerebral edema can be treated with osmotic diuretics, hyperventilation, or by treating any concomitant hypertension. An intraoperative cerebellar infarction, although uncommon, can occur due to surgical manipulation of the cerebellar vasculature, as well as from significant intraoperative hemodynamic instability and cerebellar hypoperfusion. This can result in a decrease in mental status or delayed emergence; diagnosis will need to be accomplished by neuroimaging. However, the most likely reason for a perceived delayed emergence is that inadequate time has been allowed for propofol to dissipate after a prolonged anesthetic.

DID YOU LEARN

- Why VAE is a particular concern during neurosurgery in the sitting position?
- What are the better ways to detect VAE during neurosurgery in the sitting position?
- Where the tip of a central venous catheter should be optimally positioned during neurosurgery in the sitting position?

CASE 2 Patient with a Posterior Fossa Mass Lesion

John Welker, MD, Swapna Chaudhuri, MD, PhD, and
John D. Wasnick, MD, MPH

A 45-year-old woman is to undergo surgery to remove a mass lesion in the posterior fossa. The procedure is to be done in the sitting position. She has previously been treated with a ventriculostomy for increased intracranial pressure secondary to obstructive hydrocephalus.

1. Regarding cerebral blood flow (CBF), which of the following statements is true?

   A. CBF is directly proportionate to PaO_2 between tensions of 80 and 120 mm Hg.
   B. CBF changes approximately 5 to 10 mL/100 g/mm Hg change in $PaCO_2$.
   C. Metabolic acidosis has a greater effect on CBF than respiratory acidosis.
   D. Only marked changes in PaO_2 alter CBF.

The correct answer is D. The most important extrinsic influences on CBF are respiratory gas tensions. CBF is directly proportionate to $PaCO_2$ tensions between 20 and 80 mm Hg but is not influenced by changes in oxygen tension in the normal range. Blood flow changes approximately 1 to 2 mL per 100 g of brain tissue per mm Hg change in CO_2 gas tension. Acute metabolic acidosis does not have the same effect on CBF because hydrogen ions do not cross the blood–brain barrier, whereas CO_2 does. Only marked changes in PaO_2 alter CBF.

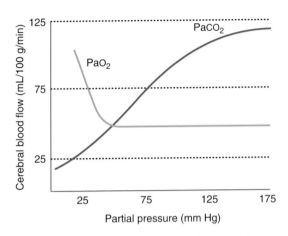

(Reproduced with permission from Butterworth JF, Mackey DC, Wasnick JD: *Morgan and Mikhail's Clinical Anesthesiology*, 6th ed. New York, NY: McGraw-Hill Education; 2018.)

2. A TEE probe is inserted after induction of general anesthesia to monitor for venous air embolism in the sitting position. The mid-esophageal bicaval view is obtained to examine the intraatrial septum for patent foramen ovale. Match the letters in the figure below with these structures: left atrium (LA), right atrium (RA), superior vena cava (SVC), and inferior vena cava (IVC).

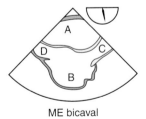

ME bicaval

(Adapted with permission from Shanewise JS, Cheung AT, Aronson S, et al. ASE/SCA guidelines for performing a comprehensive intraoperative multiplane transesophageal echocardiography examination: recommendations of the American Society of Echocardiography Council for Intraoperative Echocardiography and the Society of Cardiovascular Anesthesiologists Task Force for Certification in Perioperative Transesophageal Echocardiography, *Anesth Analg.* 1999 Oct;89(4):870-884.)

The correct answer is A (LA), B (RA), C (SVC), D (IVC). TEE and Doppler sonography are the most sensitive monitors to detect venous air embolism. TEE can rule out a patent foramen ovale that would place the patient at increased risk for a paradoxical left-sided air embolism. An abrupt reduction of $EtCO_2$ gas tension is a less sensitive monitor of air embolism secondary to the increase in alveolar dead space.

3. During the procedure, the $EtCO_2$ decreases from 35 to 20 mm Hg. The differential diagnosis includes all of the following *except*:

   A. Venous air embolism.
   B. Reduced cardiac output.
   C. Decreased dead space ventilation.
   D. Hypovolemia.

The correct answer is C. Increased dead space ventilation (V/Q = ∞) can occur in the setting of venous air embolism, reduced cardiac output, and hypovolemia. When perfusion matches ventilation, $EtCO_2$ more closely approximates arterial CO_2. Events that decrease perfusion of ventilated lungs increase dead space ventilation.

4. The surgery proceeds uneventfully, and the patient is transported to the neuroscience intensive care unit uneventfully. While there, you are assigned to complete a preoperative evaluation of a 55-year-old female scheduled for coiling of an intracranial aneurysm. The patient had a subarachnoid hemorrhage (SAH) 3 days prior. The patient currently presents with drowsiness, confusion, and mild focal deficits. This presentation corresponds to which Hunt and Hess grade for SAH?

   A. I.
   B. II.
   C. III.
   D. IV.

The correct answer is C. The Hunt and Hess scale provides a clinical severity estimate for SAH.

Hunt and Hess Grading Scale for SAH

Grade	Clinical Description
I	Asymptomatic or minimal headache and slight nuchal rigidity
II	Moderate to severe headache, nuchal rigidity, no neurological deficit other than cranial nerve palsy
III	Drowsiness, confusion, or mild focal deficit
IV	Stupor, moderate to severe hemiparesis, and possibly early decerebrate rigidity and vegetative disturbances
V	Deep coma, decerebrate rigidity, and moribund appearance

Reproduced with permission from Priebe HJ. Aneurysmal subarachnoid haemorrhage and the anaesthetist, *Br J Anaesth*. 2007 Jul;99(1):102-118.

The Fisher grading scale below provides a computed tomography (CT) scoring system for SAH.

Fisher Grading Scale of Cranial Computed Tomography (CCT)

Grade	Findings on CCT
1	No subarachnoid blood detected
2	Diffuse or vertical layers ≤1 mm
3	Localized clot and/or vertical layer >1 mm
4	Intracerebral or intraventricular clot with diffuse or no subarachnoid haemorrhage

Reproduced with permission from Priebe HJ. Aneurysmal subarachnoid haemorrhage and the anaesthetist, *Br J Anaesth.* 2007 Jul;99(1):102-118.

5. This patient is likely developing cerebral artery vasospasm and delayed cerebral ischemia (DCI). Which of the following is a worrisome sign regarding the severity of vasospasm?

   A. Decreased flow velocity (<200 cm/s) as obtained by transcranial Doppler.
   B. Lindegaard ratio <3.
   C. Lindegaard ratio >3.
   D. Brain tissue oxygen tension >20 mm Hg.

The correct answer is C. Blood velocity increases when vasospasm is present. The Lindegaard ratio compares the blood velocity of the cervical carotid artery with that of the middle cerebral artery. A ratio >3 is indicative of severe vasospasm. A brain tissue oxygen tension <20 mm Hg would also be a worrisome indicator of poor cerebral tissue perfusion. Treatment for cerebral artery vasospasm consists of nimodipine and initiation of "triple-H" therapy: hypervolemia, hemodilution, and hypertension. Recently, euvolemic hypertension has been suggested as preferable to traditional triple-H therapy.

6. The patient develops ST- and T-wave changes on the intensive care unit monitor. A bedside transthoracic echocardiogram is ordered, which demonstrates dyskinesia of the mid-segments of the left ventricle and apex. Function of the base of the heart is preserved. The most likely diagnosis for this patient is:

   A. Anterior myocardial infarction.
   B. Acute aortic dissection.
   C. Acute aortic insufficiency.
   D. Stress-induced cardiomyopathy.

The correct answer is D. Doppler echocardiography would rule out acute aortic insufficiency. An aortic dissection is detected by presence of a dissection flap in the ascending aorta and possible disruption of the aortic valvar apparatus. An anterior myocardial infarction would generally affect the distribution of the left anterior descending artery. This patient with recent SAH is at risk for takotsubo cardiomyopathy. Takotsubo cardiomyopathy occurs most frequently in postmeno-pausal women. Patients with takotsubo cardiomyopathy lack evidence of occlusive coronary artery disease but have developed ventricular dysfunction secondary to catecholamine effects on the heart.

CASE 3　Traumatic Brain Injury

Sabry Khalil, MD

A 47-year-old man presents to the emergency department following a motor vehi-cle accident. He is lethargic and combative. Blood is noticed on his face and in his mouth. He has a depressed left zygomatic fracture. His heart rate is 118 beats/min, and blood pressure is 188/98 mm Hg. Saturation is 91% on a 6-L oxygen mask. Res-pirations are shallow. Temperature is 38.5°C. Upon examination, you find a mor-bidly obese male with a thick neck wearing a hard cervical collar. No additional history is available to you. A neurosurgeon has been consulted. Laboratory data include pH 7.15, $PaCO_2$ 51 mm Hg, PO_2 68 mm Hg, hematocrit 27%, K 4.9 mEq/L, Na 147 mEq/L, BUN 42, and glucose 360 mg/dL.

1. The best course of action at this time is to:

A. Rush the patient emergently to CT scan.
B. Insert an ICP monitor.
C. Start a mannitol infusion of 0.5 g/kg.
D. Perform rapid-sequence induction and intubation with backup plans for surgical airway.

The correct answer is D. This patient has sustained major trauma with signs of traumatic brain injury (TBI). He is hypoxemic and hypercarbic, with likely impending respiratory failure. His increased $PaCO_2$ can increase both cerebral blood volume and intracranial pressure, potentially reducing cerebral perfusion pressure. Cerebral perfusion pressure is the difference between mean arterial pressure and intracranial pressure. Control of the airway using rapid-sequence induction with in-line stabilization protects against respiratory failure and aspira-tion and allows for placement of invasive ICP monitoring and radiological evalu-ation to determine the nature and extent of cerebral injury. In-line stabilization is necessary because the presence or absence of cervical spine injury has not been determined.

Radiological examination in the CT scanner is important but cannot proceed until the airway is secured in this lethargic, combative patient. ICP monitoring may be useful in guiding therapy but should not delay control of the airway. Institution of osmotic therapy with mannitol could be appropriate once diagnosis of brain injury with elevated ICP is made.

2. Based on the information in the previous question, what is the calculated serum osmolarity for this patient?

   A. >285 mmol/L.
   B. >295 mmol/L.
   C. >305 mmol/L.
   D. >315 mmol/L.

The correct answer is D. Serum osmolarity guides therapy to reduce cerebral edema. Low plasma osmolarity favors the diffusion of intravascular volume into the brain through the leaky, traumatized blood–brain barrier of the brain-injured patient. The serum osmolarity is calculated by the following equation:

$$\text{Serum osmolarity} = 2\,Na + \text{glucose}/18 + BUN/2.8$$
$$= 2 \times 147 + 360/18 + 42/2.8$$
$$= 294 + 20 + 15$$
$$= 329 \text{ mmol/L}$$

This patient is already hyperosmolar; thus, mannitol (0.5 g/kg) would likely not be employed.

3. According to the Brain Trauma Foundation (BTF), what is the recommended cerebral perfusion pressure in a patient with TBI?

   A. 40–60 mm Hg.
   B. 50–70 mm Hg.
   C. 60–80 mm Hg.
   D. 70–90 mm Hg.
   E. 80–100 mm Hg.

The correct answer is B. According to the BTF, the recommended cerebral perfusion pressure is 50 to 70 mm Hg, with an intracranial pressure less than 20 mm Hg in the brain trauma patient.

4. A CT scan shows a subdural hematoma, and the ICP is measured to be 29 mm Hg. How many secondary insults to the brain has this patient endured so far?

   A. 1.
   B. 2.
   C. 3.
   D. 4.

The correct answer is D. TBI consists of both primary and secondary insults. Primary injuries are usually focal insults related to trauma disrupting normal anatomy. Primary injuries include subdural hematoma, epidural hematoma, intra-parenchymal hemorrhage, and diffuse, nonfocal axonal injury. Secondary injuries are potentially preventable and include hypoxia (PaO_2 60 or saturation <90%), hypercarbia ($PaCO_2$ >45), hypocarbia ($PaCO_2$ <30), hyperthermia (temperature >38°C), hyperglycemia (glucose level >200), hypoglycemia (glucose level <60), intracranial hypertension (ICP >20), and hypotension (systolic blood pressure <90 mm Hg or cerebral perfusion pressure <50 mm Hg).

DID YOU LEARN?

- The importance of secondary insult management in neurotrauma.
- Neurological assessment and treatment of ICP and cerebral perfusion pressure in TBI.
- Indications for ICP monitoring.
- Calculating serum osmolarity to choose your crystalloid/diuretic.

CASE 4   Patient for Cervical Laminectomy

Ashraf N. Farag, MD, and Chase Clanton, MD

A 32-year-old woman is scheduled for a cervical laminectomy in the prone position. She reports a past medical history of asthma and factor V Leiden mutation. She occasionally self-administers an albuterol inhaler and takes 5 mg of warfarin daily. She denies any hospitalizations related to her asthma, but she had a minor pulmonary embolism when she was 15 and a transient ischemic attack (TIA) 3 years ago that left no residual neurological effects. Six months ago, she began to have right hand pain. An MRI of her cervical spine revealed that the C5-C6 disk was herniated. The patient reports that she develops a terrible rash and facial swelling after receiving codeine. Her vital signs include blood pressure 116/74 mm Hg, heart rate 69 beats/min, respiratory rate 14 breaths/min, and SpO_2 100%. A complete blood count and metabolic laboratory panel are unremarkable. An international normalized ratio obtained yesterday was 1.3. Her physical exam reveals no abnormalities.

1. The patient has a Mallampati class II airway with good neck and jaw mobility. There is no supporting device or collar around the head or neck. However, she notes that when she extends her head, her arms become weak. Based on what you know so far, the worst approach to intubation is:

A. Direct asleep laryngoscopy.
B. Direct asleep laryngoscopy with in-line stabilization.
C. Awake fiber-optic laryngoscopy (FOL).
D. Indirect asleep laryngoscopy with in-line stabilization

The correct answer is A. Approach C is the most conservative approach and would be appropriate if no further information is available. However, the stability of the patient's neck will guide decision making. An oral tracheal tube can be inserted with direct laryngoscopy under general anesthesia if the neck is stable. Review of available films and discussion with the surgeon are always warranted prior to airway management. This patient demonstrates neurological symptoms with neck motion; however, she has not been placed in a neck stabilization device. Head movement could result in spinal cord compromise.

An awake FOL will allow for a neurological exam to assess for any further injury from intubation or positioning. Asleep intubation would require in-line stabilization and would likely be most readily performed using video laryngoscopy.

2. After induction, the patient becomes very tachycardic. Looking closely at the monitor, you notice a regular rhythm and atrial flutter waves. The patient has not converted to sinus rhythm for a while now. What is the typical range of heart rates with this particular arrhythmia?

A. Atrial rate of 350–500 beats/min and a ventricular rate of 60–170 beats/min.
B. Atrial rate of 250–350 beats/min and a ventricular rate of 150 beats/min.
C. Atrial rate of 130–200 beats/min.
D. Ventricular rate of 90–120 beats/min.

The correct answer is B. It appears that this patient has developed atrial flutter. This does not always signify heart disease. This can also be a sign of hyperthyroidism or perhaps a manifestation of pulmonary embolism in this patient at risk for thrombus formation.

The atrial rate is usually 300 beats/min and the ventricular rate is 150 beats/min with a 2:1 block, making option B the correct choice here. The rhythm is regular, and the QRS complex is normal. Flutter waves are best seen in leads II and V1. The ventricular response is controlled with esmolol, and the patient returns to sinus rhythm.

3. The high airway pressure alarm goes off on the ventilator. The peak airway pressure has increased. Plateau pressure remains normal. The circuit is checked, and there are no leaks. The patient is switched to bag-mask ventilation, and breath sounds are clear bilaterally. Differential diagnosis includes which of the following?

A. Tension pneumothorax.
B. Endobronchial intubation.
C. Secretions.
D. Airway compression.
E. All of the above.

The correct answer is E. All of the above could result in an increase in peak airway pressures. Kinking of the endotracheal tube in a patient in the prone position for spinal surgery must always be considered.

Recommended Readings

Bell R, Vo A, Vexnedaroglu E, et al. The endovascular operating room as an extension of the intensive care unit: Changing strategies in the management of neurovascular disease. *Neurosurgery*. 2006;59:S3.

Bilotta F, Guerra C, Rosa G. Update on anesthesia for craniotomy. *Curr Opin Anesthesiol*. 2013;26:517.

Butterworth IV JF, Mackey DC, Wasnick JD, eds. Anesthesia for neurosurgery. In: *Morgan & Mikhail's Clinical Anesthesiology*. 6th ed. New York, NY: McGraw-Hill Education; 2018:601-620.

Dinsmore J. Anaesthesia for elective neurosurgery. *Br J Anaesth*. 2007;99:68.

Dority J, Oldham J. Subarachnoid hemorrhage: An update. *Anesthesiol Clin*. 2016;34:577.

Flexman A, Meng L, Gelb A. Outcomes in neuroanesthesia: What matters most? *Can J Anesth*. 2016;63:205.

Goyal M, Yu AY, Menon BK, et al. Endovascular therapy in acute ischemic stroke: Challenges and transition from trials to bedside. *Stroke*. 2016;47:548.

Gupta AK, Azami J. Update of neuromonitoring. *Curr Anaesth Crit Care*. 2002;13:120.

Huh J, Raghupathi R. New concepts in treatment of pediatric traumatic brain injury. *Anesthesiol Clin*. 2009;27:213.

Jinadasa S, Boone M. Controversies in the management of traumatic brain injury. *Anesthesiol Clin*. 2016;34:557.

Nadjat C, Ziv K, Osborn I. Anesthesia for carotid and cerebrovascular procedures in interventional neuroradiology. *Int Anesthesiol Clin*. 2009;47:29.

Priebe H. Aneurysmal subarachnoid haemorrhage and the anaesthetist. *Br J Anaesth*. 2007;99:102.

Quillinan N, Herson P, Traystman RJ. Neuropathophysiology of brain injury. *Anesthesiol Clin*. 2016;34:453.

Rowland M, Hadjipavlou G, Kelly M, et al. Delayed cerebral ischaemia after subarachnoid haemorrhage: Looking beyond vasospam. *Br J Anaesth*. 2012;109:315.

Sharma D, Vavilala M. Perioperative management of adult traumatic brain injury. *Anesthesiol Clin*. 2012;30:333.

Todd M. Outcomes after neuroanesthesia and neurosurgery; what makes a difference? *Anesthesiol Clin*. 2012;30:399.

CHAPTER 23

Anesthesia for Patients with Neurological & Psychiatric Diseases

| CASE 1 | Neuroleptic Malignant Syndrome |

Elizabeth Rebello, MD

You are called to the postanesthesia care unit to evaluate a 28-year-old man who underwent uneventful knee arthroscopy under sevoflurane anesthesia and now appears agitated. His past medical history includes schizophrenia and a recent knee injury, and his only medication is haloperidol. He had been given midazolam, metoclopramide, and famotidine as premedication. He is now agitated, diaphoretic, disoriented, and complains of muscle cramps. Vital signs are temperature 38.4°C, heart rate 110 beats/min, blood pressure 165/90 mm Hg, and respiratory rate 20 breaths/min. Your differential diagnosis includes malignant hyperthermia, anticholinergic toxicity, neuroleptic malignant syndrome (NMS), and serotonin syndrome.

1. A distinguishing feature that may be present with NMS, but is *not* present with serotonin syndrome, is:

   A. Hyporeflexia.
   B. Increased muscle tone.
   C. Tachycardia.
   D. Diaphoresis.

The correct answer is A. NMS, a potentially life-threatening disorder caused by an adverse reaction to medications with dopamine receptor antagonist properties or by rapid withdrawal of dopaminergic medications, is characterized by muscle rigidity, bradykinesia, hyporeflexia, hyperthermia, autonomic instability, and mental status abnormalities. Serotonin syndrome is characterized by hyperkinesia, hyperreflexia, and myoclonus. The time course is another feature that distinguishes NMS from serotonin syndrome; serotonin syndrome has a rapid onset, whereas NMS may evolve over several days. NMS must also be distinguished from malignant hyperthermia, which similarly presents with muscle rigidity, dysautonomia, and hyperthermia. However, malignant hyperthermia is often associated with a family history of the disorder and with exposure to a potent halogenated inhalational anesthetic agent with or without succinylcholine.

2. Medications that may cause NMS include all of the following *except*:

A. Haloperidol.
B. Lithium.
C. Ondansetron.
D. Metoclopramide.
E. Olanzapine.

The correct answer is C. NMS is not associated with administration of ondansetron. NMS may be caused by first-generation (haloperidol, chlorpromazine), second-generation (clozapine, olanzapine, risperidone), and third-generation (aripiprazole) antipsychotic medications. In addition, NMS has been associated with administration of metoclopramide, amoxapine, phenelzine, and lithium, and with sudden withdrawal of dopaminergic medications such as levodopa, bromocriptine, and amantadine.

3. Elevation of which laboratory value is consistent with NMS?

A. Serum iron.
B. White blood cell count (WBC).
C. Magnesium.
D. Potassium.

The correct answer is B. Clinical laboratory parameters consistent with NMS are elevations in WBC, creatine phosphokinase (CPK), and hepatic enzymes (lactate dehydrogenase, aspartate aminotransferase). The elevated WBC and CPK are thought to be due to increased muscle activity and rhabdomyolysis. In addition, serum iron is typically low in cases of NMS.

4. Treatment for neuroleptic malignant syndrome includes:

A. Diphenhydramine.
B. Cyproheptadine.
C. Promethazine.
D. Bromocriptine.

The correct answer is D. Bromocriptine, a dopaminergic agent, is the most frequent medication used to treat NMS. Treatment also consists of stopping administration of the suspected offending medication and, if NMS is due to an abrupt withdrawal of a dopaminergic medication, resuming administration of that medication. Amantadine hydrochloride and levodopa are alternate dopaminergic agents that have been used to treat NMS. Dantrolene, a muscle relaxant that works by inhibiting calcium release from the sarcoplasmic reticulum, may also be administered. Other medications that may be useful in treating NMS are benzodiazepines, which can be helpful in controlling agitation; carbamazepine; and clonidine. In cases that do not respond to standard medical care, electroconvulsive therapy has been reported to improve some of the symptoms of NMS. Patients with NMS are at increased risk of morbidity due to kidney failure and disseminated intravascular coagulation. Supportive medical therapy and aggressive hydration should be added to minimize the risk of acute kidney injury if CPK levels are highly elevated. Treatment of hyperthermia may include cooling blankets, ice packs, and iced saline gastric lavage.

DID YOU LEARN?

* The classic symptoms of NMS.
* Medications that can cause NMS.
* Factors that distinguish NMS from serotonin syndrome and malignant hyperthermia.
* The treatment of NMS.

References

Friedman L, Weinrauch LA, D'Elia JA. Metoclopramide-induced neuroleptic malignant syndrome. *Arch Intern Med.* 1987;147:1495-1497.

Gillman P. Neuroleptic malignant syndrome: Mechanisms, interactions, and causality. *Movement Disord.* 2010;25:1780-1790.

Oruch R, Pryme IF, Engelsen BA, Lund A. Neuroleptic malignant syndrome: An easily overlooked neurologic emergency. *Neuropsychiatr Dis Treat.* 2017;13:161-175.

Perry P, Wilborn C. Serotonin syndrome vs. neuroleptic malignant syndrome: A contrast of causes, diagnoses, and management. *Ann Clin Psychiatry.* 2012;24:155-162.

Strawn J, Keck P. Neuroleptic malignant syndrome. *Am J Psychiatry.* 2007;164:870-876.

Tsuchiya N, Morimura E. Postoperative neuroleptic malignant syndrome that occurred repeatedly in a patient with cerebral palsy. *Pediatr Anesth.* 2007;17:281-284.

Ware MR, Feller DB, Hall KL. Neuroleptic malignant syndrome: Diagnosis and management. *Prim Care Companion CNS Disord.* 2018;20(1):pii: 17r02185.

Young C, Kaufman B. Neuroleptic malignant syndrome postoperative onset due to levodopa withdrawal. *J Clin Anesth.* 1995;7:652-626.

CASE 2 · Serotonin Syndrome

Elizabeth Rebello, MD

A 19-year-old college student scheduled for a hysteroscopy presents to the preoperative clinic mildly agitated and disoriented, with jerking movements of her body. Her past medical history includes depression, seasonal allergies, and a recent ankle sprain. Chronic medications are sertraline (Zoloft), cetirizine (Zyrtec), and phentermine (Adipex-P, Lomaira, Suprenza), and she was recently prescribed tramadol (Ultram) for her ankle pain. You make the preliminary diagnosis of serotonin syndrome.

1. Which of the following symptoms is most consistent with serotonin syndrome?

   A. Bradycardia.
   B. Rigidity.
   C. Clonus.
   D. Hypotension.

The correct answer is C. Serotonin syndrome is a potentially fatal disorder of rapid onset caused by serotonergic medications and is characterized by the triad of altered mental status, abnormalities in neuromuscular tone, and autonomic hyperactivity. Cognitive effects may include headache, mental confusion, agitation, hallucinations, and coma; and somatic effects may include clonus, tremor, and hyperreflexia. Autonomic hyperreactivity may manifest as shivering, diaphoresis, hypertension, tachycardia, and hyperthermia. Disease severity ranges from mild to severe, and the disorder may progress to shock, seizures, acute kidney failure, coma, and death. Serotonin syndrome is a clinical diagnosis; there is no confirmatory laboratory test. Bradycardia, rigidity, and hypotension are not characteristics of serotonin syndrome. The Hunter Serotonin Toxicity Criteria may be used to aid in the diagnosis and consist of any one of the following groupings of clinical signs in the presence of a serotonergic agent:

- Hypertonia, temperature $>38°C$ ($100.4°F$), and ocular clonus or inducible clonus
- Ocular clonus with agitation or diaphoresis
- Spontaneous clonus
- Tremor and hyperreflexia
- Inducible clonus with agitation or diaphoresis

2. Medications that can cause serotonin syndrome include all the following *except*:

   A. Ondansetron.
   B. Lorazepam.
   C. St. John's wort.
   D. Meperidine.

The correct answer is B. A high dose of a single serotonergic agent, with or without other medications that increase serotonin, can predispose a patient to serotonin syndrome. The table below lists medications that may predispose a patient to serotonin syndrome.

Medications That May Predispose a Patient to Serotonin Syndrome

Antidepressants	Monoamine oxidase inhibitors (phenelzine, selegiline)
	Tricyclic antidepressants (amitriptyline, desipramine, nortriptyline, doxepin)
	Selective serotonin reuptake inhibitors (SSRIs) (citalopram, paroxetine, sertraline, fluoxetine)
	Other (buspirone, trazodone, mirtazapine)
Opioids	
CNS stimulants	Phentermine
	Cocaine
	Methylphenidate
Anticonvulsants	Carbamazepine, valproic acid
Over-the-counter cough medications	Dextromethorphan
Antibiotics	Linezolid
Herbal supplements	St. John's wort
	Yohimbe
	Nutmeg
	Ginseng
Antiemetics	Ondansetron
	Metoclopramide

The next table provides the mechanisms by which medications may increase serotonin.

Mechanisms for Increasing Serotonin

1. Decreasing serotonin breakdown (monoamine oxidase inhibitors, linezolid)
2. Decreasing serotonin reuptake (SSRIs, dextromethorphan, methadone, fentanyl, tramadol, meperidine, tricyclic antidepressants, cocaine, St. John's wort)
3. Increasing serotonin precursors (buspirone)
4. Increasing serotonin release (cocaine, methylphenidate, buspirone, lithium)

3. Both serotonin syndrome and neuroleptic malignant syndrome (NMS; a severe life-threatening reaction caused by medications with dopamine receptor-antagonist properties or by the rapid withdrawal of dopaminergic medications) are associated with autonomic dysfunction and altered mental status. A distinguishing feature that may be present with serotonin syndrome, but *not* with NMS, is:

A. Hyperkinesia.
B. Bradykinesia.
C. Lead pipe rigidity.
D. Slow onset.

The correct answer is A. Hyperkinesia and myoclonus are characteristic of serotonin syndrome, but rigidity and bradykinesia are associated NMS. The time course is another feature that distinguishes serotonin syndrome from NMS: serotonin syndrome has a rapid onset, in contrast to NMS, which may evolve over several days.

4. Treatment for serotonin syndrome consists of:

   A. Diphenhydramine.
   B. Cyproheptadine.
   C. Promethazine.
   D. Bromocriptine.

The correct answer is B. Treatment for serotonin syndrome consists of discontinuing the offending medication and administration of a serotonin antagonist such as cyproheptadine, which is only available in oral form. In addition, a benzodiazepine may be given for agitation. Antipyretic therapy with acetaminophen is not recommended because the increase in temperature is due to muscular, rather than hypothalamic, activity. In addition, measures to control hyperthermia and autonomic instability should be in place, such as cooling blankets, placement of an arterial line, and possible administration of β-blockade medication. If the overdose is within an hour of presentation, gastric lavage and administration of activated charcoal may be utilized.

DID YOU LEARN?

- The classic symptoms of serotonin syndrome.
- Medications that can cause serotonin syndrome.
- Factors that distinguish serotonin syndrome from NMS.
- The treatment of serotonin syndrome.

Recommended Reading

Butterworth IV JF, Mackey DC, Wasnick JD, eds. Anesthesia for patients with neurologic and psychiatric disease. In: *Morgan & Mikhail's Clinical Anesthesiology*. 6th ed. New York, NY: McGraw-Hill Education; 2018:621-636.

References

Bijl D. The serotonin syndrome. *Neth J Med*. 2004;62:309-313.
Bouer E, Shannon M. The serotonin syndrome. *N Engl J Med*. 2005;352:1112-1120.
Dunkley E, Isbister G, Sibbritt D, et al. The Hunter serotonin toxicity criteria: Simple and accurate diagnostic decision rules for serotonin toxicity. *QJM*. 2003;96:635-642.
Fraswe J, South M. Life-threatening fluvoxamine overdose in a 4-year-old child. *Intensive Care Med*. 1999;25:548.

Iqbal M, Basil M, Kaplan J, et al. Overview of serotonin syndrome. *Ann Clin Psychiatry.* 2012;24: 310-318.

Perry P, Wilborn C. Serotonin syndrome vs. neuroleptic malignant syndrome: A contrast of causes, diagnoses, and management. *Ann Clin Psychiatry.* 2012;24:155-162.

Rastogi R, Swarm R, Patel TA. Opioid association with serotonin syndrome. Implications to the practitioners. *Anesthesiology.* 2011;115:1291-1298.

Shaikh ZS, Malins TJ. Serotonin syndrome: Take a closer look at the unwell surgical patient. *Ann R Coll Surg Engl.* 2011;93:569-572.

CHAPTER 24

Anesthesia for Patients with Neuromuscular Disease

CASE 1   Patient with Myasthenia Gravis Scheduled for Ambulatory Surgery

Jennifer Wu, MD, MBA

A 70-year-old man with myasthenia gravis is scheduled to have foot surgery at a freestanding ambulatory surgery center in 4 days. The preoperative nurse called him by phone and flagged his case for review by the anesthesiologist. He has no other medical conditions. His medications include pyridostigmine 90 mg orally (PO) every 3 h and prednisone 10 mg PO daily.

1. Which of the following characterizes myasthenia gravis?

    A. Muscle weakness that improves with repeated effort.
    B. Fatigability of skeletal muscle.
    C. Rigidity after exposure to inhalation anesthetics.
    D. Delayed muscle relaxation.
    E. Unpredictable relapsing and remitting symptoms caused by demyelination.

The correct answer is B. *Myasthenia gravis* is an autoimmune disorder characterized by weakness and easy fatigability of skeletal muscle due to autoimmune destruction of postsynaptic acetylcholine receptors at the neuromuscular junction. The proximal muscles are affected, and there are periods of exacerbations and remissions. Option A describes *Lambert–Eaton myasthenic syndrome*, which is a paraneoplastic syndrome that causes proximal muscle weakness and is often associated with small-cell lung carcinoma or other malignancies. Option C describes *malignant hyperthermia,* which is a muscle disease that is triggered by inhalation anesthetics or succinylcholine, resulting in tachycardia, hyperthermia, hypercarbia, and rigidity. Option D describes *myotonic dystrophy,* which is a slowing of relaxation after muscle contraction. Unlike myasthenia gravis, the weakness with myotonic dystrophy occurs in the distal muscles. Option E describes *multiple sclerosis,* which is a neurological rather than a neuromuscular disease. Demyelination occurs in the brain and spinal cord.

2. Assuming that you plan to use regional anesthesia, what will you instruct the patient to do with his medications preoperatively?

   A. Take no medications.
   B. Take a stress dose of prednisone on the morning of surgery with a sip of water.
   C. Take the pyridostigmine as scheduled on the morning of surgery with a sip of water.
   D. Take prednisone and pyridostigmine as scheduled on the morning of surgery with a sip of water.
   E. Double the usual pyridostigmine dose on the morning of surgery with a sip of water.

The correct answer is D. Patients may continue the scheduled regimen of prednisone and pyridostigmine (an acetylcholinesterase inhibitor) on the morning of surgery. Patients who are controlled on an oral regimen of pyridostigmine may experience weakness if they skip their usual morning dose. Some clinicians will omit the morning dose in patients who can tolerate missing a dose and who will require muscle relaxation during surgery (eg, for abdominal surgery). This patient will not require muscle relaxation. Oral medications may be taken with a sip of water 1 to 2 h prior to the anticipated start of surgery. Option B suggests taking a stress dose of oral corticosteroid medication. Although a stress dose of a corticosteroid will be administered, it will be given intravenously at the beginning of surgery. Option E is incorrect, as there is no indication to double the dose of pyridostigmine. Additional acetylcholinesterase inhibitors, such as edrophonium or neostigmine, can be administered intravenously if necessary.

3. The patient arrives at the freestanding ambulatory surgery center on the day of surgery and refuses regional anesthesia. Relatively speaking, what is the best anesthetic plan?

   A. General anesthesia and endotracheal intubation with propofol and succinylcholine.
   B. General anesthesia and endotracheal intubation with propofol, a defasciculating dose of rocuronium, and succinylcholine.
   C. General anesthesia with endotracheal intubation with propofol and rocuronium.
   D. General anesthesia with a face mask.

The correct answer is A. General anesthesia with an endotracheal tube is considered by many to be safer than a laryngeal mask airway (LMA) in patients with myasthenia gravis because these patients are believed to be at increased risk for aspiration. Nevertheless, many clinicians would select an LMA in this case. Very few clinicians would undertake such a general anesthetic using a face mask only. Succinylcholine is safe to use, although the patient may require a larger dose of 2 mg/kg intravenously and have prolonged relaxation for an additional 5 to 10 min. Option B is incorrect because a patient may have profound muscle relaxation with even a small defasciculating dose of rocuronium.

4. The patient is extubated and brought to the postanesthesia care unit (PACU). He becomes weaker. The anesthesiologist gives edrophonium, and the weakness improves for about 5 min. What was the cause of the weakness?

   A. Myasthenic crisis.
   B. Cholinergic crisis.
   C. Opioid overdose.
   D. Residual muscle relaxant.

The correct answer is A. Weakness that improves with the administration of the short-acting acetylcholinesterase inhibitor edrophonium is caused by myasthenic crisis. Treatment is supportive care and administration of a longer-acting acetylcholinesterase inhibitor such as pyridostigmine. Option B, cholinergic crisis, occurs when excessive acetylcholinesterase inhibitors are administered. Treatment with edrophonium would exacerbate cholinergic crisis. Opioid overdose and residual muscle relaxation can occur in the PACU but would not be improved with edrophonium.

DID YOU LEARN?

- How to differentiate myasthenia gravis from other disorders.
- What preoperative instructions to give a patient with myasthenia gravis.
- How to safely administer anesthesia for a patient with myasthenia gravis.
- How to evaluate postoperative weakness in a patient with myasthenia gravis.

Recommended Reading

Butterworth IV JF, Mackey DC, Wasnick JD, eds. Anesthesia for patients with neuromuscular disease. In: Morgan & Mikhail's Clinical Anesthesiology. 6th ed. New York, NY: McGraw-Hill Education; 2018:637-650.

References

Morgan GE, Mikhail MS, Murray MJ. *Clinical Anesthesiology*. New York, NY: McGraw-Hill/Lange; 2013.

Abel M, Eisenkraft JB. Anesthetic implications of myasthenia gravis. *Mt Sinai J Med.* 2002;69:31-37.

Blichfeldt-Lauridsen L, Hansen BD. Anesthesia and myasthenia gravis. *Acta Anaesthesiol Scand.* 2012;56(1):17-22.

CHAPTER 25

Kidney Physiology & Anesthesia

CASE 1 | Postoperative Oliguria

Lori A. Dangler, MD, MBA

You are called to evaluate a 66-year-old man in the postanesthesia care unit (PACU) following right femoral-popliteal bypass surgery performed under general anesthesia. His past medical history is notably for a 40-pack-year history of smoking and peripheral vascular disease. He has been recovering for about 30 min, and the nurse reports that he has "made very little urine" since arriving in the PACU and you note a measured output of only 5 mL in the last 30 min.

1. What is considered the best definition of oliguria in an adult?

   A. <1 mL/kg/h.
   B. <100 mL/24 h.
   C. <0.5 mL/kg/h.
   D. An increase in serum creatinine >1 mg/dL from baseline.

The correct answer is C. Oliguria is commonly defined as <0.5 mL/kg/h in the adult. For children weighing less than 10 kg, oliguria is defined as <1 mL/kg/h. Anuria is often defined as <100 mL/24 h. Acute kidney injury (AKI) is characterized by an acute increase in serum creatinine of >1 mg/dL from baseline in combination with diminished urinary output.

You perform a focused history and chart review that includes noting the time elapsed since the operation, the absence of surgical- or anesthetic-related problems or complications, and the absence of any periods of intraoperative hypotension, and you check intraoperative fluid balances. You discover that the patient received radiocontrast dye for imaging studies both prior to this surgical procedure and also intraoperatively. You also perform a focused physical exam, finding no indication of occult hemorrhage or bladder distention, and note the urine's appearance in the collection bag, which seems to be concentrated. You review the patient's course with his PACU nurse and review the PACU fluids flowsheet. The patient is alert and oriented. He is afebrile, with a heart rate 105 beats/min, blood pressure 100/60 mm Hg, and SpO$_2$ 96% on room air.

2. What is your most important next step?

   A. Order a 500-mL IV fluid bolus.
   B. Ask the nurse to flush the Foley urinary drainage catheter.
   C. Place a central venous catheter to assess volume status.
   D. Administer furosemide (Lasix) 40 mg intravenously (IV).

The correct answer is B. Tachycardia in combination with oliguria is most likely secondary to hypovolemia, which can result in inadequate kidney perfusion. Your approach should include ensuring adequate IV access and ordering an IV fluid bolus while continuing with your evaluation. However, your first concern with acute oliguria is to make sure that the urinary drainage catheter is not obstructed. Only after verifying bladder catheter patency, assessing the patient's hemodynamic status, correcting any hypovolemia, and obtaining urine for diagnostic studies should one consider using drugs such as furosemide to promote renal tubular flow and urine output.

The urinary drainage catheter is patent, and the patient has received 500 mL of Ringer's lactate. There is no further increase in the amount of urine output after another 30 min have elapsed.

3. What initial laboratory study or studies will most help you isolate the cause of the oliguria?

   A. Complete blood count.
   B. Serum creatinine kinase (CK).
   C. Serum Na$^+$ and creatinine, and urine Na$^+$ and creatinine.
   D. Urine myoglobin.

The correct answer is C. Initial laboratory evaluation in this situation commonly includes a urine microscopic exam and calculation of the *fractional excretion of sodium* (FE$_{Na}$). The FE$_{Na}$ is calculated as follows:

$$FE_{Na} = 100 \times \frac{Sodium_{urinary} \times Creatinine_{plasma}}{Sodium_{plasma} \times Creatinine_{urinary}}$$

A microscopic examination of the urine showing epithelial casts in the sediment is taken as the gold standard for the diagnosis of acute tubular necrosis. However, the FE_{Na} is a measure of the reabsorptive function of the tubules and may provide more specific information concerning kidney functional status, differentiating prerenal conditions from AKI. Additional studies such as complete blood count, CK, and urine myoglobin may be ordered as indicated.

You continue to receive updates from the recovery nurse, and despite the patient receiving another 500-mL IV fluid challenge, there is still scant urine output; however, the patient's heart rate has decreased to 97 beats/min and his blood pressure is currently 110/72 mm Hg. You believe the patient is now hemodynamically stable. Laboratory results have returned that allow you to calculate the FE_{Na}, which is 4%.

4. How do you interpret an FE_{Na} of 4%?

   A. Prerenal oliguria.
   B. AKI.
   C. Postrenal obstructive oliguria.
   D. It is indeterminate; further testing is needed.

The correct answer is B. Oliguria is traditionally classified into three categories. *Prerenal* oliguria is characterized by a decrease in kidney blood flow as a result of a low cardiac output and/or inadequate renal perfusion pressure. It is typically associated with a FE_{Na} <1% and a urine$_{Na}$ <20. Acute, *intrinsic* kidney injury (AKI) results from an insult to the kidney itself that has adversely impacted the glomeruli, interstitium, and/or tubules. AKI is associated with a FE_{Na} >1% and urine$_{Na}$ >40. The *postrenal* category includes obstructive processes in the kidney outflow tracts and is not diagnosed by the FE_{Na} calculation, but by physical examination, point-of-care ultrasound, or magnetic resonance or computed tomography imaging.

The consulting nephrologist agrees with your diagnosis of AKI. The IV radio-contrast dye in combination with advanced age, peripheral vascular disease, and hypovolemia likely resulted in the patient's AKI.

DID YOU LEARN?

- Definition of oliguria.
- General approach to assessing a patient with oliguria.
- Primary categorization of oliguria: prerenal, renal, and postrenal disorders.
- Importance of the FE_{Na} in the differential diagnosis of acute oliguria.

Recommended Readings

Butterworth IV JF, Mackey DC, Wasnick JD, eds. Kidney physiology & anesthesia. In: *Morgan & Mikhail's Clinical Anesthesiology*. 6th ed. New York, NY: McGraw-Hill Education; 2018:651-674.

Butterworth IV JF, Mackey DC, Wasnick JD, eds. Anesthesia for patients with kidney disease. In: *Morgan & Mikhail's Clinical Anesthesiology*. 6th ed. New York, NY: McGraw-Hill Education; 2018:675-694.

References

Chenitz KB, Lane-Fall MB. Decreased urine output and acute kidney injury in the post anesthesia care unit. *Anesthesia Clin*. 2012;30:513-526.

Goren O, Matot I. Perioperative acute kidney injury. *Br J Anaesth*. 2015;115:ii3-ii14.

KDIGO Workgroup. AKI definition. *Kidney Int*. 2012;2(suppl):19-36.

Kellum J, Bellomo R, Ronco C. Does this patient have acute kidney injury? An AKI checklist. *Intens Care Med*. 2016;42:96-99.

Marino PL. *Marino's The ICU Book*, 4th ed. Chapter 35. Philadelphia, PA: Lippincott Williams & Wilkins, 2013.

Weisbord SD, Palevsky PM. Contrast-associated acute kidney injury. *Crit Care Clin*. 2015;31:725-735.

CHAPTER 26

Anesthesia for Patients with Kidney Disease

CASE 1 — Patient with Renal Cell Carcinoma for Nephrectomy and Inferior Vena Cava Thrombectomy

Jagtar Singh Heir, DO

A 73-year-old woman with recently diagnosed renal cell carcinoma (RCC) presents for nephrectomy and inferior vena cava (IVC) thrombectomy. The patient has a history of poorly controlled hypertension, type 2 diabetes, anemia, a horseshoe kidney, and chronic kidney disease. The patient has coronary artery disease (CAD) and had two sequential drug-eluting stents placed in her right coronary artery 3 months ago. Laboratory data include hemoglobin of 8.2 g/dL, serum creatinine of 1.6 mg/dL, and elevated alkaline phosphatase (AP), aspartate aminotransferase (AST), and total bilirubin values. Physical examination reveals right upper quadrant tenderness, hepatomegaly, and a palpable abdominal mass. As you evaluate this patient in advance of her surgery, you are concerned about the potential for paraneoplastic syndromes and their anesthetic implications.

1. What types of changes may occur secondary to abnormal hormonal production in paraneoplastic syndromes?

   A. Hypercalcemia.
   B. Elevated plasma and urine metanephrines.
   C. Elevated parathyroid hormone.
   D. Stauffer syndrome.
   E. All of the above.

The correct answer is E. Paraneoplastic syndromes (PNS) occur often with malignant disease, and they can cause both structural and functional changes in regions anatomically remote from the tumor itself. One of the most common effects of PNS is hypercalcemia due to excess parathyroid hormone, bone metastases, and/or elaboration of tumor-associated interleukin factors. Other PNSs include polycythemia, hyperaldosteronism, polymyositis, dermatomyositis, Cushing syndrome, syndrome of inappropriate antidiuretic hormone secretion, Lambert–Eaton myasthenic syndrome, carcinoid syndrome, and Stauffer syndrome. *Stauffer syndrome* is often associated with renal cell carcinoma and is characterized by elevation of serum liver enzymes (AST, alanine aminotransferase, and AP), γ-globulins, and bilirubin. The hepatic abnormalities in Stauffer syndrome are humorally mediated and not due to tumor infiltration of the liver itself or to intrinsic liver disease.

The classic triad of flank pain, hematuria, and palpable mass is present in fewer than 15% of patients with RCC. It is important to investigate signs and symptoms of paraneoplastic syndromes that may be associated with this cancer, as this can lead to earlier diagnosis and more effective treatment. Appropriate laboratory tests may be suggested by the history and physical findings. For example, if the patient complains of headaches and is noted to have hypertension, the plasma and urine catecholamine metabolites metanephrine and vanillylmandelic acid (VMA) may be ordered to rule out pheochromocytoma. In many clinical scenarios, the severity of the PNS follows the course of the cancer, and successful cancer treatment can lead to resolution of the syndrome, whereas return of the PNS may be a harbinger of tumor recurrence.

2. In a patient with multiple risk factors for intracoronary stent thrombosis, what drug choices (in addition to aspirin) would be helpful in reducing the chances of stent thrombosis?

A. Additional aspirin.
B. Enoxaparin.
C. A glycoprotein IIb/IIIA inhibitor.
D. Subcutaneous heparin 5000 U.
E. Nonsteroidal anti-inflammatory drugs (NSAIDs).

The correct answer is C. Coronary artery stent thrombosis is a devastating complication, associated with a mortality of 45% or greater. This patient has several risk factors that put her at increased risk for coronary stent thrombosis: diabetes, chronic kidney disease, cancer, and multiple coronary artery stents. Cancer patients often exhibit a prothrombotic state due to certain interleukins and tissue factors, increased platelet activity, and abnormal angiogenesis. Since one of the patient's stents was placed within the past year, complete stent endothelialization may not have occurred, further increasing her chances of stent thrombosis.

Patients adhering to a recommended antiplatelet regimen may still be susceptible to stent thrombosis due to inadequate response to the antiplatelet regimen as a result of genetic polymorphism, receptor upregulation, relative underdosing of medication, and/or drug interactions. Increasing, or repeating, the aspirin dose would be reasonable if the patient's usual course of aspirin had been disrupted, as higher doses may be more efficacious in that situation. Currently, however, there are no studies that demonstrate that a larger aspirin dose is superior to a lower dose, particularly in the perioperative setting. Despite being commonly used as "bridging" therapy in this scenario, neither heparin nor enoxaparin has any anti-platelet activity. Subcutaneous heparin has a wide range of bioavailability, and there is no assurance that it would achieve a therapeutic effect in this patient. Periop-erative enoxaparin would preclude use of an epidural catheter for postoperative analgesia. Efforts at bridging therapy have been attempted with intravenous (IV) NSAIDs but have not proven beneficial in preventing stent thrombosis.

High-risk patients have a reduced incidence of cardiac complications when receiving glycoprotein IIb/IIIA inhibitors such as tirofiban. These short-acting medications can be interrupted preoperatively and restarted postoperatively.

Approximately 2 h into the case, an estimated 600-mL blood loss has been replaced with 2 units of packed red blood cells (PRBCs). However, the patient continues to require intermittent boluses of IV phenylephrine to maintain adequate blood pres-sure. In addition, adequate monitoring of the ECG is increasingly difficult due to surgical manipulation of the patient and frequent electrocautery interference.

3. What is the next appropriate step?

    A. Initiate norepinephrine infusion.

    B. Transfuse additional blood.

    C. Perform transesophageal echocardiogram (TEE) examination.

    D. Send cardiac enzymes and troponins for analysis.

    E. Obtain an arterial blood gas.

The correct answer is C. Sudden, unexplained hypotension and/or hypoxemia is defined as a Category I indication for use of intraoperative TEE, meaning it is supported by the strongest evidence or expert opinion. TEE can yield a great deal of clinically useful data in this scenario, including ventricular function, vol-ume status, the presence or absence of thrombi in the IVC and heart, valvular function, and estimates of filling pressures and cardiac output. Initiation of a norepinephrine infusion without assessment of volume status or systemic vascu-lar resistance would be inappropriate, as would transfusion of additional blood without first ascertaining the current volume or hemoglobin status. In patients with tumor invasion of the IVC, many clinicians use TEE routinely in every case to determine the upper extent of the tumor thrombus. Additional labora-tory evaluations, such as cardiac enzymes and arterial blood gas determination, although potentially useful, would also be time consuming. Initiation of TEE is the most useful step at this point in time with this particular patient, as it will rapidly yield the most clinically relevant data impacting subsequent hemody-namic management.

Upon release of the Pringle clamp and suprahepatic IVC clamp, the patient exhibits sudden hypotension and a decrease in SpO_2. The following figures show the results.

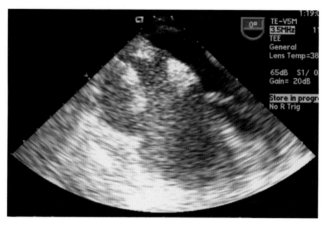

Mid-esophageal four-chamber view.

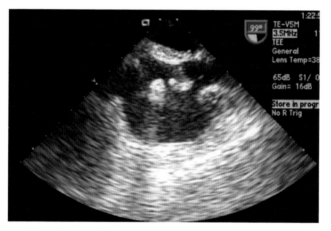

Mid-esophageal bicaval view of right atrium.

4. What is the most reasonable next step?

A. Consult with the cardiac surgeon and prepare for cardiopulmonary bypass.
B. Initiate thrombolytic therapy.
C. Reapply the IVC clamps.
D. Administer epinephrine.
E. Administer bolus IV calcium and sodium bicarbonate.

The correct answer is A. The TEE has numerous useful functions in this situation in addition to those already discussed: It can assist the surgeon with proper IVC clamping, monitor for pulmonary emboli (air, thrombus), and detect a patent foramen ovale.

A large right atrial thrombus is noted in the mid-esophageal four-chamber and mid-esophageal bicaval views. The most likely event in this scenario is tumor embolism during resection. The most appropriate next step is to communicate this finding to the urologist and cardiac surgeon so that steps can be taken to initiate cardiopulmonary bypass if the surgeon cannot retrieve the embolus. Although resuscitative drugs such as epinephrine, calcium, and sodium bicarbonate may be acutely required, IV heparin must be administered immediately in preparation for initiation of cardiopulmonary bypass.

Clamping of the hepatic pedicle, also known as the Pringle clamp, is a maneuver that occludes the hepatic artery, portal vein, and common bile duct. It is done to reduce bleeding, as the liver often has to be mobilized during an IVC thrombectomy. Reapplying the IVC clamps would be appropriate only if another thrombus or remnant of the thrombus is visualized by the TEE. Furthermore, reapplying the IVC clamps may worsen the situation, as preload would be further decreased. Heparin has no thrombolytic properties; however, administering thrombolytic agents during major vascular surgery will increase hemorrhage and worsen the clinical situation.

DID YOU LEARN?

- Clinical implications of PNSs.
- Risk factors associated with stent thrombosis and strategies to reduce the incidence of acute stent thrombosis.
- Clinically useful information that TEE can yield in a sudden hypotensive/hypoxemic intraoperative scenario.
- Specific application and use of TEE in an IVC thrombectomy case.

Recommended Reading

Butterworth IV JF, Mackey DC, Wasnick JD, eds. Anesthesia for patients with kidney disease. In: *Morgan & Mikhail's Clinical Anesthesiology*. 6th ed. New York, NY: McGraw-Hill Education; 2018:675-694.

References

American Society of Anesthesiologists and Society of Cardiovascular Anesthesiologists Task Force on Transesophageal Echocardiography. Practice guidelines for perioperative transesophageal echocardiography. An updated report by the American Society of Anesthesiologists and the Society of Cardiovascular Anesthesiologists Task Force on Transesophageal Echocardiography. *Anesthesiology*. 2010;112(5):1084-1096.

Bricker JL, Young JV, Butterworth J. The patient with a tumor invading the vena cava. Chapter 12 in Cohen NH, ed. *Medically Challenging Patients Undergoing Cardiothoracic Surgery*. Philadelphia, PA: Wolters Kluwer; 2009:303-326.

Couture P, Denault AY, McKenty S, et al. Impact of routine use of intraoperative transesophageal echocardiography during cardiac surgery. *Can J Anesth*. 2000;47:20-26.

Iakovou I, Schmidt T, Bonizzoni E, et al. Incidence, predictors, and outcome of thrombosis after successful implantation of drug-eluting stents. *JAMA*. 2005;293:2126-2130.

Jaffe R, Strauss BH. Late and very late thrombosis of drug-eluting stents. Evolving concepts and perspectives. *J Am Coll Cardiol*. 2007;50(2):119-127.

Newsome LT, Kutcher MA, Ghandi SK, et al. A protocol for the perioperative management of patients with intracoronary drug-eluting stents. *APSF Newsletter*, Winter 2006-2007.

Nguyen TA, Diodati JG, Pharand C. Resistance to clopidrogel: A review of the evidence. *J Am Coll Cardiol*. 2005;45(8):1157-1164.

Palapattu GS, Kristo B, Rajfer J. Paraneoplastic syndromes in urologic malignancy: The many faces of renal cell carcinoma. *Rev Urol*. 2002;4(4):163-170.

CHAPTER 27

Anesthesia for Genitourinary Surgery

CASE 1   Patient for Prostatectomy

Kallol Chaudhuri, MD, PhD

A 62-year-old obese patient with a history of adenocarcinoma of the prostate underwent robot-assisted laparoscopic radical prostatectomy under general anesthesia. The patient was placed in steep Trendelenburg position for the procedure, which lasted about 8 h. Intraoperative course and emergence from anesthesia were uneventful. However, upon awakening from anesthesia in the postanesthesia care unit, the patient complained of dimness of vision in both eyes. The visual loss was not accompanied by any pain or discomfort, and his vital signs were within normal limits.

1. Compared to open retropubic prostatectomy, which of the following statements is *most likely* true regarding robot-assisted laparoscopic prostatectomy?

   A. It provides poor visualization of the operative field.
   B. There is a decreased need for postoperative analgesics.
   C. Patients have a longer length of hospital stay after the surgery.
   D. The operative time is significantly less than with the open procedure.

The correct answer is B. When compared to open retropubic prostatectomy, laparoscopic robot-assisted radical prostatectomy has some important advantages, including better visualization of the surgical field, less blood loss, decreased need for intraoperative blood transfusion, less postoperative pain, less scaring, and shorter length of hospital stay.

2. All of the following are common concerns regarding anesthetic management for robot-assisted radical prostatectomy *except*:

A. Major blood loss.
B. Difficulty in accessing the intravenous lines during surgery.
C. Reduced pulmonary compliance.
D. Obstructed view of patient's airway during surgery.

The correct answer is A. The primary concerns with robotic surgery are limited access to the patient's airway, to intravascular lines, and to monitoring devices during the procedure. Adequate intravascular access and appropriate and reliable hemodynamic monitoring (including invasive arterial pressure monitoring) should be considered prior to docking of the robot. Additional concerns of robotic surgery are related to the complications of the steep Trendelenburg position with or without lateral decubitus and from the pneumoperitoneum required for this procedure. In general, major blood loss is unusual during this procedure.

3. Which of the following complications is *most likely* to be observed during the postoperative period in patients operated in steep Trendelenburg position?

A. Cerebral ischemia.
B. Myocardial infarction.
C. Acute renal failure.
D. Respiratory distress.

The correct answer is D. Physiological changes from the steep Trendelenburg position, along with ventilatory difficulties due to the additive effect of pneumoperitoneum, are major concerns during anesthetic management of robot surgery. Complications associated with the position include edema of the face and upper airway, reduction of pulmonary compliance, increased risk of barotrauma, postextubation respiratory distress, postoperative visual loss, compartment syndrome, and brachial plexus injury.

4. What is the most common pathophysiology associated with perioperative visual loss?

A. Corneal abrasion.
B. Ischemic optic neuropathy.
C. Macular degeneration.
D. Central retinal artery occlusion.

The correct answer is B. Perioperative visual loss (POVL) is a devastating complication reported most commonly in patients after spine surgery in the prone position. However, it has also been reported with head and neck surgery, cardiac bypass surgery, major vascular surgery, and prolonged robotic surgery in the head-down position. POVL occurs secondary to ischemic optic neuropathy, perioperative glaucoma, or cortical hypotension and embolism.

References

Kla KM, Lee LA. Perioperative visual loss. *Best Pract Res Clin Anesthesiol.* 2016;30:69-77.

Paranjape S, Chhabra A. Anesthesia for robotic surgery. *Trends Anesth Crit Care.* 2015;4:25-31.

Pathirana S, Kam PC. Anaesthetic issues in robotic-assisted minimally invasive surgery. *Anaesth Intens Care.* 2018;46:1.

CASE 2 Transurethral Resection of Prostate

Glorimar Medina-Rivera, MD, MBA

A 70-year-old Hispanic man scheduled for a transurethral resection of the prostate (TURP) has arrived in the holding area. He is pleasant but very anxious. He has had no previous surgeries and takes several medications for high blood pressure and insulin for type 2 diabetes mellitus. Vital signs include blood pressure 158/91 mm Hg and heart rate 87 beats/min. SpO$_2$ is 100%, and fingerstick fasting blood glucose is 247 mg/dL. The ECG shows an old myocardial infarction. He reports moderate back and neck pain due to a car accident several years ago. After discussing the case with the surgeon, you learn that a solution of glycine 1.5% will be used and the expected duration of the procedure will be 2 h.

1. What would be the preferred anesthetic technique for this case?

   A. General anesthesia.
   B. Spinal anesthesia (sensory level T6).
   C. Saddle block (sensory level L1).
   D. MAC.

The correct answer is B. The optimal anesthetic technique for this patient is one that will allow early recognition of TURP syndrome. Neuraxial blockade in an awake patient allows early detection of mental status changes and, therefore, earlier correction of the problem if it presents. Saddle block or MAC anesthesia would be inadequate for this surgical procedure.

You administer a hyperbaric bupivacaine spinal anesthetic with supplemental O_2 2 L/min by nasal cannula. One hundred minutes into the procedure, the patient reports feeling "uncomfortable," is unable to further describe his discomfort, and starts moving his arms. Vital signs are blood pressure 99/51 mm Hg, heart rate 97 beats/min, respiratory rate 22 breaths/min, and SpO_2 94%. Sensory blockade level is T6 bilateral. The ECG is unchanged.

2. Of the following, which is the most likely cause of these symptoms?

A. High spinal.
B. Unrecognized psychiatric disorder.
C. Evolving myocardial ischemia.
D. TURP syndrome.
E. Autonomic hyperreflexia.

The correct answer is D. Large quantities of hypotonic irrigating fluid used for TURP procedures can be systemically absorbed during resection of the prostate gland through the prostate's rich venous plexus. The absorbed volume may average 20 mL/min, and the total amount absorbed depends on the duration of the procedure and the pressure of the irrigation fluid. Large amounts of absorbed irrigation fluid may produce multiple problems, collectively called TURP syndrome, including hyponatremia, hypo-osmolality, and volume overload. TURP syndrome is compatible with this clinical scenario, and the other potential diagnoses can be readily ruled out.

Manifestations of TURP Syndrome

Hyponatremia
Hypo-osmolality
Fluid overload
Congestive heart failure
Pulmonary edema
Hypotension
Hemolysis
Solute toxicity
Hyperglycinemia (glycine)
Hyperammonemia (glycine)
Hyperglycemia (sorbitol)
Intravascular volume expansion (mannitol)

TURP, transurethral resection of the prostate.
Reproduced with permission from Butterworth JF, Mackey DC, Wasnick JD: *Morgan and Mikhail's Clinical Anesthesiology*, 6th ed. New York, NY: McGraw-Hill Education; 2018.

A high spinal would likely have presented earlier in the anesthetic, and your examination of the patient has ruled out this condition. The patient has no history of psychiatric disorders, making this diagnosis unlikely. There is no ECG evidence of myocardial ischemia. Autonomic hyperreflexia is a condition of reactive autonomic hyperactivity resulting in marked hypertension and is most commonly seen with spinal cord injury above the T6 level.

A less likely possibility not listed is accidental bladder perforation, which would be a more prominent consideration for the rare patient having transurethral resection of the bladder under spinal anesthesia.

3. After placing a right radial arterial line, point-of-care testing reveals pH 7.26, PCO_2 51, PO_2 62, $[Na^+]$ 131, hemoglobin 10.2 g/dL, and glucose 223 mg%. The best initial pharmacological intervention at this point is:

A. Diphenhydramine 25 mg intravenously (IV).
B. Phenylephrine 100 µg IV.
C. Normal saline 9% 500 mL IV bolus.
D. Furosemide 20–40 mg IV.
E. Regular insulin 15 units IV.

The correct answer is D. Treatment of volume overload in TURP syndrome consists of fluid restriction when evidence suggests the amount of excess volume is relatively minor, and administration of a loop diuretic when symptoms and/or signs indicate significant overload. Marked hyponatremia (<120 mEq/L) is relatively infrequent, and in such cases, 3% sodium chloride may be slowly infused until the $[Na^+]$ rises to 120 mEq/L.

There is no indication for diphenhydramine in this situation, and it is unlikely that the patient's relatively minor hypotension or hyperglycemia is causing his symptoms.

4. Interdisciplinary communication is critical for the best management of TURP syndrome patients. At the conclusion of this case, you discuss different TURP management options for future patients with the surgical team. Of the following options, which one would be the most important in minimizing the risk of TURP syndrome?

A. Patient selection.
B. Hanging the irrigating fluid higher than 60 cm above the patient.
C. Blood pressure management.
D. Duration of surgery.

The correct answer is D. The most important step in minimizing the risk of TURP syndrome is to limit the duration of the procedure. If the pressure of the irrigating fluid exceeds venous pressure, intravascular absorption of irrigation fluid via prostate venous sinuses is more likely to occur. Therefore, increasing the irrigation fluid infusion pressure by hanging the fluid higher would be counterproductive. A decrease in venous blood pressure would also increase the absorption of fluid. There are not any preexisting medical conditions that will predispose or protect a patient from TURP syndrome.

DID YOU LEARN?

- Recognition of TURP syndrome manifestations.
- Implications of anesthetic options for TURP.
- Management of TURP syndrome.
- Options to minimize the risk of TURP syndrome.

Recommended Reading

Butterworth IV JF, Mackey DC, Wasnick JD, eds. Anesthesia for genitourinary surgery. In: *Morgan & Mikhail's Clinical Anesthesiology.* 6th ed. New York, NY: McGraw-Hill Education; 2018:695-714.

References

Cornu JN, Herrmann T, Traxer O, et al. Prevention and management following complications from endourology procedures. *Eur Urol Focus.* 2016;2:49.

Hawary A, Mukhtar K, Sinclair A, et al. Transurethral resection of the prostate syndrome: Almost gone but not forgotten. *J Endourol.* 2009;12:2013.

Ishio J, Nakahira J, Sawai T, et al. Change in serum sodium level predicts clinical manifestations of transurethral resection syndrome: A retrospective review. *BMJ Anesthesiol.* 2015;15:52.

Nakahira J, Sawai T, Fujiwara A, et al. Transurethral resection syndrome in elderly patients: A retrospective observational study. *BMC Anesthesiol.* 2014;14:30.

CHAPTER 28
Hepatic Physiology & Anesthesia

CASE 1	Postoperative Jaundice

Sabry Khalil, MD, and Marina Gitman, MD

A 42-year-old obese woman underwent an open cholecystectomy under a general anesthetic with desflurane. Past medical history includes type 2 diabetes mellitus, seizure disorder, sickle cell disease, and hyperlipidemia. Her medications include simvastatin, folic acid, oral contraceptive pills, valproic acid, hydroxyurea, and metformin. Intraoperatively, she received 2 units of packed red blood cells to maintain a hemoglobin level of 10 g/dL. On postoperative day 4, the patient developed jaundice. During a subsequent morbidity and mortality conference discussion, the differential diagnosis of the postoperative jaundice included inhalation anesthetics.

1. Which of the following is a correct match regarding etiology of jaundice?

    A. Desflurane – obstructive jaundice.
    B. Oral contraceptive pills – hepatocellular jaundice.
    C. Sickle cell crisis – prehepatic jaundice.
    D. Obesity – hemolytic jaundice.

The correct answer is C. Types of jaundice include prehepatic (hemolytic), hepatocellular, and posthepatic/obstructive. Halogenated anesthetics rarely cause centrilobular necrosis, with jaundice accompanied by marked elevations of aminotransferases taking several weeks to months to develop. Oral contraceptive pills may cause cholestatic jaundice with increased levels of alkaline phosphatase. Sickle cell disease is a common cause of cholelithiasis, which carries the risk of common bile duct obstruction; however, in the setting of surgery and transfusion, hemolytic jaundice is a more logical possibility (prehepatic type). Obesity can cause nonalcoholic fatty liver disease with the associated elevation of aminotransferases; however, it is unlikely to cause hemolytic jaundice.

2. Which of the following is true regarding anesthesia and the development of jaundice?

A. Desflurane is less likely than sevoflurane to produce postanesthesia jaundice.
B. Modern halogenated anesthetics do not cause jaundice.
C. Total intravenous anesthesia could be a better possible option for patients with a history of halogenated anesthetic-induced hepatotoxicity.
D. Autoimmune hepatitis usually presents on postoperative day 1.

The correct answer is C. The incidence of fulminant hepatitis due to halogenated anesthetics is directly proportional to the degree of hepatic metabolism, which decreases from halothane to enflurane to isoflurane to desflurane, with sevoflurane considered the least likely to undergo metabolism. Early clinical features of injury include nonspecific symptoms, such as fever and malaise, and can take several days to weeks to appear. The use of halogenated inhalation anesthetics for those rare patients with a documented history of anesthetic-induced liver injury is not advised when there are multiple good options for total intravenous anesthesia.

3. Which of the following is correct regarding hepatic flow?

A. The hepatic artery is the major contributor of hepatic blood flow.
B. Hepatic blood flow represents approximately 15% of cardiac output.
C. Total hepatic blood flow is such that a decrease in either hepatic arterial flow or portal venous flow results in a compensatory increase in the other.
D. The hepatic artery is a branch of the superior mesenteric artery.

The correct answer is C. Hepatic blood flow represents about 30% of cardiac output, with 75% from the portal vein and 25% from the hepatic artery. Hepatic blood flow is regulated through intrinsic and extrinsic mechanisms. The intrinsic mechanism is termed the hepatic arterial buffer response (HABR). For example, if portal blood flow decreases, the hepatic artery flow increases, and vice versa. The hepatic artery is a branch of the celiac artery.

4. Which of the following laboratory values strongly suggest the potential need for surgical and/or endoscopic intervention?

A. Increased unconjugated bilirubin, normal aminotransferases, and normal alkaline phosphatase.
B. Increased conjugated bilirubin, markedly increased amniotransferases, and slightly increased alkaline phosphatase.
C. Increased conjugated bilirubin, slightly increased aminotransferases, and markedly increased alkaline phosphatase.
D. None of the above.

The correct answer is C. Option A is the typical laboratory finding of hemolytic jaundice, while option B is the typical finding of hepatocellular jaundice. Option C represents posthepatic or obstructive jaundice, evidenced by a marked increase in alkaline phosphatase. Potential etiology is obstruction of the common bile duct by stone during removal of the gallbladder or iatrogenic injury of the common bile duct.

DID YOU LEARN?

- Relationship between sickle cell disease and postoperative jaundice.
- Laboratory findings in obstructive jaundice.
- Presentation of volatile anesthetic-associated liver injury.

Recommended Readings

Barton CA. Treatment of coagulopathy related to hepatic insufficiency. *Crit Care Med.* 2016;44:1927.

Bona R. Hypercoagulable states: What the oral surgeon needs to know. *Oral Maxillofac Surg Clin N Am.* 2016;28:491.

Boral BM, Williams BJ, Boral LI. Disseminated intravascular coagulation. *Am J Clin Pathol.* 2016;146:670.

Butterworth IV JF, Mackey DC, Wasnick JD, eds. Hepatic physiology & anesthesia. In: *Morgan & Mikhail's Clinical Anesthesiology.* 6th ed. New York, NY: McGraw-Hill Education; 2018:715-732.

Cohen MJ, Christie SA. Coagulopathy of trauma. *Crit Care Clin.* 2017;333:101.

Goobie SM, Haas T. Perioperative bleeding management in pediatric patients. *Curr Opin Anaesthesiol.* 2016;29:352.

Hackl C, Schlitt HJ, Renner P, et al. Liver surgery in cirrhosis and portal hypertension. *World J Gastroenterol.* 2016;22:2725.

Kandiah PA, Olson JC, Subramanian RM. Emerging strategies for the treatment of patients with acute hepatic failure. *Curr Opin Crit Care.* 2016;22:142.

Peyvandi F, Garagiola I, Biguzzi E. Advances in the treatment of bleeding disorders. *J Thromb Haemost.* 2016;14:2095.

Tapper EB, Jiang ZG, Patwardhan VR. Refining the ammonia hypothesis: A pathology-driven approach to the treatment of hepatic encephalopathy. *Mayo Clin Proc.* 2015;90:646.

Wijdicks EFM. Hepatic encephalopathy. *N Engl J Med.* 2016;375:1660.

Wikkelsø A, Wetterslev J, Møller AM, et al. Thromboelastography (TEG) or rotational thromboelastometry (ROTEM) to monitor haemostatic treatment in bleeding patients: A systemic review with meta-analysis and trial sequential analysis. *Anaesthesia.* 2017;72:519.

Williams B, McNeil J, Crabbe A, et al. Practical use of thromboelastometry in the management of perioperative coagulopathy and bleeding. *Transfus Med Rev.* 2017;31:11.

CHAPTER 29

Anesthesia for Patients with Liver Disease

CASE 1 | Patient with Liver Disease and Incarcerated Hernia: Preoperative Assessment and Anesthetic Management

Michael Ramsay, MD, FRCA

You are asked to consult on a 60-year-old man with a history of alcoholic hepatic cirrhosis who is now posted for emergent laparotomy for an incarcerated abdominal hernia.

1. As you are walking to see the patient in the preoperative holding area, what are your initial thoughts?

A. The patient has been admitted from home, and the perioperative risk—although increased—should not be high.
B. He might have a coagulopathy, and if the international normalized ratio (INR) is elevated, he will need preoperative fresh frozen plasma infused.
C. A preoperative echocardiogram report shows a left-ventricular ejection fraction (LVEF) of 55%. Therefore, his cardiac status is excellent.
D. This patient is at high risk for increased morbidity and mortality, and this may be assessed by calculating the Child–Turcotte–Pugh (CTP) or Model for End-Stage Liver Disease (MELD) score.

The correct answer is D. Patients who present for emergency surgery with coexisting alcoholic liver disease are at increased risk for both morbidity and mortality.

Hepatic dysfunction includes impairment of the synthetic actions of the liver that include protein synthesis, maintenance of coagulation system integrity, metabolism of drugs and nutrients, conversion of ammonia to urea and detoxification of other toxic substances, and filtration of the portal venous blood. The function of all major organs may become impaired in the setting of hepatic dysfunction, resulting in hepatorenal syndrome, hepatopulmonary syndrome, portopulmonary hypertension, encephalopathy, and cirrhotic cardiomyopathy—all further complicated by ascites, varices, and muscle wasting. The cirrhotic cardiomyopathy may be missed because the LVEF may be increased, as the patient will have a low systemic vascular resistance. A careful cardiac assessment with echocardiography may demonstrate systolic and diastolic dysfunction, together with impaired conduction. There is also downregulation of β-adrenergic receptors. Therefore, increased doses of β-adrenergic drugs may be necessary to maintain hemodynamics when compared to a normal patient.

An elevated INR indicates liver dysfunction but does not predict bleeding in a cirrhotic patient. The INR was a test designed to monitor the effects of the drug warfarin, but when used to assess liver disease, it merely indicates the level of dysfunction. The liver synthesizes both clotting factors and anticoagulating factors, and these latter factors are not measured by the INR. A patient with an INR of 3.0 may be hypercoagulable or have a bleeding tendency. A viscoelastic test is necessary to assess the state of coagulation.

Two predictive models exist that may assist in assessment of surgical risk in the patient with chronic liver disease: the CTP score and the MELD score. The CTP score allocates up to 3 points depending on the severity of derangement in ascites, hepatic encephalopathy, total bilirubin, serum albumin, and INR. Class A patients have a CTP score of 5 to 6 points and a perioperative mortality of 10%. Class B patients have a CTP score of 7 to 9 points and a surgical mortality risk of 30%. Class C patients have a CTP score of 10 to 15 points and a mortality risk of greater than 80%. The criticisms of the CTP score are that two parameters—encephalopathy and ascites—are subjective and that it does not take into account kidney function. The MELD score is considered more objective, and its variables include serum creatinine, INR, and serum bilirubin. This model has been demonstrated to accurately predict mortality at 3 months for a patient with end-stage liver disease (ESLD). The MELD score adequately predicts patients' increased risk of postoperative complications after umbilical hernia repair and may be used as a guide to clinical decision making for general surgery in the cirrhotic patient.

A new assessment, which is the fragility of the patient, is now being considered. *Fragility* is a state of decreased physiological reserve and a loss of resilience, both mental and physical. It is strongly associated with perioperative mortality and is assessed by measuring grip strength, walking speed, or thickness of the psoas muscle on a computed tomography (CT) scan examination.

Is it unusual to encounter abdominal hernias in ESLD patients? What are the implications of this condition? Patients with ascites as a result of cirrhosis and portal hypertension have an estimated 20% risk of developing an umbilical hernia. In ESLD patients, umbilical hernias that proceed to incarceration and emergent surgery have a perioperative mortality of 20%. For uncomplicated umbilical hernias in this patient population, careful consideration of the potential perioperative mortality compared to conservative treatment is needed, with guidance from the CTP or MELD scores.

2. Which of the following is an anesthetic management concern?

A. The presence of multiorgan dysfunction.
B. The alcoholic patient will be resistant to many anesthetic agents.
C. The alcoholic patient will be very sensitive to many anesthetic agents.
D. The patient has a high fragility score, which means a loss of resilience.
E. All of the above.

The correct answer is E. Preoperative assessment involves the examination of a debilitated patient with potential for multiple organ system dysfunction. The major concerns in ESLD include muscle wasting, ascites, pleural effusions, chronic kidney disease, cardiomyopathy, respiratory compromise, electrolyte derangements, encephalopathy, coagulopathy, and altered drug pharmacokinetics and pharmacodynamics. A history of alcoholism adds another factor in the variable response to anesthesia. The alcoholic patient early in the disease course may be resistant to anesthetic agents, but as the liver disease progresses, such patients become much more sensitive. The presence of encephalopathy, which is a sign of severe deterioration, provides an indication of where the alcoholic patient may be on this clinical continuum.

Pleural effusions and ascites adversely impact spontaneous ventilation and may prevent the patient lying flat until ventilation is controlled. Hepatopulmonary syndrome may be present, with intrapulmonary shunts causing hypoxia when breathing room air. This is one of the few conditions in which hypoxia improves with the patient lying flat. Portopulmonary hypertension may exist in a few patients, and management is best guided by transesophageal echocardiography. There is a small risk of variceal bleeding on passage of a transesophageal scope, but the benefits outweigh the risk.

3. Which of the following is true about the management of coagulation?

A. Epidural anesthesia is absolutely contraindicated in cirrhotic patients.
B. Postoperative venous thromboembolism precautions should be withheld until the INR is back to normal.
C. The incidence of postoperative pulmonary embolism is very low.
D. The incidence of pulmonary embolism is high if preventive measures are not taken.

The correct answer is D. The coagulopathy of liver cirrhosis is characterized by the impaired synthesis of coagulation factors, resulting in increased INR and decreased coagulation inhibitor factors (protein C, protein S, and antithrombin III). The state of the coagulation system is best assessed by viscoelastic technology such as thromboelastography (TEG) and rotational thromboelastometry (ROTEM). These technologies can assess the real-time activity of the coagulation system and demonstrate fibrinolysis and disseminated intravascular coagulation, if they exist. Low platelet counts may not necessitate platelet transfusions, as the existing platelets may be more easily activated because of an increased von Wille-brand multimer, enhanced by an ADAMTS13 deficiency. Again, viscoelastic test-ing of coagulation will detect this.

Preoperative sedation is challenging in the patient with ESLD. Hepatic encepha-lopathy has been associated with increased γ-aminobutyric acid (GABA) neu-rotransmitter in the brain. This may be potentiated by the administration of benzodiazepine drugs, precipitating hepatic coma.

A modified rapid-sequence induction technique should be used to secure the airway, as these patients are at increased risk for aspiration. Maintaining liver per-fusion is vital to minimize the risk of acute liver failure. Adequate maintenance of systemic blood pressure and oxygenation are important, but surgical retraction may also be a major factor in adversely impacting liver perfusion. A balanced electrolyte solution not containing lactate is preferable for intravenous fluids so as to not to exacerbate lactic acidosis. A large-bore venous cannula is advisable, as a large varix may be entered by the surgeon, resulting in significant hemorrhage. The choice of anesthetic agent is not as important as maintaining hemodynamic stability.

Postoperative recovery in an intensive care unit should be considered so that liver decompensation can be detected early and prompt interventions made. Many patients with liver cirrhosis who need surgery are referred to centers that have a liver transplant program in place that could be activated if the liver acutely decompensates.

DID YOU LEARN?

- The anesthetic and perioperative implications of caring for a surgical patient with liver cirrhosis.
- How to assess the perioperative risk associated with surgery and anesthesia on a cirrhotic patient.
- That the INR is merely a measure of liver impairment and does not predict the degree of coagulopathy present.
- The incidence of venous thromboembolism is elevated postoperatively in the cirrhotic patient, and preventive measures should be in place.
- Consideration should be given to transferring patients to a liver trans-plant surgery center for their surgery so that if the liver fails, they can be potential transplant candidates.

References

Aloia TA, Geerts WH, Clary BM, et al. Venous thromboembolism prophylaxis in liver surgery. *J Gastrointest Surg.* 2016;20:221-229.

Biancofiore G, Blasi A, De Boer MT, et al. Perioperative hemostatic management in the cirrhotic patient: A position paper on the behalf of the Liver Intensive Care Group of Europe (LICAGE). *Minerva Anestesiol.* 2019;85(7):782-798.

Im GY, Lubezky N, Facciuto MF, Schiano TD. Surgery in patients with portal hyper-tension: A preoperative checklist and strategies for attenuating risk. *Clin Liver Dis.* 2014;18:477-505.

Ramsay M. Anesthesia for liver transplantation. In: Busuttil RW, Klintmalm GB, eds. *Transplantation of the Liver,* 3rd ed. Philadelphia, PA: Elsevier Saunders; 2015.

Ramsay M, Trotter J. Editorial: The INR is only one side of the coagulation cascade: It's time to watch the clot. *Anaesthesia.* 2016;71:611-626.

Wanderer JP Nathan N. To clot or not to clot: Understanding coagulopathy in liver disease. *Anesth Analg.* 2018;126:2.

Zielsdorf SM, Kubasiak JC, Janssen I, Myers JA, Luu MB. A NSQIP analysis of MELD and perioperative outcomes in general surgery. *Am Surg.* 2015;81:755-759.

CASE 2 Patient with Portopulmonary Hypertension Presenting for Liver Transplantation

Michael Ramsay, MD, FRCA

A 45-year-old man with sclerosing cholangitis and liver cirrhosis was called in from home for liver transplantation. The donor organ will be available in approximately 1 h. The patient has a MELD score of 32, weight of 75 kg, and height of 178 cm. In reviewing his pretransplantation assessment, you note a transthoracic echocardiogram from 12 months ago that reported a left-ventricular ejection fraction (LVEF) of 60% but was otherwise unremarkable.

1. As you plan your anesthetic, what are your initial thoughts on cardiovascular assessment and intraoperative management?

A. The patient has the cardiac function of an athlete and needs no further workup.

B. The patient is coming directly to the operating room, so there is no time or need for further assessment of cardiac status.

C. You decide the only cardiac monitoring needed is an ECG, intraarterial blood pressure cannula, and a central venous pressure (CVP) line.

D. You will initially review the chest radiograph for signs of right heart failure and obtain a transthoracic echocardiogram.

E. You will place the patient under anesthesia but assess cardiac hemodynamics with a CVP, pulmonary artery catheter, and transesophageal echocardiograph before allowing surgery to begin.

The correct answer is D. Major cardiovascular and hemodynamic changes may have taken place during the course of a year in a patient with liver cirrhosis. If there is pressure put on you to proceed quickly because of time constraints, an explanation of the potential risks without this basic information should be given. If this patient was discovered to have developed moderate or severe pulmonary hypertension since the last evaluation, the safest course would be to defer the transplantation, use the organ for a different recipient, and initiate treatment for portopulmonary hypertension (POPH).

Initial assessment revealed a heavily jaundiced and somewhat cachectic male with marked ascites and moderate dyspnea. Laboratory data include hematocrit 29%, hemoglobin 9.5 g/dL, and platelet count 25,000/μL. Serum creatinine is 2.4 mg/dL, and INR is 2.5. The patient had undergone a transjugular intrahepatic portosystemic shunt (TIPS) procedure 3 months ago.

Induction of general anesthesia and intubation was uneventful and followed placement of a radial arterial catheter. A pulmonary artery catheter was inserted and revealed pulmonary artery pressures of 90/50 mm Hg, with mean pulmonary artery pressure (MPAP) of 63 mm Hg. The pulmonary capillary wedge pressure (PCWP) was elevated at 22 cm H_2O, and the pulmonary vascular resistance (PVR) was calculated to be 450 dynes·s·cm^{-5} with a cardiac output (CO) of 3.6 L/min. A transesophageal echocardiogram (TEE) probe was placed and revealed a markedly dilated right ventricle and right atrium. The surgery was postponed, and the donor organ used for a backup recipient.

2. What would have been the risks of proceeding with the liver transplantation in this patient?

A. Loss of the donor graft because of venous congestion.
B. Death of the recipient because of right-ventricular failure.
C. A stormy intra- and postoperative course managing right heart failure and a failing graft.
D. The need for extracorporeal membrane oxygenation (ECMO).
E. The risks are dependent on right-ventricular function and the degree of POPH.
F. All of the above.

The correct answer is F. The patient was transferred to the intensive care unit for recovery from anesthesia and for management of the newly diagnosed, severe POPH. The precipitating factor for this patient may have been the TIPS procedure, which is associated with increased CO and increased right-ventricular filling pressures that are poorly tolerated.

What is POPH, and why is it so important in this patient? POPH is a serious complication of portal hypertension that may or may not be accompanied by liver cirrhosis. It is found in approximately 6.5% of liver transplantation candidates and occurs when there is obstruction to arterial flow in the pulmonary arterial bed. Initially, this may be due to vasoconstriction and thus will be acutely reversible with pulmonary vasodilators such as inhaled nitric oxide; however, it becomes progressively less reversible over time due to proliferation of pulmonary arteriolar endothelium and smooth muscle, which may be further complicated by platelet aggregation. Mediators associated with the development of POPH include increased circulating endothelin-1 and estradiol levels, and they accompany a deficiency of prostacyclin synthase in pulmonary endothelial cells.

3. How is POPH differentiated from other causes of increased pulmonary artery pressures?

   A. There is a hyperdynamic cardiac state with a normal PVR.
   B. There is volume overload with an elevated PCWP.
   C. There is an increase in PVR and transpulmonary gradient.
   D. The patient has cirrhotic cardiomyopathy.

The correct answer is C. The definition and severity of POPH are based on hemodynamic data obtained from pulmonary artery catheterization and echocardiography. POPH is defined as an MPAP above 25 mm Hg, a PVR greater than 240 dynes·s·cm^{-5}, and a transpulmonary gradient greater than 12 mm Hg. In many definitions, the PCWP of 15 mm Hg or less is included in the definition, but this may not always be true in the liver transplant population, as the occurrence of volume overload is often present, together with ventricular dysfunction that will cause an elevation in the PCWP, as occurred in the case described above. The most important value is the PVR, as this influences the work of the right ventricle, which may become dysfunctional and cause graft congestion, leading to graft loss and mortality in the liver transplantation patient. Therefore, careful assessment of cardiac function by TEE is essential, and signs of right ventricle (RV) failure should suggest delaying transplantation and optimizing the hemodynamics by medical therapy.

POPH is associated with a 1-year survival rate of 35% to 46% without treatment. As the disease progresses, the cardiac index begins to decline as the ventricles fail and the right heart distends. Liver transplantation alone may not reverse POPH, but the addition of vasodilator therapy will improve outcomes.

There are three hemodynamic patterns that may be seen in liver transplant candidates that may result in pulmonary hypertension and must be differentiated. The most common presentation is the hyperdynamic, high-CO state, which is often found in the cirrhotic patient, and the key differential measurement is the normal PVR. The second hemodynamic pattern is volume overload, which may occur with true POPH, and the key values are normal PVR and elevated PCWP. The third presentation is true POPH, with an elevated PVR and transpulmonary gradient.

The patient described had true POPH in association with volume overload. Liver transplantation with a MPAP of 63 mm Hg carries a mortality risk approaching 100% due to likely cardiac and graft failure. The data reported would stratify the risk of mortality as at least 50% if the MPAP is above 35 mm Hg. The key to assessing the risk is assessing the RV function by TEE. If the RV is strong, hypertrophied, and not dilated, the risk of failure is much less than if it is found to be widely dilated.

4. Which of the following statements is correct?

   A. POPH is an indication for liver transplantation.
   B. Liver transplantation, if clinically feasible, will always reverse POPH.
   C. POPH is always associated with liver cirrhosis.
   D. Medical therapy can reduce POPH to a level that can allow liver transplantation to safely occur, but will be required to be continued after transplantation.

The correct answer is D. This patient was considered too high a risk to undergo liver transplantation—MPAP 63 mm Hg, PVR 450 dynes·s·cm^{-5}, with a markedly dilated right heart—therefore, medical therapy was instituted in an effort to reverse the degree of pulmonary hypertension, improve right heart function, and reinstitute the patient as a liver transplant candidate. The therapies available include the prostanoids, phosphodiesterase-5 (PDE-5) inhibitors, and endothelin receptor antagonists. The goal of therapy is to reverse the hemodynamics of POPH, especially the PVR, and allow the right heart function to strengthen and improve such that the patient can undergo and survive the rigors of liver transplantation, especially reperfusion when the CO may increase and acutely increase MPAP. Liver transplantation may or may not reverse the pathological changes of POPH such that therapy may have to continue after successful liver transplantation.

Prostacyclin analogues such as intravenous (IV) epoprostenol possess vasodilator, antithrombotic, and antiproliferative properties. Inhaled iloprost and IV and subcutaneous treprostinil have been reported to have favorable hemodynamic effects. PDE-5 inhibitors prevent the metabolism of cyclic guanosine monophosphate, which mediates the vascular effects of nitric oxide. Oral sildenafil may improve functional capacity, decrease PVR and MPAP, and increase CO in patients with POPH. Bosentan, an oral dual endothelin receptor antagonist, may lead to improvements in exercise capacity and hemodynamics in POPH. A small group of patients have been reported to have been successfully treated with the selective endothelin receptor antagonist ambrisentan, demonstrating improved functional class, increased CO, and a mean reduction in PVR of 61%.

A new endothelin receptor antagonist, macitentan, shows promise of efficacy.

What is the most appropriate methodology for subsequent reconsideration for liver transplantation candidacy? The patient was reevaluated for liver transplantation 6 months after combined therapy with a PDE-5 inhibitor and a selective endothelin receptor antagonist. A TEE revealed good function in both right and left ventricles, with an LVEF of 55%. A pulmonary artery catheter demonstrated pulmonary artery pressures of 50/25 mm Hg with a MPAP of 35 mm Hg. The PVR was reduced to 220 dynes·s·cm^{-5}. This patient now met safe criteria for liver transplantation, and a successful liver transplant was performed. The initial pulmonary artery pressures after reperfusion were elevated to 60/35 mm Hg with a MPAP of 40 mm Hg and a CO of 8 L/min. A TEE showed good RV function, and over the next few days, the pulmonary artery pressures normalized, but medical therapy needed to be continued.

DID YOU LEARN?

- POPH is an unusual but dangerous complication of portal hypertension.
- If POPH is found during the evaluation of a liver transplantation candidate, it should be carefully characterized by TTE and the placement of a pulmonary artery catheter and the PVR calculated.
- Liver transplantation should be deferred and medical therapy instituted in patients with an MPAP >35 mm Hg, a PVR >240 dynes·s·cm^{-5}, and evidence on echocardiogram of right-ventricular dysfunction.
- POPH is not an indication for liver transplantation. It may progress after liver transplantation.

References

Cartin-Ceba R, Krowka MJ. Portopulmonary hypertension. *Clin Liver Dis.* 2014;18:421-438.

Dalia AA, Flores A, Chitilian H, et al. A comprehensive review of transesophageal echocardiography during liver transplantation. *J Cardiothorac Vasc Anesth.* 2018;32:1815-1824.

DuBrock HM, Channick RN, Krowka MJ. What's new in the treatment of portopulmonary hypertension? *Expert Rev Gastroenterol Hepatol.* 2015;9:983-992.

Krowka MJ. Management of pulmonary complications in pretransplant patients. *Clin Liver Dis.* 2011;15:765-777.

Krowka MJ, Fallon MB, Kawut SM, et al. International Liver Transplant Society practice guidelines: Diagnosis and management of hepatopulmonary syndrome and portopulmonary hypertension. *Transplantation.* 2016;100:1440-1452.

Ramsay M. Portopulmonary hypertension and right heart failure in patients with cirrhosis. *Curr Opin Anaesthesiol.* 2010;23:145-150.

Verma S, Hand F, Armstrong MJ, et al. Portopulmonary hypertension: Still an appropriate consideration for liver transplantation? *Liver Transpl.* 2016;22:1637-1642.

CASE 3 — Patient with End-Stage Liver Disease

Marina Gitman, MD, and Sabry Khalil, MD

A 63-year-old obese man with ESLD from alcoholic cirrhosis with a MELD score of 32 presents to the operating room for an exploratory laparotomy for small bowel obstruction. Past medical history includes well-controlled hypertension, non–insulin-dependent diabetes, and chronic kidney disease. Past surgical history includes an open right hemicolectomy and a recent transjugular intrahepatic portosystemic shunt (TIPS) placement for refractory ascites. He has no allergies and currently takes metoprolol and metformin. ESLD has been complicated by frequent episodes of hepatic encephalopathy, upper gastrointestinal bleeding, refractory ascites, and hepatopulmonary syndrome. Preoperative vital signs are temperature 37.1°C, heart rate 105 beats/min, blood pressure 95/52 mm Hg, respiratory rate 20 breaths/min, and SpO$_2$ 91% on 4 L/min nasal cannula. On exam, he is alert and oriented but has difficulty remembering yesterday's events and appears jaundiced and deconditioned. Cardiovascular exam is normal, and breath sounds are slightly diminished bilaterally. Hemoglobin level is 8.5 g/dL, platelet count is 48,000/μL, and INR is 2.4.

1. Which of the following is true regarding the MELD score for this patient?

   A. It is calculated using the patient's bilirubin level, albumin level, INR, and the severity of encephalopathy and ascites.

   B. It accurately predicts 30-day post-liver transplant survival.

   C. Sodium level is used for the calculation of the MELD score.

   D. A MELD score of 32 predicts that this patient's 90-day in-hospital mortality rate is 25%.

The correct answer is C. CTP score, not MELD score, is calculated using the patient's bilirubin level, albumin level, INR (prothrombin time), and severity of encephalopathy and ascites. Historically, a MELD score was calculated using the patient's levels of creatinine, bilirubin, and INR. It was originally described in 2000 as a predictor of 90-day mortality of patients with ESLD who underwent a TIPS; and in 2002, it was adapted for prioritization of patients with ESLD on the liver transplantation recipient waiting list. A MELD score of 30 to 39 in a hospitalized patient corresponds to an 83% mortality rate. Hyponatremia (Na <126 mEq/L) is an independent predictor of mortality in patients with ESLD, and in 2016, a sodium level was added to the calculation of the MELD score.

2. All of the following have the potential to worsen hepatic encephalopathy *except*:

   A. Gastrointestinal bleeding.
   B. Rifaximin.
   C. TIPS.
   D. Infection.

The correct answer is B. Gastrointestinal bleeding, dehydration, infection, and TIPS all have the potential to exacerbate hepatic encephalopathy. Rifaximin is an antibiotic with poor oral bioavailability that is used to treat the intestinal bacterial overgrowth that is responsible for overproduction of ammonia that contributes to hepatic encephalopathy.

3. Which of the following best describes the typical hemodynamic changes associated with ESLD?

   A. Cirrhotic cardiomyopathy is defined by an increased contractile response to stress.
   B. Increased systemic vascular resistance (SVR), decreased CO, and decreased mixed venous oxygen concentration (SvO$_2$).
   C. Common alterations to vital signs include bradycardia and hypertension.
   D. Sympathetic activation and hyperdynamic circulation with dysregulation of β-adrenergic receptors.

The correct answer is D. Cirrhotic cardiomyopathy is defined by a decreased contractile response to stress, reduced diastolic relaxation, and electrophysiological abnormalities such as a prolonged QT interval. Sympathetic activation and a hyperdynamic circulation, evidenced by an increase in CO, decrease in SVR, and an increase in SvO$_2$, result in dysregulation of β-adrenergic receptors that can lead to a blunted response to stress as well as β-adrenergic drugs.

4. Which of the following is true regarding this patient's coagulation status?

A. Fresh frozen plasma (FFP) should be administered in order to decrease INR to below 1.5 to prevent intraoperative bleeding.
B. Production of all clotting factors is decreased except for factor VII, which is increased.
C. Preferred methods of assessment of coagulation status in ESLD include conventional tests such as INR and PTT (partial thromboplastin time).
D. A decrease in the levels of proteins C and S and an increase in the level of clotting factor VIII may result in a prothrombotic state, increasing the risk for thromboembolic phenomena.

The correct answer is D. Typically, ESLD results in decreased levels of almost all of the clotting factors. However, the levels of anticoagulant proteins C and S are also decreased, but clotting factor VIII and von Willebrand factor are increased. This rebalancing of hemostasis will not always manifest clinically as bleeding but can also tip toward a prothrombotic side. Conventional tests of coagulation such as INR or PTT do not adequately assess coagulation as a whole, while dynamic tests such as thromboelastography (TEG) or thromboelastometry (ROTEM) provide a more accurate assessment and can help guide treatment. For these reasons, prophylactic correction of INR to a certain number with FFP is not indicated and may be potentially detrimental. Instead, dynamic tests of coagulation together with the assessment of the full clinical picture should guide transfusion of FFP and other clotting factors.

Recommended Readings

Forkin KT, Colquhoun DA, Nemergut EC, et al. The coagulation profile of end-stage liver disease and considerations for intraoperative management. *Anesth Analg.* 2018; 126(1):46-61.

Gitman M, Albertz M, Nicolau-Raducu R, et al. Cardiac diseases among liver transplant candidates. *Clin Transplant.* 2018;32(7):e13296.

Kamanth PS, Wiesner RH, Malinchoc M, et al. A model to predict survival in patients with end-stage liver disease. *Hepatology.* 2001;33(2):464-470.

Machicao VI. Model for end-stage liver disease—sodium score: The evolution in the prioritization of liver transplantation. *Clin Liver Dis.* 2017;21(2):275-287.

Malinchoc M, Kamath PS, Gordon FD, et al. A model to predict poor survival in patients undergoing transjugular intrahepatic portosystemic shunts. *Hepatology.* 2000;31(4): 864-871.

Northup P, Reutemann B. Management of coagulation and anticoagulation in liver transplantation candidates. *Liver Transpl.* 2018;24(8):1119-1132.

Ramsay M. Anesthesia for patients with liver disease. In: Butterworth IV JF, Mackey DC, Wasnick JD, eds. *Morgan & Mikhail's Clinical Anesthesiology.* 6th ed. New York, NY: McGraw-Hill Education; 2018:733-752.

Suraweera D, Sundaram V, Saab S. Evaluation and management of hepatic encephalopathy: Current status and future. *Gut Liver.* 2016;10(4):509-519.

CHAPTER 30

Anesthesia for Patients with Endocrine Disease

CASE 1 | Patient for Kidney Transplantation

Sarah Armour, MD

A 50-year-old man with type 1 diabetes is scheduled for kidney transplantation. His blood glucose on the morning of surgery is 225 mg/dL. He was hemodialyzed the day before. A blood sample was obtained this morning revealing that his potassium is 3.5 mM and his sodium is 144 mM.

1. An infusion of 0.45% saline and 2 units/h of regular insulin are started in the preoperative holding area. What effect would this have on his blood glucose and electrolytes?

   A. Extracellular potassium will increase, glucose will decrease, and sodium will decrease.
   B. Extracellular potassium will decrease, glucose will decrease, and sodium will decrease.
   C. Intracellular potassium will increase, glucose will increase, and sodium will decrease.
   D. Extracellular potassium will decrease, glucose will decrease, and sodium will increase.

The correct answer is B. Insulin causes an intracellular shift of potassium, therefore lowering the potassium level in the blood. The insulin will lower the blood glucose level, and the hypotonic 0.45% normal saline solution will cause the sodium to decrease.

CASE 2 — Patient with Elevated Creatinine Concentration

Sarah Armour, MD

A 50-year-old man with type 1 diabetes and chronic kidney disease is undergoing coronary artery bypass surgery. He does not yet require dialysis, and his preoperative creatinine is 1.8 mg/dL. After weaning from bypass, his blood glucose is 375 mg/dL.

1. Extreme perioperative hyperglycemia during cardiac surgery has been associated with all of the following *except*:

   A. Increased mortality.
   B. Poor wound healing.
   C. Infection.
   D. Worse neurological outcome.
   E. All of the above are correct, so there is no exception.

The correct answer is D. Hyperglycemia has been associated with hyperosmolarity, infection, poor wound healing, and increased mortality. Severe hyperglycemia has been shown to worsen neurological outcome after cerebral ischemia and will likely adversely affect neurological and neuropsychological outcomes following cardiac surgery. However, relevant clinical trials have failed to identify worse outcomes with loose versus tight control of blood glucose during CABG surgery. Studies confirming outcome benefits to control of blood sugar in cardiac surgery have largely focused on the intensive care unit (ICU). The only relevant clinical trial examining tighter versus looser control of intraoperative blood glucose failed to identify any neurological or neuropsychological benefit but did not directly address the risks of extreme hyperglycemia.

2. The likely best blood glucose management in patients like this includes:

   A. "Tight" control with a target of <150 mg/dL during surgery.
   B. A target of <180 mg/dL during surgery and postoperatively.
   C. Avoidance of morning insulin dose on the day of surgery to avoid hypoglycemia during surgery.
   D. Treatment of intraoperative hyperglycemia with subcutaneous regular insulin according to a sliding scale.

The correct answer is B. Several clinical trials have sought to determine the best range within which to maintain blood glucose during critical illness. The best available evidence from these ICU studies suggests that the goal of intraoperative management should be to maintain blood glucose below 180 mg/dL while avoiding hypoglycemia. There no convincing evidence that "tight" control of blood glucose (<150 mg/dL) in the operative setting is preferable to below 180 mg/dL, and some ICU studies even suggest that "tight" control leads to worse outcomes.

Maintaining blood glucose below 180 mg/dL in patients undergoing cardiopulmonary bypass decreases infectious complications. Because the absorption of subcutaneous insulin can be unpredictable during surgery due to changes in tissue blood flow, IV insulin is much preferred.

3. A few months later, the patient presents with abdominal pain, constipation, worsening muscle weakness, and memory loss. He is found to have a serum calcium level of 16 mg/dL. A neck sonogram shows parathyroid hyperplasia. He is scheduled for a neck dissection for parathyroidectomy. Appropriate perioperative therapy for hypercalcemia could include all of the following choices *except*:

A. Hydration with saline.
B. Avoiding hypoventilation.
C. Diuresis with furosemide.
D. Diuresis with hydrochlorothiazide.

The correct answer is D. Removal of all four parathyroid glands is often required in patients with parathyroid hyperplasia. These patients often present with symptoms of severe hypercalcemia with polyuria, polydipsia, abdominal pain, muscle weakness, ECG changes (shortened QT interval, widened T waves), and cognitive impairment. In patients with hypercalcemia due to hyperparathyroidism, attempts should be made to decrease the serum calcium to acceptable values to reduce the risk of perioperative cardiac arrhythmias. Anesthetic management should therefore include hydration with normal saline and diuresis with furosemide (loop diuretics promote calcium loss), avoidance of hypoventilation (acidosis increases ionized calcium), and careful use of neuromuscular blockers guided by a twitch monitor since the response to neuromuscular blockers is unpredictable with hypercalcemia. Hydrochlorothiazide leads to an increase in calcium reabsorption and should be avoided.

DID YOU LEARN?

- Pharmacological effects of insulin.
- Adverse effects of hyperglycemia in critical illness.
- Management of hyperglycemia.

References

Butterworth J, Wagenknecht LE, Legault C, et al. Attempted control of hyperglycemia during cardiopulmonary bypass fails to improve neurologic or neurobehavioral outcomes in patients without diabetes mellitus undergoing coronary artery bypass grafting. *J Thorac Cardiovasc Surg.* 2005;130(5):1319.

Reddy P, Duggar B, Butterworth J. Blood glucose management in the patient undergoing cardiac surgery: A review. *World J Cardiol.* 2014;6(11):1209-1217.

Thompson BM, Stearns JD, Apsey HA, et al. Perioperative management of patients with diabetes and hyperglycemia undergoing elective surgery. *Curr Diab Rep.* 2016;16:2.

CASE 3 — Patient Following Motor Vehicle Accident

Sarah Armour, MD

A 41-year-old man presents for an exploratory laparotomy following a motor vehicle accident. An abdominal ultrasound was suggestive of splenic rupture. He states that his primary care physician has suspected him of having hypertension, but that his blood pressure has been inconsistently elevated when he has been examined. There is no other relevant past medical history. The patient received 2 L of lactated Ringer's solution in the emergency department before being brought to the surgical suite. Immediately before induction of anesthesia, his blood pressure was 145/85 mm Hg. When the abdomen was opened, the blood pressure fell to 105/65 mm Hg. With manipulation of abdominal contents near the bifurcation of the aorta, his blood pressure abruptly increased to 185/110 mm Hg. The helpful medical student working with you suggests that light anesthesia could be the culprit (despite the end-tidal concentration of desflurane being 8.5%). One hundred micrograms of fentanyl and 100 mg of propofol were injected intravenously. Nevertheless, the blood pressure now reads 190/115 mm Hg. You now inject 5 mg of metoprolol intravenously. Curiously, the patient becomes more hypertensive following treatment with metoprolol.

1. What is the most likely cause of worsening hypertension following administration of metorprolol in the above clinical scenario?

   A. Essential hypertension.
   B. Faulty arterial line reading.
   C. Unopposed stimulation of α-receptors.
   D. Unopposed stimulation of β-receptors.

The correct answer is C. This patient has presented with a history and signs that are highly suggestive of pheochromocytoma. Pheochromocytomas are catecholamine-secreting tumors derived from chromaffin cells. Patients typically present with a triad of hypertension, palpitations, and diaphoresis. Nevertheless, pheochromocytoma is the etiology of hypertension in fewer than 0.1% of cases. Although these tumors are usually found in the adrenal medulla, they can be found in a variety of locations including the organ of Zuckerkandl at the aortic bifurcation. Surgical manipulation of the tumor can release a catecholamine surge that leads to hypertension and possible arrhythmias. Under ideal circumstances, patients with pheochromoctoma will be treated with selective α-adrenergic blockers, such as phenoxybenzamine or prazosin, for 10 to 14 days prior to surgical procedures. Our patient, however, needs immediate surgery and has received no treatment. Catecholamines act on both α- and β-receptors. If a selective β-adrenergic antagonist such as metoprolol is given prior to adequate treatment with an α-adrenergic antagonist, the unopposed stimulation of the α-receptors can lead to worsening of hypertension.

2. The blood pressure is now 210/120 mm Hg. Which of the following would most immediately address the hypertension given the circumstances?

A. Phenoxybenzamine.
B. Phentolamine.
C. Nitroprusside.
D. Esmolol.
E. Fentanyl.

The correct answer is C. Blood pressure of 210/100 mm Hg is a hypertensive crisis that needs immediate treatment to reduce the risk of myocardial ischemia or cerebrovascular accident. Nitroprusside is a fast-acting direct vasodilator that can be used to immediately bring the blood pressure down to a more acceptable value. Alternatives to nitroprusside for rapid control of blood pressure would include clevidipine and nicardipine. Phenoxybenzamine is an α-blocker recommended for preoperative treatment of patients with pheochromocytoma. It is only available for oral administration, eliminating it as a choice for an anesthetized patient in the operating room. Phentolamine is a selective α-adrenergic antagonist and is available in an intravenous form. However, it has a relatively slow onset of action, limiting its utility in emergent situations where immediate control of blood pressure is required. Careful titration of phentolamine could be useful once the blood pressure has been reduced to a level that does not place the patient in immediate danger. Selective β-blockers should be avoided at this time due to the possible risk of worsening hypertension from unopposed stimulation of the α-receptors. β-Blockers can be used following α-blockade if there is a concern about tachycardia or arrhythmias. Fentanyl is not an antihypertensive agent despite its widespread use as such during general anesthesia, and it is likely to be effective only when inadequate depth of anesthesia is a concern.

3. The surgeon elects to resect the pheochromocytoma. Following ligation of the tumor's venous supply, the patient becomes hypotensive. What is the most likely etiology of his hypotension?

A. Hypovolemia.
B. Withdrawal of endogenous catecholamines.
C. Myocardial dysfunction.
D. Both A and B.
E. None of the above.

The correct answer is D. Hypovolemia and acute withdrawal of catecholamines are thought to be the most likely causes of hypotension following resection of a pheochromocytoma. Most patients with pheochromocytoma (and probably all who have not received preoperative α-blockade) have decreased circulating blood volume, necessitating careful fluid resuscitation. Had the patient received an adequate course of an α-adrenergic blocker over the 10 to 14 days prior to resection, the volume status would most likely have been at least partially corrected, and unusually large volumes of intravenous fluid likely would be unnecessary. In addition, following ligation of the tumor's venous supply, there is an acute decrease of catecholamine concentrations in blood, commonly causing hypotension. We recommend having a norepinephrine infusion available. Postoperative hypotension is less likely if the patient was adequately α-blocked and volume-resuscitated.

4. The blood pressure is now 65/40 mm Hg. Which of the following would be the best immediate response?

A. Administer epinephrine intravenously.
B. Inject ephedrine intravenously.
C. Administer a bolus of 0.9% saline.
D. Initiate a norepinephrine infusion and administer a fluid bolus.

The correct answer is D. Hypotension following resection of a pheochromocytoma is likely due to a combination of hypovolemia and acute withdrawal of catecholamines. Given that this patient was injured in a motor vehicle collision, other causes of hypotension, including bleeding, myocardial dysfunction, pneumothorax, tamponade, and so on, must be ruled out. A blood pressure of 65/40 mm Hg needs immediate attention. While fluid resuscitation may improve blood pressure, administering norepinephrine may be necessary. Fluid resuscitation is continued if hypovolemia is thought to be the cause of hypotension. Epinephrine is recommended in a code situation. Ephedrine causes indirect release of catecholamines and is best avoided in patients with pheochromocytoma.

DID YOU LEARN?

- Preoperative treatment of patient with pheochromocytoma.
- Intraoperative treatment of hypertension caused by pheochromocytoma.
- Causes of hypotension following resection of pheochromocytoma.
- Treatment of hypotension following resection of pheochromocytoma.

Recommended Reading

Butterworth IV JF, Mackey DC, Wasnick JD, eds. Anesthesia for patients with endocrine disease. In: *Morgan & Mikhail's Clinical Anesthesiology.* 6th ed. New York, NY: McGraw-Hill Education; 2018:753-772.

Reference

Naranjo J, Dodd S, Martin YN. Perioperative management of pheochromocytoma. *J Cardiothorac Vasc Anesth.* 2017;31:1427-1439.

CHAPTER 31

Anesthesia for Ophthalmic Surgery

CASE 1 | Retrobulbar Block Complications

Ravish Kapoor, MD, and Dan S. Gombos, MD, FACS

You are scheduled to provide anesthesia for a hyperopic 70-year-old man undergoing bilateral cataract surgery. The only positive findings on preoperative evaluation are a history of osteoarthritis, for which the patient takes daily naproxen, and a chronic dry cough. There are no known drug allergies, and the patient has maintained NPO status since midnight. After speaking with the patient in the preoperative holding area, you administer midazolam 1 mg intravenously (IV) and transport him on a stretcher to the operating room. Then, 2 L/min nasal cannula oxygen is applied, and the following vital signs are observed: heart rate 70 beats/min, blood pressure 129/73 mm Hg, SpO_2 98%, and respiratory rate 12 breaths/min.

The ophthalmologist plans on performing a retrobulbar block with procaine due to a shortage of other local anesthetics (LAs). He asks that you administer intravenous diphenhydramine 20 min prior to the block, which is an unusual request for him, but you oblige.

1. Why did the surgeon likely request the prophylactic administration of diphenhydramine for this patient?

A. The surgeon wants extra sedation for the patient during surgery.
B. There is an increased risk of allergic reactions with ester LAs.
C. Diphenhydramine is a potent antiemetic.
D. Diphenhydramine will hasten the retrobulbar block.

The correct answer is B. True allergic reactions to LAs are rare and are more likely attributable to the preservative methylparaben or to sulfite antioxidants contained in the solution than to the local anesthetic itself. Ester LAs such as procaine and benzocaine that are metabolized to p-aminobenzoic acid (PABA) are associated with a greater incidence of allergic reactions than other local anesthetics. Giving diphenhydramine, an H_1-blocker, could counteract any potential histamine release–associated allergic reactions.

2. After the patient receives fentanyl 50 μg IV, the surgeon asks the patient to look straight ahead in order to perform the block on the right eye. What is the purpose of requesting the patient to look in this particular direction for the block?

   A. Less risk for damage to the optic nerve.
   B. Better distribution of LA.
   C. Faster onset of LA.
   D. Increased duration of LA.

The correct answer is A. Injections should be made with the globe in "primary" gaze, so that the optic nerve remains in its normal position behind the globe. In the past, it has been advised to request the patient to look "supranasally," but this position has since been shown to place the needle near the ophthalmic artery, superior orbital vein, and the posterior pole of the globe. Injection into the nerve can cause optic nerve atrophy, and penetration of the optic nerve sheath can cause subarachnoid spread of the LA directly into the central nervous system (CNS). Signs of spread into the CNS include dysarthric speech, convulsions, respiratory depression, and/or cardiac arrest. Intravascular injection can also cause convulsions, particularly if the injection is intraarterial. Patients should be carefully monitored after injection, and resuscitation equipment should be readily available. A straight-ahead gaze position has not been shown to improve spread of LA, and the position of the eye during the block does not affect the onset or duration of the LA. However, injection of hyaluronidase, a hydrolyzer of connective tissue polysaccharides, is frequently added to enhance spread of LA.

3. While the block is being performed, you notice that the heart rate suddenly drops to the 30s. You quickly react by administering atropine IV, and the heart rate increases. What is the afferent to efferent neural pathway responsible for this bradycardic episode?

   A. Trigeminal nerve → ciliary nerves → ciliary ganglion → trigeminal ganglion → dorsal nucleus of vagus nerve → vagus nerve.
   B. Optic nerve → ciliary nerves → retinal ganglion → dorsal nucleus of vagus nerve → vagus nerve.
   C. Oculomotor nerve → oculomotor ganglion → vagus ganglion → vagus nerve.
   D. Abducens nerve → ciliary nerves → ciliary ganglion → dorsal nucleus of vagus nerve → vagus nerve.

The correct answer is A. The *oculocardiac reflex* consists of both an afferent and efferent limb. Pressure on the orbital structures, traction on the extraocular muscles, or even ocular pain can trigger an afferent impulse via the ophthalmic branch of the trigeminal nerve. The impulses travel through the ciliary nerves to the ciliary ganglion and then pass to the trigeminal (Gasserian) ganglion. The efferent limb starts in the dorsal nucleus of the vagus and travels to the sinoatrial node and then the atrioventricular (AV) node of the heart. The oculocardiac reflex can produce sinus bradycardia, but also has been reported to cause a variety of dysrhythmias, including junctional or AV block, bigeminy, ectopic beats, ventricular tachycardia or fibrillation, and asystole. It is particularly common with strabismus surgery in pediatric patients. The initial treatment is to ask the surgeon to pause stimulation. Hypercarbia, hypoxia, and light general anesthesia can increase the potential for, or the intensity of, the reflex. If needed, atropine can be administered IV to treat symptomatic or severe bradycardia. Although a retrobulbar block may help to prevent the reflex during surgery, the administration of the block itself has the potential to trigger the reflex.

4. The patient's heart rate returns to 70 beats/min and the nurse preps the eye for surgery with ophthalmic betadine solution. The surgeon steps out of the operating room to answer a phone call, and the patient yells: "The light has faded in my right eye, doc!" What do you do?

    A. Check pupillary reactivity to light.
    B. Delay surgery and send patient for a STAT computed tomography.
    C. Provide reassurance that this is a common occurrence after retrobulbar block.
    D. None of the above.

The correct answer is C. Amaurosis, or temporary painless vision loss, may occur with retrobulbar injections due to the optic nerve becoming blocked. Patients should be warned of the possibility of loss of light perception, especially if the block is on the only functioning eye, and also be reassured that even if light perception is retained, it does not imply that the block is not working.

The ophthalmologist returns and reassures the patient that temporary vision loss is normal after a retrobulbar block, and after another dose of midazolam IV, the patient relaxes and the incision is made.

The surgery on the right eye takes only 15 min, and the patient still appears to be sedated and comfortable. Therefore, the surgeon begins to perform a block on the left eye. During injection, you hear the patient clear his throat and move slightly, but the surgeon proceeds to completely administer the LA. Drapes are subsequently applied and the surgeon starts to look through the microscope. He notices minimal venous bleeding, states that the patient has a retrobulbar hemorrhage likely due to patient movement, and aborts the surgery and applies a pressure dressing on the eye.

5. What are possible *acute* consequences of a retrobulbar hemorrhage?

 A. Increased intraocular pressure.
 B. Central retinal artery occlusion.
 C. Optic nerve atrophy.
 D. Both A and B.

The correct answer is D. Retrobulbar hemorrhage is the most common complication associated with performing a retrobulbar block. It is usually venous in origin, but can be arterial and can manifest as proptosis, ecchymosis, chemosis, or increased intraocular pressure. Optic nerve atrophy may also present later as microvasculature of the optic nerves becomes occluded. A hematoma can lead to central retinal artery occlusion. Various patient-related risk factors for retrobulbar hemorrhage include older age, history of anticoagulant or nonsteroidal anti-inflammatory drug use, preexisting coagulopathy, previous eye surgery, and pathology of the globe such as extreme myopia. Extreme myopia also poses the risk for ocular penetration/globe perforation. The experience of the individual performing the block is an important factor in minimizing the risk of retrobulbar hemorrhage, and management can range from conservative treatment (ocular massage) to surgical intervention (canthotomy/cantholysis), as needed.

DID YOU LEARN?

- Complications associated with retrobulbar blocks.
- Mechanism and management of the oculocardiac reflex.
- Risk factors and consequences of retrobulbar hemorrhage.

Recommended Readings

Butterworth IV JF, Mackey DC, Wasnick JD, eds. Anesthesia for ophthalmic surgery. In: *Morgan & Mikhail's Clinical Anesthesiology.* 6th ed. New York, NY: McGraw-Hill Education; 2018:773-786.

Cote CJ, Lerman J, Anderson B, eds. *A Practice of Anesthesia for Infants and Children,* 5th ed. Philadelphia, PA: Saunders Elsevier; 2013:688-89.

CHAPTER 32

Anesthesia for Otolaryngology– Head & Neck Surgery

CASE 1	Young Woman Scheduled for Subtotal Thyroidectomy

Gang Zheng, MD

A 28-year-old woman with a history of hyperthyroidism presents for subtotal thyroidectomy. She discontinued her oral antithyroid therapy 2 years ago, and 1 month ago, she developed dysphagia and hoarseness. She denies any other major medical or surgical problems. There are no signs of hyperthyroidism after completion of 8 weeks of methimazole (MMI) therapy. Her serum T_3 and T_4 are normal with a low serum thyroid-stimulating hormone (TSH). She just completed 7 days of oral potassium iodide (SSKI) in preparation for her thyroidectomy. The patient is cachectic with an enlarged and mobile thyroid gland and Graves ophthalmopathy. Her airway examination is normal other than an enlarged neck circumference. The heart rate is 68 beats/min and regular, and the remainder of her physical examination is unremarkable. ECG reveals normal sinus rhythm.

1. Which of the following is a correct statement regarding perioperative management of a hyperthyroid patient?

   A. A suppressed value of TSH is *not* an indication to postpone the surgery as long as T_3 and T_4 are normal.
   B. Since SSKI has antithyroid properties, other antithyroid agents, such as MMI or propylthiouracil (PTU), should be discontinued after initiating SSKI therapy.
   C. Should emergency surgery be necessary in the setting of uncontrolled hyperthyroidism, PTU and MMI have no therapeutic value.
   D. Thyroid storm is primarily a laboratory diagnosis suggested by markedly elevated serum T_4 and T_3 values.

The correct answer is A. Normal TSH is not always achieved after 8 weeks of therapy, especially in a patient with prolonged hyperthyroidism; as long as T_3 and T_4 are normalized, surgery may proceed. All antithyroid agents should be continued until the morning of surgery due to their relatively short half-lives. Even with short-term use, oral antithyroid drugs still have therapeutic value during emergency surgery through inhibition of peripheral deiodination of T_4 and T_3, and they may be given via nasogastric tube during the surgical procedure. The diagnosis and treatment of thyroid storm are primarily based upon clinical findings, and there are no definitive T_3 and T_4 values indicative of this diagnosis.

2. All of the following regarding the patient's intraoperative management are correct *except*:

   A. A patient with hyperthyroidism is susceptible to exaggerated sympathetic nervous system responses during anesthetic induction.
   B. A hyperthyroid patient may develop muscle disease, resulting in reduced requirement for nondepolarizing muscle relaxant.
   C. A patient with hyperthyroidism does not typically exhibit increased volatile anesthetic requirement.
   D. Thyroid storm often presents with bradycardia and hypertension.

The correct answer is D. Tachyarrhythmias and marked increases in cardiac output during thyroid storm can quickly progress to cardiovascular collapse and shock. *Hypotension*, but not hypertension, is a major clinical sign of thyroid storm. Maintaining adequate anesthetic depth is important during surgery in order to avoid exaggerated sympathetic nervous system (SNS) response, and drugs that stimulate the SNS should be used with great caution. Hyperthyroid patients commonly develop muscle weakness and muscle wasting secondary to thyrotoxic myopathy (hyperthyroid myopathy), and thereby exhibit reduced nondepolarizing muscle relaxant requirement. Hyperthyroid patients usually do not have increased volatile anesthetic requirements.

3. The patient is extubated after meeting criteria for tracheal extubation and immediately develops respiratory stridor. Each of the following is included in the differential diagnosis of postextubation respiratory stridor *except*:

   A. Laryngospasm.
   B. Paradoxical vocal cord movement.
   C. Bilateral superior laryngeal nerve injury.
   D. Bilateral recurrent laryngeal nerve injury.

The correct answer is C. The superior laryngeal nerve (SLN), a branch of the vagus nerve, supplies a motor branch (the external branch of the SLN) to the cricothyroid muscle, which tenses the vocal cords and aids in phonation. Bilateral SLN injury causes voice fatigue and altered voice pitch, but not respiratory stridor.

Paradoxical vocal cord movement is episodic vocal cord dysfunction caused by inappropriate vocal cord closure. Respiratory strider is a common symptom, and this condition may mimic asthma. The patient may quickly develop signs of hypoxia following tracheal extubation. Reassurance, slow deep breathing, and a small dose of midazolam often control the symptoms. The recurrent laryngeal nerve (RLN) controls vocal cord abduction and adduction, and the patient with bilateral RLN injury will develop respiratory stridor. Immediate tracheal reintubation is indicated in this situation.

DID YOU LEARN?

- In the perioperative management of the hyperthyroid patient, it is very important to continue antithyroid medications until the day of surgery. Even short-term use of antithyroid medications for emergent surgery is useful.
- TSH normalization is often delayed following T_3 and T_4 correction, and a suppressed TSH alone should not be an indication for delaying surgery.
- Thyroid storm is a clinical diagnosis, and the treatment should be based upon clinical findings.
- Anticholinergic and β-agonist medications may induce exaggerated cardiac responses in hyperthyroid patients.
- The differential diagnosis and treatment of postextubation respiratory stridor.

Recommended Readings

Farling PA. Thyroid disease. *Br. J Anesth.* 2000;85:15-28.
Furman WR, Robertson AC. Anesthesia for patients with thyroid disease and for patients who undergo thyroid or parathyroid surgery. https://www.uptodate.com/contents/anesthesia-for-patients-with-thyroid-disease-and-for-patients-who-undergo-thyroid-or-parathyroid-surgery. Accessed June 17, 2019.
Malhotra S, Sodhi V. Anaesthesia for thyroid and parathyroid surgery. Continuing Education in Anaesthesia. *Crit Care Pain.* 2007;7:55-58.

CASE 2 — A 56-Year-Old Woman Scheduled for Parathyroidectomy

Gang Zheng, MD

You have been asked to see a 56-year-old, 72-kg woman scheduled for parathyroidectomy. She previously had been in good health with no prior surgical history and now presents with somnolence, abdominal pain, polyuria, and mood swings. She takes no medication with exception of occasional oral hydrocodone for abdominal cramping. Physical examination reveals blood pressure 155/95 mm Hg and mild, generalized hypotonia. Laboratory findings reveal hemoglobin of 9 g/dL and a total serum calcium concentration of 13.5 mg/dL.

1. All of the following may commonly be present in a patient with hyperparathyroidism *except*:

   A. Polydipsia.
   B. Nausea and vomiting.
   C. Shortened PR interval and prolonged QT interval on ECG.
   D. Renal insufficiency.

The correct answer is C. Polydipsia, nausea, and vomiting are the common characteristics of symptomatic hypercalcemia, usually seen in patients with a total serum calcium concentration ≥12 mg/dL. Patients who are clinically symptomatic also often present with multiple organ involvement. Some of the common anesthetic-related issues include dehydration, hyperchloremic metabolic acidosis, generalized muscle weakness, and ECG changes (*prolonged* PR and *shortened* QT intervals). These patients will need to be medically managed to decrease their hypercalcemia and improve their overall medical condition. Persistent hypercalcemia promotes urolithiasis and hinders urine concentration ability. However, hyperparathyroid patients often present with asymptomatic hypercalcemia found via routine laboratory studies. Asymptomatic patients usually do not need treatment for their hypercalcemia prior to parathyroidectomy.

You decide to treat your patient's hypercalcemia preoperatively with intravascular saline and a loop diuretic. You begin with an infusion of 1 L of normal saline over the next hour, to be followed with an initial dose of furosemide 20 mg intravenously.

2. All of the following are correct statements regarding this patient's volume status and fluid diuresis therapy, *except*:

   A. The major reasons for intravascular volume depletion in cases of hypercalcemia are vomiting, polyuria, and urinary sodium loss.
   B. Loop diuretics can be added to the regimen after the patient's volume status is corrected.
   C. Thiazide diuretics can be added to the regimen after patient's volume status is corrected.
   D. Bisphosphonates can be used for life-threatening hypercalcemia.

The correct answer is C. Thiazide diuretics increase calcium reabsorption in the distal renal tubule and thus are not used to treat hypercalcemia. The major reasons for hypercalcemia-related intravascular volume depletion are vomiting, polyuria, and urinary sodium loss, and the purpose of normal saline intravenous infusion in patients with normal cardiac function is both restoration of normal intravascular volume and promotion of diuresis-induced urinary calcium excretion. Serum electrolytes must be carefully monitored during intravascular saline and diuretic therapy because serum potassium, chloride, and magnesium levels may fall along with the serum calcium level. Loop diuretics promote urinary excretion of calcium along with electrolytes and water, but should be administered only after adequate intravascular volume and urine output have been restored. Bisphosphonates are potent inhibitors of osteoclast activity and thus are commonly used to treat pronounced hypercalcemia, especially hypercalcemia of malignancy.

3. You are concerned about possible postoperative complications related to parathyroid surgery. The signs and symptoms of acute hypocalcemia after parathyroid surgery include all of the followings *except*:

   A. Positive Chvostek's sign or Trousseau's sign.
   B. Hoarseness.
   C. Inspiratory stridor.
   D. Perioral paresthesias.

The correct answer is B. Hoarseness without respiratory stridor indicates unilateral recurrent laryngeal nerve injury. Hypocalcemia following parathyroid surgery is a major postoperative complication. Although parathyroid hormone has a short half-life (1–3 min), the symptoms of hypoparathyroidism usually take several hours or longer to develop (typically, 1–2 days following surgery). Unless all parathyroid glands are removed, impaired blood supply to remaining parathyroid gland(s) is the principal cause of postoperative hypoparathyroidism and hypocalcemia. Most of such hypocalcemia is clinically silent; however, acute, symptomatic hypocalcemia may require urgent treatment. Patients with symptomatic hypocalcemia often present with perioral paresthesias, and a positive Chvostek's sign (ipsilateral contraction of facial muscles following gentle percussion over facial nerve) and Trousseau's sign (carpal spasm induced by ischemia induced with a blood pressure cuff or a tourniquet) are typical findings with bedside examination.

Although it is uncommon, transient impairment of speech and/or inspiratory stridor may present in the patient with severe hypocalcemia due to irritability of intrinsic laryngeal muscles. This should not be confused with hoarseness. Intravenous calcium should be administered to acutely symptomatic hyperparathyroid patients; otherwise, oral calcium supplementation is sufficient. Inspiratory stridor induced by *paradoxical vocal cord dysfunction*, in which the vocal cords close during inhalation, may mimic the effects of severe hypocalcemia; however, in the former situation, other signs of hypocalcemia, such as Chvostek's sign or Trousseau's sign, are absent. This condition is often related to anxiety and may be treated with reassurance and/or a benzodiazepine.

DID YOU LEARN?

- Hypercalcemia is the primary cause of clinical symptoms in a patient with hyperparathyroidism, but most hyperparathyroid patients have a silent clinical course.
- Surgery need not be postponed in cases of asymptomatic hypercalcemia; patients with symptomatic hypercalcemia should be medically optimized prior to surgery.
- Hydration with intravenous normal saline to restore intravascular volume followed by an intravenous loop diuretic is sufficient to manage symptomatic, but not life-threatening, hypercalcemia.
- Postoperative hypocalcemia is a common problem after parathyroid surgery.
- Oral calcium therapy is adequate for patients with asymptomatic hypocalcemia.
- Intravenous calcium should be administered to patients who present with signs or symptoms of hypocalcemia.

Recommended Readings

Butterworth IV JF, Mackey DC, Wasnick JD, eds. Anesthesia for Otolaryngology–Head and Neck Surgery. In: *Morgan & Mikhail's Clinical Anesthesiology*. 6th ed. New York, NY: McGraw-Hill Education; 2018:787-802.

Hagberg CA. *Benumof's Airway Management: Principles and Practice*, 2nd ed. St. Louis, MO: Mosby; 2007:1154.

Hines RL, Marschall KE. *Anesthesia and Co-existing Disease*, 7th ed. New York, NY: Elsevier; 2017.

Silva BC, Cusano NE, Bilezikian JP. Primary hyperparathyroidism. *Best Pract Res Clin Endocrinol Metab*. 2018;32(5):593-607.

CHAPTER 33

Anesthesia for Orthopedic Surgery

| CASE 1 | Total Shoulder Arthroplasty |

Ryan Derby, MD, MPH, and Edward R. Mariano, MD, MAS

You are the anesthesiologist for a neurologically intact 72-year-old ASA III woman, 70 kg, with a history of severe osteoarthritis of her left shoulder, essential hypertension treated with lisinopril, and remote history of transient ischemic attack (TIA), who is scheduled to undergo a left total shoulder arthroplasty in the beach chair position (BCP). Preinduction vital signs are noninvasive blood pressure (NIBP) 165/75 mm Hg, mean arterial pressure (MAP) 105 mm Hg, heart rate (HR) 75 beats/min, oxygen saturation (SpO$_2$) 97%, and respiratory rate 14 breaths/min. An interscalene block with perineural catheter placement is performed prior to surgery. Prior to induction of general anesthesia, the primary surgeon requests "controlled hypotension" during the operation. Specifically, the surgeon requests that you reduce the patient's blood pressure during surgery to a MAP of 55 mm Hg to minimize blood loss. After uneventful induction and intubation with standard ASA monitors, including NIBP on her right arm, and following placement of the patient in the BCP, her vital signs are now NIBP 100/40 mm Hg (MAP 60 mm Hg), HR 82 beats/min, SpO$_2$ 100%, and respiratory rate 12 breaths/min.

1. Your next action is to:

   A. Begin a nitroglycerine infusion with a MAP goal of 55 mm Hg.
   B. Increase your volatile anesthetic concentration.
   C. Administer 500 mL of 5% dextrose in water solution.
   D. Administer phenylephrine 100 μg intravenously (IV) with an explanation to the surgeon.

The correct answer is D. The measured NIBP on the right arm may grossly overestimate the cerebral perfusion pressure, and this patient is also at risk of malperfusion because of her history of TIA. The most appropriate immediate step is to raise her blood pressure in order to optimize cerebral perfusion.

BCP for shoulder surgery has been associated with decreases in cerebral oxygen saturation of over 20% in up to 80% of patients. Stroke, blindness, brain death, or other severe neurological dysfunction after surgery in the BCP have been reported, highlighting the need to accurately measure the blood pressure at the level of the brain. Although hypotension and decreases in cerebral perfusion are common, catastrophic neurological morbidity after BCP is infrequent and poorly defined. However, this does not diminish the need for careful attention to blood pressure monitoring.

Evidence suggests that the lower limit of cerebral autoregulation pressure in awake, supine, normotensive patients ranges from a MAP of 57 to 91 mm Hg, with the lower limit generally estimated to be 70 mm Hg. Blood pressure measured in the arm may overestimate cerebral perfusion pressure due to the difference in pressures between the brain and blood pressure measurement sites at different heights attributable to gravity. The difference in blood pressure (mm Hg) is equal to the height of a column of water (cm H_2O) multiplied by a conversion factor (1 cm H_2O = 0.74 mm Hg). Because there may be large differences in the measured blood pressure and actual cerebral perfusion pressure, it is important to account for this difference in measurements, especially for this patient who is at risk for cerebral ischemia. Furthermore, the cerebral autoregulation curve is shifted to the right in patients with chronic arterial hypertension. In these patients, cerebral blood flow is dependent on higher arterial pressure relative to the average patient; therefore, a MAP of 60 mm Hg measured by NIBP at the arm level may be well below the lower limit of autoregulation and may be too low to adequately perfuse this patient's brain.

The risk of neurological adverse outcomes associated with BCP may be minimized by avoiding general anesthesia, performing surgery in the lateral decubitus position, using regional anesthesia techniques such as interscalene blocks and lower extremity sequential compression devices, and maintaining a MAP >70 mm Hg. Additionally, NIBP should be measured on the upper arm and not on the leg, and an arterial line is recommended in high-risk patients warranting more precise monitoring; when used, the arterial line transducer should be zeroed at the level of the patient's external auditory meatus, which approximates the level of the circle of Willis.

You explain to the surgeon why this patient requires maintenance of a higher MAP during surgery and are able to achieve a MAP of 75 mm Hg as measured by NIBP using intermittent phenylephrine boluses and initiation of a phenylephrine infusion. The surgeon asks you how to best monitor this patient in order to ensure adequate cerebral perfusion and avoid postoperative neurological complications.

2. You explain that the best monitoring strategy is:

A. Invasive blood pressure monitoring with the transducer leveled at the patient's external auditory meatus.
B. Invasive blood pressure monitoring with the transducer leveled at the patient's heart.
C. Twelve-lead electroencephalogram (EEG) to assess for hemispheric ischemia.
D. Monitoring of jugular venous bulb pressures.
E. No one monitor has been shown to be superior to others in preventing postoperative neurological complications.

The correct answer is E. All of these modalities have been used to monitor for cerebral ischemia, but no single modality has effectively prevented gross neurological injury after surgery in the BCP.

Cerebral oximetry, 12-lead EEG, and jugular venous bulb pressure monitoring have all shown utility in detecting a decrease in cerebral perfusion or hemispheric ischemia. However, decreases in cerebral saturation have not necessarily correlated with long-term adverse neurological outcomes. Invasive blood pressure monitoring allows for tighter control of systemic blood pressure with vasoactive medications and is indicated when closer monitoring of blood pressure is required (eg, controlled hypotension) or for a patient who is at particularly high risk for cerebral ischemia. In these instances, measuring arterial blood pressure at the level of the external auditory meatus is most appropriate.

As the surgeon is closing, she remarks that the patient was able to move her fourth and fifth digits prior to induction, despite more than 30 min having elapsed since the interscalene block was placed using 20 mL of 1.5% mepivacaine. She is concerned that the patient will have a "patchy" block postoperatively with inadequate pain control and requests that you replace the catheter while the patient is still under general anesthesia.

3. Your next step is to:

A. Keep the catheter and assess the patient in the postanesthesia care unit (PACU).
B. Discontinue the interscalene catheter and replace it prior to emergence.
C. Discontinue the interscalene catheter and order hydromorphone patient-controlled analgesia (PCA).
D. Discontinue the catheter and replace it with an axillary perineural catheter.

The correct answer is A. Sparing in the distribution of C8 and T1 is an expected finding with interscalene blocks and does not indicate a failed or patchy block in this patient. The best approach is to assess pain in the PACU following emergence from general anesthesia. This is true even if the intraoperative physiological response to surgical stimulation suggests that the block may not completely cover the surgical site.

Interscalene brachial plexus blocks are often used for shoulder surgery. Interscalene blocks are performed at the level of the nerve roots and trunks and frequently spare C8 and T1. Sparing of the C8 and T1 nerve roots results in preserved neurological function of peripheral nerves derived from them, including the ulnar nerve. It is important to include brachial plexus blockade and perineural catheter placement in the analgesic regimen for total shoulder arthroplasty, as they can improve shoulder range of motion with physical therapy the day after surgery in addition to providing profound pain relief. An axillary block is inadequate for shoulder analgesia because it is too distal in the brachial plexus, missing blockade of the suprascapular and axillary nerves.

Although the performance of peripheral nerve block procedures in patients under general anesthesia is often debated, we suggest that this practice be used only in those circumstances where benefits clearly outweigh risks (eg, pediatric patients). Our caution arises from case reports of catastrophic nerve injury and even paraplegia from interscalene blocks performed under general anesthesia; however, these case reports uniformly describe poor technique in performing the block. If replacing the interscalene catheter is warranted in this patient, the appropriate time to perform it is when the patient is sufficiently awake to be able to participate in the procedure.

On postoperative day (POD) 2, the interscalene catheter is discontinued; on POD 4, the patient remarks that she has uncomfortable numbness and tingling in her left thumb, index, and middle fingers on the operative side. The surgeon asks you to evaluate and treat the patient for nerve block–related nerve injury.

4. Your next course of action is to:

A. Inform the surgeon that the injury is not due to the interscalene catheter.
B. Inform the surgeon that a persistent paresthesia likely represents a compressive hematoma that should be explored emergently.
C. Perform a physical exam of the affected areas and reassure the patient.
D. Immediately request a neurology consultation.

The correct answer is C. The most appropriate course of action when faced with this issue is to carefully examine and document all neurological deficits, continue to monitor the deficit to ensure that it does not worsen or progress to include motor dysfunction, and reassure the patient that the majority of neurological symptoms improve with time.

There are many causes of perioperative neurological symptoms, including patient factors and factors related to both surgery and anesthesia. Indeed, symptoms of postoperative median nerve compression at the carpal tunnel that disappear over a period of days have been reported. Block-related nerve injury may result from direct needle trauma, intraneural injection, compressive hematoma, or the neurotoxic properties of local anesthetics. The incidence of block-related nerve injury is poorly defined, but estimated to be approximately 4 in 10,000 patients. The variation in incidence depends upon the specific block procedure performed, the approach, the needle type, and other issues. However, evidence suggests that the incidence of peripheral nerve injury in patients receiving a peripheral nerve block is no greater than in nonblock patients. General anesthesia alone, younger age, and American Society of Anesthesiologists (ASA) physical status less than III are associated with higher incidence of peripheral nerve injury. The large majority of block-related paresthesias resolve within 6 months with conservative treatment. Surgery-related nerve injury can also occur, and the etiology may include one or more of the following: direct nerve damage during surgical dissection, compression or stretch from retractors or hematomas, vascular injury, humeral shaft fractures, and cement extrusion. The incidence of surgical procedure-related nerve injury has been estimated at anywhere between 1% and 4.3%, with reverse shoulder replacements (when the plastic cup or socket is fixed to the proximal humerus and the ball is fixed to the glenoid) associated with a greater incidence.

It is important to identify emergent scenarios, such as a compressive hematoma, which may imminently threaten limb function. Nerve injury requiring immediate evaluation and intervention should be suspected whenever sensory or motor function or a dysesthesia progressively worsens. When symptoms or physical signs suggest severe injury or when there is no improvement in neurological function, a neurology or neurosurgery consultation may be warranted, with nerve conduction studies, electromyography, and even consideration for surgical repair.

DID YOU LEARN?

- Effects of BCP on cerebral perfusion and intraoperative management considerations.
- Different methods of monitoring cerebral oxygen saturation and their ability to predict postoperative cognitive sequela.
- Appropriate regional anesthesia block for coverage of shoulder surgery.
- Appropriate evaluation of postoperative neuropathy.

Recommended Readings

Butterworth IV JF, Mackey DC, Wasnick JD, eds. Cardiovascular monitoring. In: *Morgan & Mikhail's Clinical Anesthesiology*. 6th ed. New York, NY: McGraw-Hill Education; 2018:81-118.

Butterworth IV JF, Mackey DC, Wasnick JD, eds. Noncardiovascular monitoring. In: *Morgan & Mikhail's Clinical Anesthesiology*. 6th ed. New York, NY: McGraw-Hill Education; 2018:119-138.

Mariano ER. Anesthesia for orthopedic surgery. In: Butterworth IV JF, Mackey DC, Wasnick JD, eds. *Morgan & Mikhail's Clinical Anesthesiology*. 6th ed. New York, NY: McGraw-Hill; 2018:803-818.

References

Barrington MJ, Watts SA, Jamrozik K, et al. Preliminary results of the Australasian Regional Anaesthesia Collaboration: A prospective audit of more than 7000 peripheral nerve and plexus blocks for neurologic and other complications. *Reg Anesth Pain Med.* 2009;34(6):534-541.

Ilfeld BM, Morey TE, et al. Joint range of motion after total shoulder arthroplasty with and without a continuous interscalene nerve block: A retrospective, case-controlled study. *Reg Anesth Pain Med.* 2005;30(5):429-433.

Kwak HJ, Lee D, Lee YW, et al. The intermittent sequential compression device on the lower extremities attenuates the decrease in regional cerebral oxygen saturation during sitting position under sevoflurane anesthesia. *J Neurosurg Anesthesiol.* 2011;23:1-5.

Ladermann A, Lubbeke A, Melis B, et al. Prevalence of neurologic lesions after total shoulder arthroplasty. *J Bone Joint Surg Am.* 2011;93(14):1288-1293.

Murphy GS, Greenberg SB, Szokol JW. Safety of beach chair position shoulder surgery: A review of the current literature. *Anesth Analg.* 2019;129:101-118.

Neal JM, Barrington MJ, Brull R, et al. The second ASRA Practice Advisory on neurologic complications associated with regional anesthesia and pain medicine: Executive summary 2015. *Reg Anesth Pain Med.* 2015;40(5):401-430.

Rohrbaugh M, Kentor ML, Orebaugh SL, Williams B. Outcomes of shoulder surgery in the sitting position with interscalene nerve block: A single-center series. *Reg Anesth Pain Med.* 2013;38:28-33.

Songy CE, Siegel ER, Stevens M, et al. The effect of the beach-chair position angle on cerebral oxygenation during shoulder surgery. *J Shoulder Elbow Surg.* 2017;26(9):1670-1675.

Yajnik M, Kou A, Mudumbai SC, et al. Peripheral nerve blocks are not associated with increased risk of perioperative peripheral nerve injury in a Veterans Affairs inpatient surgical population. *Reg Anesth Pain Med.* 2019;44(1):81-85.

CASE 2   Hip Fracture in a Patient with Dementia

Ryan Derby, MD, MPH, and Edward R. Mariano, MD, MAS

You are called to evaluate a confused 70-year-old fisherman in the emergency department for urgent fixation of an intertrochanteric hip fracture sustained when he slipped while hauling in his net. He denies any loss of consciousness or other injuries with the fall. He has not seen a physician in over 30 years and claims that he is "healthy as a whale" with no medical problems. He states that he has been in his normal state of health but has been "feeling his age of late" and moving slower than usual. He is oriented to person but incorrectly answers that the year is 1976 and that he is at the wharf. He denies chest pain, shortness of breath, and orthostasis, but he endorses mild dyspnea with exertion. His vital signs are NIBP 170/80 mm Hg, MAP 110 mm Hg, HR 95 beats/min, SpO$_2$ 97%, respiratory rate 14 breaths/min, and verbal pain score 7 out of 10 (10 being the worst possible pain). An electrocardiogram (ECG) reveals normal sinus rhythm with left atrial enlargement. Physical exam is pertinent for the following: he appears older than his stated age and is in moderate discomfort; airway exam shows intact dentition,

Mallampati II classification, and full cervical range of motion; pulmonary examination is normal, and cardiac exam reveals a strong pulse with regular rhythm and a grade IV/VI systolic ejection murmur at the right upper sternal border. The surgeon would like to proceed as soon as possible to the operating room for definitive treatment of the fracture with intramedullary nailing of the femur. However, when you interview the patient, he refuses to have the surgery, stating he does not understand why he needs it.

1. Your first course of action is to:

   A. Proceed to the operating room because fixation of a hip fracture is emergent and associated with better outcomes.
   B. Ask for a psychiatry consult to formally evaluate the patient for competence.
   C. Perform your own assessment to determine whether the patient has the capacity to make an informed decision.
   D. Seek out the patient's next of kin as a surrogate decision maker.

The correct answer is C. Determining whether a patient is competent to make an informed medical decision is critical in balancing a patient's autonomy with protecting patients with impaired mental faculties from making harmful decisions regarding their medical care. This is often difficult to assess, and there are few formal practice guidelines. Furthermore, time does not always allow for judicial review or psychiatric evaluation of a patient's competence, so the anesthesiologist must frequently rely on his or her own assessment. The above scenario warrants an immediate assessment of the patient's competence, as he is refusing what seems to be reasonable care given the severity of his injury. Moreover, he is not oriented to place, time, or his circumstances. Because of the urgent (although not emergent) nature of this situation, it may not be reasonable to seek an official psychiatric or legal consultation, which could result in an unwarranted delay.

It is important to remember that a diagnosis of a psychiatric disorder does not necessarily indicate that a patient is incompetent. However, some mental disorders such as acute schizophrenia and severe depression have been associated with a reduction in at least one element of decision making in nearly 50% of patients.

Standards for legal competence vary but generally agree that a competent person should be able to perform the following:

1. Communicate a decision.
2. Understand the relevant information.
3. Appreciate the situation and its consequences.
4. Reason through alternatives.

If the anesthesia provider deems a patient to be incompetent based on the above criteria, a surrogate decision maker or advanced directive must be identified. When a surrogate decision maker or an advance directive is not available to clarify the patient's wishes, states give decision-making powers to family members with the following typical order of priority: spouse, adult children, parents, siblings, and other relatives. In instances when these are not available and time permits, a court resolution should be sought.

Scores of less than 19 on the Mini Mental State Examination have also been associated with a high likelihood of incompetence, and scores greater than 23 are associated with competence. Other psychometric tests such as the MacArthur Competence Assessment Tool for Treatment have also been developed in attempting to standardize the assessment of a patient's decision-making capacity.

All efforts should be made to address any underlying causes of a patient's impaired decision-making capacity.

2. You determine that the patient is incompetent to make medical decisions for himself based on his lack of orientation and inability to understand relevant information pertaining to his situation and the potential consequences. You are able to contact his wife and coordinate a detailed discussion of risks and benefits with the patient, his wife, and the surgeon; all parties agree to proceed with the surgery. The surgeon applauds your efforts to obtain informed consent and then asks if you are ready to proceed to the operating room. You respond:

   A. "We can proceed immediately now that we have consent."
   B. "We need to wait at least 6 h from the patient's last meal."
   C. "The patient cannot be safely taken to the operating room until his blood pressure is optimized and on stable medications."
   D. "I would like to get a bedside echocardiogram before proceeding."

The correct answer is D. Careful cardiac evaluation in patients undergoing non-cardiac surgery is essential. This is especially true in patients with preexisting cardiac disease or a poor history that is suggestive of underlying disease. Cardiovascular complications account for up to 50% of deaths following noncardiac surgery and are closely related to preexisting cardiac disease. Your patient's prominent murmur and vague symptoms of recent decrease in functional capacity are worrisome for undiagnosed aortic stenosis. He might also be having myocardial ischemia. The location of the murmur in the right upper sternal border is especially concerning for aortic stenosis, which, depending on its severity, will have an important impact on the type of anesthesia selected (general anesthesia versus neuraxial) and the monitoring used (invasive arterial blood pressure, transesophageal echocardiography). Given that a better assessment of the patient's underlying cardiac disease may have important implications for the patient's prognosis, it is important to obtain thorough preoperative evaluation.

In general, the purpose of preoperative cardiac testing should be to determine whether the patient's condition can or should be further optimized prior to surgery. These criteria are different for elective versus emergent surgery. In emergent cases, preoperative testing may not be possible. For your patient who is in stable condition, while it is important to proceed to the operating room as expeditiously as possible, postponing the case until after cardiac evaluation is performed may help intra- and postoperative management. The American College of Cardiology (ACC), in collaboration with the American Heart Association (AHA), has created guidelines related to evaluation of patients with cardiac disease undergoing non-cardiac surgery that can help guide your decision to obtain preoperative cardiac evaluation. Active cardiac conditions identified by the ACC/AHA guidelines that are associated with major cardiac risk and warranting management prior to all elective surgeries include:

- Unstable coronary disease (myocardial infarction within 7 days, or within 1 month with myocardium at ongoing risk for ischemia; unstable angina).
- Decompensated heart failure.
- Significant arrhythmias.
- Severe valvular heart disease.

The ACC/AHA guidelines suggest a stepwise approach to preoperative evaluation and make the following recommendations:

- Patients in need of emergent surgery should proceed directly to the operating room.
- Patients with active cardiac disease (as identified above) should be evaluated by a cardiologist and treated according to ACC/AHA guidelines.
- Patients undergoing low-risk procedures should proceed to surgery.
- Patients with poor exercise tolerance (<4 metabolic equivalents) and no known risk factors should proceed to surgery.

Thus, your patient should receive at minimum a preoperative cardiac evaluation given his emergent need for surgery and history and physical examination findings compatible with an active cardiac condition. A bedside echocardiogram can be accomplished efficiently and interpreted either by a cardiologist or another appropriately trained physician. The purpose of the study is to determine the etiology of the patient's murmur. Clearly one would treat severe aortic stenosis quite differently from severe mitral regurgitation. The echocardiogram could also determine whether the patient has impaired systolic or diastolic ventricular function. The patient may have undiagnosed coronary artery disease (CAD). However, it would *not* be in this patient's interests for the team to delay open reduction and internal fixation of the hip fracture for a CAD workup. Stenting would only delay the surgery and require antiplatelet therapy, and there is no symptomatic indication for coronary bypass surgery. Multiple studies have associated worse outcomes with delays in repair of hip fractures.

A single elevated blood pressure reading without a history of hypertension and in the setting of other causes, such as pain, does not warrant postponing surgery when urgent fracture fixation is necessary. Similarly, although NPO status is important and should be observed, it is not the most important reason for postponing surgery in this case.

The bedside echocardiogram reveals mild-to-moderate aortic stenosis with a valve area of 1.5 cm^2, concentric left ventricular hypertrophy, no evidence of wall motion abnormalities, and mildly decreased ejection fraction of 45%. Immediately prior to going to the operating room, you review the medications administered to the patient and see that he received low-molecular-weight heparin (LMWH) 30 mg subcutaneously in the emergency department.

3. You decide to:

    A. Continue with your plan for spinal anesthesia.

    B. Postpone surgery for 11 h until it is safe to perform neuraxial anesthesia.

    C. Perform general anesthesia.

    D. Obtain STAT coagulation studies (partial thromboplastin time [PTT] and prothrombin time [PT]/international normalized ratio [INR]) and proceed with neuraxial anesthesia only if they are normal.

The correct answer is C. Hemorrhagic complications following spinal or epidural anesthesia are exceedingly rare but potentially catastrophic. The incidence of spinal hematoma is estimated to be 1 in 220,000 spinal anesthetics but may be higher for epidural anesthetics, especially given the increase in routine use of novel anticoagulants for both inpatients and those presenting for elective surgery. Thus, it is important to weigh the risks of hemorrhagic complications with the potential benefits that neuraxial anesthesia provides. The American Society of Regional Anesthesia and Pain Medicine (ASRA) has published guidelines for the use of neuraxial regional anesthesia in the patient receiving antithrombotic therapy and has also published a smartphone app for such guidance. These consensus guidelines are based on the best available evidence accumulated by experts in the field and are reviewed periodically to address new data and emerging trends in anticoagulation use.

Although the incidence of spinal hematoma is estimated to be low, an increase in complications following the introduction of LMWH in the United States in 1993 spurred a close examination of neuraxial practices in this setting. Many of these cases involved intraoperative or early postoperative administration of LMWH and concomitant antiplatelet therapy. Other factors associated with risk of spinal hematoma include increasing patient age and spinal cord abnormalities such as spinal stenosis, preexisting coagulopathy, difficult or traumatic needle placement, and placement of an indwelling catheter, especially in the presence of ongoing anticoagulation. Hemorrhage occurs most frequently in the epidural space, most likely because of the prominent epidural venous plexus, which explains why epidural catheter removal in the presence anticoagulation may also be associated with an increased risk of bleeding complications.

LMWH differs pharmacologically from unfractionated heparin and therefore requires different considerations. Importantly, LMWH has a prolonged half-life, is not reversible by protamine, and lacks a monitor for its anticoagulant effect. Plasma concentrations are increased in patients with kidney disease.

Current ASRA consensus guidelines regarding the management of patients undergoing spinal or epidural anesthesia while receiving perioperative LMWH include the following:

- Needle placement should occur 10 to 12 h after last LMWH dose for patients who receive once-daily dosing.
- In patients receiving a larger or more frequent dose than once per day, needling should be delayed at least 24 h to ensure normal hemostasis.

- Patients receiving LMWH 2 h prior to surgery for deep venous thrombosis prophylaxis should not receive neuraxial anesthesia, as this is the time of peak anticoagulation activity.
- In patients receiving twice-daily postoperative dosing, the first administration should be delayed at least 24 h after surgery, and any indwelling catheters should be discontinued prior to first dose.
- Administration of LMWH should be delayed at least 2 h after removal of indwelling catheters.
- In patients receiving once-daily postoperative dosing, indwelling neuraxial catheters may safely be maintained; however, they should be removed no earlier than 10 h after the last dose of LMWH.
- The presence of blood during spinal or epidural placement does not necessitate cancelling the surgery; however, the first dose of LMWH should be given at least 24 h after needling.

Our patient's last dose of LMWH was <10 h prior, which falls outside ASRA guidelines. It is therefore unacceptable to proceed with a spinal anesthetic based on coagulation issues, particularly in a patient with moderate aortic stenosis and dementia.

The patient is scheduled as the first case of the day, and you successfully perform a general anesthetic; intraoperatively, you maintain a total intravenous anesthetic with propofol and ketamine infusions. The surgery is completed uneventfully, and your patient is transferred to the postanesthesia care unit for recovery in stable condition. You are called back to evaluate the patient for severe pain and elect to insert an epidural catheter 15 h after his last dose of enoxaparin to provide regional analgesia consistent with your hospital's enhanced recovery pathway. The next morning, once-daily dosing of LMWH is initiated. The following morning, you round on your patient and find him lying comfortably in bed. The patient complains of mild hip pain and remarks that he has been unable to get up to use the restroom because his legs continue to be weak. Otherwise, he has no complaints.

4. Your next move is to:

A. Prescribe a nonsteroidal anti-inflammatory for his back pain.
B. Increase his IV dose of PRN hydromorphone for improved analgesia.
C. Encourage the patient to ambulate to decrease his risk of thromboembolic events.
D. Order a STAT magnetic resonance image (MRI) of his lumbar spine.

The correct answer is D. Arguably, the most catastrophic complication from a lumbar puncture is spinal hemorrhage resulting in permanent neuronal injury and paralysis. The incidence of spinal hematoma has been estimated to be 1 in 220,000 spinal and 1 in 150,000 epidural anesthetics. These numbers, calculated from large retrospective analyses by Tryba and colleagues in 1993, likely underestimate the overall incidence; the true incidence today may be higher in the setting of more routine use of novel anticoagulants in the perioperative period.

Spinal hematomas are associated with increased age, epidural placement, preexisting or iatrogenic coagulopathies, traumatic needling, and early initiation of deep venous thrombosis prophylaxis such as LMWH.

The classic presentation of a spinal hematoma includes sharp radiating radicular pain in the back, worsening motor and sensory weakness that lasts longer than the expected neuraxial block duration, and urinary retention. In a closed-claims analysis of neuraxial complications, however, the majority of patients presented with motor weakness, whereas fewer complained of back pain as a presenting symptom. Thus, any such patient with progressive weakness should prompt an immediate workup for spinal hematoma, even when back pain is absent. Closed-claims analysis has shown that, although symptoms are often reported within the first postoperative day, more than 24 h may often elapse prior to actual diagnosis.

Finally, neuraxial recovery likely is only possible with prompt diagnosis and treatment with emergent laminectomy and evacuation of hematoma. While only 38% of patients report good or partial recovery from spinal hematoma, spinal cord ischemia tends to be reversible if treatment occurs within 8 h of onset of neurological symptoms. The poorest outcomes are seen when treatment occurs more than 24 h after initial symptoms.

Thus, the appropriate management of this patient with prolonged lower extremity weakness in the setting of neuraxial block and LMWH prophylaxis is immediate radiographic imaging (MRI or computed tomography) to evaluate for an epidural hematoma and to notify the neurosurgical team and operating room staff to be on standby for prompt surgical treatment if warranted.

DID YOU LEARN?

- How to appropriately assess and obtain informed consent from a patient with an abnormal mental status.
- The preoperative evaluation and management of the patient with a newly recognized cardiac murmur.
- The ASRA guidelines for the use of neuraxial anesthesia in patients receiving LMWH.
- The evaluation and management of a potential epidural hematoma.

Recommended Readings

Butterworth IV JF, Mackey DC, Wasnick JD, eds. Anesthesia for patients with cardiovascular disease. In: *Morgan & Mikhail's Clinical Anesthesiology*. 6th ed. New York, NY: McGraw-Hill Education; 2018:381-440.

Butterworth IV JF, Mackey DC, Wasnick JD, eds. Preoperative assessment, premedication, & perioperative documentation. In: *Morgan & Mikhail's Clinical Anesthesiology*. 6th ed. New York, NY: McGraw-Hill Education; 2018:295-306.

Butterworth IV JF, Mackey DC, Wasnick JD, eds. Spinal, epidural, & caudal blocks. In: *Morgan & Mikhail's Clinical Anesthesiology*. 6th ed. New York, NY: McGraw-Hill Education; 2018:959-996.

Mariano ER. Anesthesia for orthopedic surgery. In: Butterworth IV JF, Mackey DC, Wasnick JD, eds. *Morgan and Mikhail's Clinical Anesthesiology*. 6th ed. New York, NY: McGraw-Hill; 2018:803-818.

References

Appelbaum PS. Assessment of patients' competence to consent to treatment. *N Engl J Med.* 2007;347:1834-1840.

Fleisher LA, Fleischmann KE, Auerbach AD, et al. 2014 ACC/AHA guideline on perioperative cardiovascular evaluation and management of patients undergoing noncardiac surgery: A report of the American College of Cardiology/American Heart Association Task Force on practice guidelines. *J Am Coll Cardiol.* 2014;64(22):e77-e137.

Grisso T, Appelbaum PS. *Assessing Competence to Consent to Treatment: A Guide for Physicians and Other Health Professionals.* New York, NY: Oxford University Press; 1998.

Horlocker TT, Vandermeulen E, Kopp SL, et al. Regional anesthesia in the patient receiving antithrombotic or thrombolytic therapy: American Society of Regional Anesthesia and Pain Medicine Evidence-Based Guidelines (Fourth Edition). *Reg Anesth Pain Med.* 2018;43(3):263-309.

Lee LA, Posner K, Domino KB, Caplan RA, Cheney FW. Injuries associated with regional anesthesia in the 1980's and 1990's. *Anesthesiology.* 2004;101:143-152.

Moen V, Dahlgren N, Irestedt L. Severe neurological complications after central neuraxial blockades in Sweden 1990-1999. *Anesthesiology.* 2004;101:950-959.

Nishimura RA, Otto CM, Bonow RO, et al. 2017 AHA/ACC focused update of the 2014 AHA/ACC guideline for the management of patients with valvular heart disease: A Report of the American College of Cardiology/American Heart Association Task Force on clinical practice guidelines. *J Am Coll Cardiol.* 2017;70(2):252-289.

Sturman ED. The capacity to consent to treatment and research: A review of standardized assessment tools. *Clin Psychol Rev.* 2005;25:954-974.

CASE 3 | Total Hip Arthroplasty with Fat Embolism

Ryan Derby, MD, MPH, and Edward R. Mariano, MD, MAS

An 88-year-old, 70-kg, ASA III man presents with a subcapital fracture of his right hip from a ground-level fall and is scheduled for a total hip arthroplasty. His vital signs are NIBP 115/75 mm Hg, HR 90 beats/min, SpO_2 90% on oxygen 4 L/min by nasal cannula, and respiratory rate 16 breaths/min, with 3/10 pain localized to his right hip. His medical history is significant for diabetes, hypertension treated with metoprolol, coronary artery disease (CAD) with prior myocardial infarction (MI), status post a remote coronary angioplasty now managed only with aspirin, and moderate functional capacity. Prior to his fall, he was able to walk on flat ground and climb two flights of stairs without shortness of breath or exertional dyspnea. Physical exam is unremarkable with the exception of signs related to his fracture. ECG reveals normal sinus rhythm with Q waves in the anterolateral leads. Transthoracic echocardiography demonstrates mild left ventricular hypertrophy, an ejection fraction of 45%, and no valvular abnormalities or evidence of pulmonary artery thrombus. Chest radiograph is normal, without evidence of fractured ribs, pleural effusion, or pneumothorax. Laboratory evaluation reveals hemoglobin 14 g/dL, platelet count 110,000, creatinine 0.8 mg/dL, fingerstick blood glucose 155 mg/dL, INR of 1.0, and no electrolyte abnormalities. He is comfortable and able to maneuver in his bed despite his injury. After reviewing his medical history and laboratory findings, you are asked by the patient to recommend the type of anesthesia that is associated with the fewest complications.

1. You recommend:

    A. Opioid-free general anesthesia with volatile anesthetics alone.
    B. General anesthesia with opioids and volatile anesthetics.
    C. Neuraxial anesthesia (spinal or combined spinal/epidural).
    D. Local anesthesia.

The correct answer is C. Elderly surgery patients undergoing total joint arthroplasty are at especially high risk for postoperative morbidity and warrant special attention to prevent and promptly address any complications. Local anesthesia is not a valid technique for this surgery. Neuraxial anesthesia has been shown to improve outcomes in patients undergoing elective total hip surgery when compared to general anesthesia alone, with decreases in 30-day mortality, intraoperative blood loss, deep venous thrombosis, pulmonary complications, non-MI cardiac-related complications, infection, and operative time. These advantages make neuraxial anesthesia, with or without general anesthesia, the preferred anesthetic technique for elective total hip and knee arthroplasty. However, patient comorbidities such as aortic stenosis, CAD, coagulopathy, electrolyte disorders, anemia, and hypovolemia, along with intraoperative concerns such as blood loss and procedural complexity and duration, must be thoroughly considered when contemplating anesthetic management options. The hip fracture patient population is difficult to study, and results from studies examining morbidity and mortality in this setting are inconclusive. Evidence suggests that neuraxial anesthesia may have advantages over general anesthesia when facilities regularly employ this technique for more than 20% to 25% of cases.

Hip fracture patients pose a special challenge and require thoughtful consideration of their comorbidities. Patients are usually elderly and commonly have comorbidities including CAD, chronic obstructive pulmonary disease (COPD), chronic heart failure, and diabetes. Additionally, they may present in a hypovolemic state—hemoconcentrated from poor oral intake or inadequate intravenous rehydration, but anemic from occult bleeding—and atelectatic from prolonged immobility. They may also suffer from other trauma-related issues such as fat embolism or deep venous thrombosis (DVT) with embolic disease. Fat embolism occurs more frequently in long bone fractures and may explain preoperative hypoxemia, heart failure, and/or right heart strain.

This patient is appropriate for a neuraxial anesthesia technique, as he does not have evidence of aortic stenosis, his coagulation status is acceptable, and he is able to comfortably position himself in the lateral decubitus position for administration of a spinal or epidural anesthetic. However, his relatively low SpO_2 with supplemental oxygen is concerning, so elective airway management prior to operation and mechanical ventilation throughout the procedure are recommended.

2. The anesthesiologist performing the case is concerned about the patient's relatively low SpO_2 with supplemental oxygen and asks you for the likely etiology and advice on how to manage it. You reply that the most likely explanation for the patient's increased supplemental oxygen requirement is:

    A. Fat embolism.
    B. Aspiration.
    C. COPD.
    D. Atelectasis.

The correct answer is A. Fat embolism is common in long bone fractures and generally presents as mild hypoxemia that may progress to fat embolism syndrome, a less frequent, but often fatal, condition. Treatment of fat embolism consists of supportive care and early fixation of the fracture in order to reduce the risk of additional embolism, fat embolism syndrome, and pulmonary complications. Supportive treatment includes supplemental oxygen and continuous positive airway pressure to prevent hypoxemia. This patient has mild hypoxemia but no signs of fat embolism syndrome; however, prompt fixation of his fracture is warranted. It would also be prudent to obtain an arterial blood gas in this patient to assess the severity of his hypoxemia. Aspiration is unlikely to have occurred as this patient did not experience any loss of consciousness or airway reflexes. COPD and atelectasis are potential causes of the patient's hypoxemia but unlikely to account for the clinical picture seen in a patient with no prior history or pertinent chest radiograph findings.

Fat embolism syndrome typically presents 72 h after long bone or pelvic fracture with the classic triad of dyspnea, confusion, and petechiae. The etiology is related to circulating fat globules released into the circulation through tears of the medullary vessels in the fractured bone. Increased blood free fatty acid levels have a direct toxic effect on the pulmonary capillary–alveolar membrane, leading to release of vasoactive amines and prostaglandins and resulting in systemic capillary damage. This may manifest as acute respiratory distress syndrome and/or as neurological symptoms such as stupor, confusion, agitation, or coma.

Diagnosis of fat embolism syndrome is suggested by the overall clinical scenario and by petechiae found on the axillae, conjunctiva, and upper chest. Coagulation abnormalities are occasionally present, and pulmonary involvement is suggested by severe hypoxemia, respiratory failure, and diffuse pulmonary opacities on chest radiograph. Acute manifestations of fat embolism syndrome under general anesthesia may present as a decline in end-tidal CO_2 concentration and arterial oxygen saturation or as an increase in pulmonary artery pressures identified by pulmonary artery catheter or transesophageal echocardiography, with ECG evidence of ischemia and right-sided heart strain.

3. The procedure is performed without complications under spinal anesthesia. After returning to the surgical ward, the patient suddenly becomes tachypneic and tachycardic, and his oxygen requirements increase to 10 L/min by non-rebreather mask in order to maintain SpO_2 of 85%. ECG shows new T-wave changes in V_1–V_3, new Q wave in lead III, and right bundle-branch block. The rapid response team is called to the bedside. Which of the following tests would confirm the most likely diagnosis in this scenario?

A. Serial blood troponins.
B. Spiral computed tomography (CT) scan of the chest.
C. Transthoracic echocardiogram.
D. Chest radiograph

The correct answer is B. Pulmonary embolism (PE) is the most likely life-threatening etiology in this patient, and a spiral CT of the chest is the appropriate diagnostic test. This diagnosis is suggested by the abrupt onset of symptoms and physical signs, sudden hypoxemia, and right heart strain seen on ECG in this orthopedic patient who is already at risk for PE. The other tests listed may help confirm our suspicion and rule out other diagnoses, but the diagnosis of PE should not be delayed by them. A hemodynamically significant PE will likely show right ventricular dysfunction on a transthoracic echocardiogram, but this would not be diagnostic.

Thromboembolic events such as deep vein thromboses (DVT) and PE are major sources of morbidity and mortality in orthopedic patients. Patients undergoing hip or knee replacement or surgery for lower extremity trauma are at greatest risk and experience DVT rates of 40% to 60%. The incidence of PE following hip surgery has been reported to be as high as 17%. Risk factors include obesity, use of a tourniquet, lower extremity trauma, procedures lasting more than 30 min, age above 60 years, and prolonged immobilization. The underlying mechanism for the formation of thrombi is associated with Virchow's triad: venous stasis, hypercoaguable state due to systemic inflammatory responses to surgery, and vascular intimal changes from trauma and surgery.

Neuraxial anesthesia alone or combined with general anesthesia may reduce thromboembolic complications, particularly in the era before routine DVT prophylaxis.

4. The patient is transferred to the intensive care unit for closer monitoring. Over the next 24 h, the nurses become concerned about worsening confusion, daytime sleepiness, combativeness, and agitation. You are asked to come to the bedside and evaluate the patient. The most likely etiology is:

A. Infection.
B. Stroke.
C. Side effects of opioid analgesics.
D. Anemia.
E. All of the above.

The correct answer is E. The etiology of postoperative delirium (POD) is multifactorial and may be difficult to diagnose. It is important to first rule out life-threatening causes such as stroke and anemia and reversible causes such as infection before considering cognitive testing.

POD is common among elderly patients undergoing orthopedic procedures and warrants special consideration. Up to 20% of patients over 60 years old presenting for elective total joint arthroplasty have evidence of preoperative cognitive impairment. Metanalysis suggests that patients with perioperative diagnosis of cognitive impairment and POD are associated with much greater risk of in-hospital and 1-year mortality. Patients who are particularly prone to POD included those with reduced preoperative neurocognitive test scores, reduced functional status, and preoperative "frailty." The occurrence of POD is independent of the type of anesthesia or surgery. There are many potential causes of POD, but predisposing factors include increased age, male gender, psychiatric disease, poor nutrition, smoking, poor functional status, diabetes, atrial fibrillation, prior cerebral vascular accidents or transient ischemic attacks, and atherosclerosis. Precipitating perioperative factors include hip fracture, emergency surgery, intraoperative hyperthermia, blood transfusion, anemia, hypoxemia, sedation and pain management complications, infections, alcohol or other substance withdrawal, and electrolyte abnormalities. Elderly patients are also particularly susceptible to sleep–wake disturbances. Risk stratification of elderly patients using validated tests such as the Mini Mental State Examination has been suggested to identify patients as particular risk of POD and adverse outcomes.

DID YOU LEARN?

- Selection of anesthetic technique for patients undergoing total hip arthroplasty.
- Pathophysiology of fat embolism and management.
- Presentation and differential diagnosis of thromboembolic events.
- Evaluation of postoperative mental status changes.

Recommended Readings

Butterworth IV JF, Mackey DC, Wasnick JD, eds. Geriatric anesthesia. In: *Morgan & Mikhail's Clinical Anesthesiology*. 6th ed. New York, NY: McGraw-Hill Education; 2018:929-942.
Mariano ER. Anesthesia for orthopedic surgery. In: Butterworth IV JF, Mackey DC, Wasnick JD, eds. *Morgan & Mikhail's Clinical Anesthesiology*. 6th ed. New York, NY: McGraw-Hill; 2018:803-818.

References

Agnelli G, Becattini C. Acute pulmonary embolism. *N Engl J Med.* 2010;363:266-274.
Cao SJ, Chen D, Yang L, Zhu T. Effects of an abnormal mini-mental state examination score on postoperative outcomes in geriatric surgical patients: A meta-analysis. *BMC Anesthesiol.* 2019;19:74.

Leung JM, Tsai T, Sands L. Preoperative frailty in older surgical patients is associated with early postoperative delirium. *Anesth Analg.* 2011;112(5):1199-1201.

McIsaac DI, Wijeysundera DN, Huang A, Bryson GL, van Walraven C. Association of hospital-level neuraxial anesthesia use for hip fracture surgery with outcomes: A population-based cohort study. *Anesthesiology.* 2018;128(3):480-491.

Memtsoudis SG, Sun X, Liu S, Banerjee S, et al. Perioperative comparative effectiveness of anesthetic technique in orthopedic patients. *Anesthesiology.* 2013;118:1046-1058.

Neuman MD, Rosenbaum PR, Ludwig JM, Zubizarreta JR, Silber JH. Anesthesia technique, mortality, and length of stay after hip fracture surgery. *JAMA.* 2014;311(24):2508-2517.

Rudolph J, Marcantonio E. Postoperative delirium: Acute change with long-term implications. *Anesth Analg.* 2011;112(5):1202-1211.

Saleh J, El-Othmani MM, Saleh KJ. Deep vein thrombosis and pulmonary embolism considerations in orthopedic surgery. *Orthop Clin North Am.* 2017;48(2):127-135.

CHAPTER 34
Obstetric Anesthesia

CASE 1   Acute Hemorrhage in Patient Undergoing Cesarean Section with Spinal Anesthesia

Michael A. Frölich, MD, MS, and Mark Powell, MD

You are relieving your colleague at 19:00 hours as you start your call duties. You meet in the operating room to take over the anesthetic management of a 23-year-old patient undergoing cesarean section. She presented in active labor with a history of two prior cesarean sections. The patient has a history of bronchial asthma, for which she uses an albuterol inhaler once or twice per day as needed. The patient weighs 85 kg, and her airway examination is unremarkable. She received a bupivacaine spinal anesthetic and has a 20-gauge intravenous (IV) line in her right arm. One- and 5-min neonatal APGAR scores are 7 and 9. Obstetricians are unable to remove the placenta, which has grown through the myometrium and report unexpected bleeding. The patient's blood pressure is 89/43 mm Hg, her heart rate is 124 beats/min, and her oxygen saturation (SpO_2) is 96% on 3 L oxygen per nasal cannula. She is complaining of mild nausea.

1. Your next action is to:

   A. Increase the oxygen flow to the nasal cannula to 5 L.
   B. Give 4 mg of ondansetron IV.
   C. Administer crystalloid fluids and start a 16-gauge IV.
   D. Administer 10 units of oxytocin slowly IV.

The correct answer is C. This patient is at immediate risk of uterine bleeding, and adequate IV access for volume resuscitation is the most urgent consideration. The obstetrician has described findings consistent with the diagnosis of *placenta increta* (invasion of the myometrium by the placenta) or *placenta percreta* (placental penetration of the entire myometrium). These conditions interfere with placental separation and removal and also with postpartum uterine contraction. They are major causes of postpartum hemorrhage.

Increased oxygen administration is of marginal benefit. Mild nausea may be related to uterine exteriorization or to an acute decline in blood pressure. Ondansetron will not improve either of these conditions. Oxytocin given at a time when obstetricians are attempting to remove the placenta is of uncertain benefit.

Your colleague is facile in starting a second IV. He also starts an arterial line for blood pressure monitoring and anticipated frequent laboratory blood sampling. The arterial waveform is as follows:

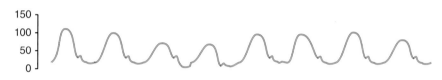

2. The arterial blood pressure tracing above reflects:

   A. Hypercalcemia.
   B. Hypovolemia.
   C. Mitral stenosis.
   D. Hypercontractility.

The correct answer is B. This patient is hypovolemic from acute blood loss. There are three clues in the arterial waveform: the low blood pressure itself, marked respiratory variation, and low position of the dicrotic notch. The position of the dicrotic notch correlates with the systemic resistance. A notch appearing low in the diastolic portion of the pressure tracing indicates a low vascular resistance, as seen in a hypovolemic state.

The obstetrician tells you that an emergent hysterectomy is necessary and that she will call her colleague trained in gynecological oncology to assist. The spinal anesthetic level is still adequate, but the patient is becoming increasingly restless, attempts to move around, and complains of increasing nausea.

3. The most appropriate next step is to:

   A. Induce general anesthesia using rapid-sequence induction with ketamine and succinylcholine.
   B. Give incremental doses of propofol to sedate the patient.
   C. Provide mask ventilation with a 50% oxygen/nitrous oxide mixture.
   D. Give 100 μg of fentanyl IV for added patient comfort.

The correct answer is A. At this point it has become clear that the patient will be undergoing an emergent abdominal operation that is associated with major blood loss. Ketamine is a good choice in the hypovolemic obstetric patient with asthma, as it maintains vascular resistance and is a bronchodilator. She shows signs of hypovolemia on the monitor and physical signs of decreased cerebral perfusion (restlessness). She is at risk for further hemodynamic compromise and her protective airway reflexes may be depressed during hemorrhagic shock.

Although a continuation of the spinal anesthetic is conceivable if the patient can be immediately stabilized and surgery can be completed expeditiously, the more likely immediate outcome in this case is further acute hemorrhage requiring massive transfusion. The administration of propofol to a hypotensive, awake patient is unwise. The two analgesic options (nitrous oxide and fentanyl) are not indicated, as pain is an unlikely source of the patient's restlessness.

The emergent hysterectomy is underway and the surgical blood loss at this point is an estimated 3000 mL, but surgeons indicate that further blood loss should be minimal. Her anesthesia is maintained with isoflurane/N_2O at 0.75 mean alveolar concentration (MAC) and IV fentanyl (total dose 150 μg). In addition, the patent has received 4 units of packed red blood cells, 2 units of fresh frozen plasma, 3000 mL of lactated Ringer's solution, and 1 g of cefazolin. A central venous line was placed and the central venous pressure, after proper calibration, is 12 mm Hg. Oxytocin is infusing at a rate of 20 units/h. Her blood pressure is 78/37 mm Hg.

4. The most likely cause of the observed hypotension is:

   A. Oxytocin.
   B. Hypocalcemia.
   C. Excessively deep anesthesia.
   D. Hypovolemia.

The correct answer is B. Severely hemorrhaging patients transfused with several units of packed red cells, fresh frozen plasma, and lactated Ringer's solution are likely to exhibit hypotension and cardiac hypocontractility secondary to acute hypocalcemia, primarily related to calcium binding by citrate preservative in blood products (citrate toxicity). Oxytocin at a rate of 20 units/h and a volatile agent at 0.75 MAC are unlikely causes of hypotension. Based on the central venous pressure and volume replacement, her volume status is unlikely to be low.

DID YOU LEARN?

- The differential diagnosis of nausea in the patient undergoing a cesarean section.
- The correct identification of hypovolemia on an arterial blood pressure tracing.

- The most appropriate management of intraoperative postpartum hemorrhage.
- The differential diagnosis of hypotension in the patient with acute surgical blood loss.

References

Ruiter L, Kazemier BM, Mol BWJ, Pajkrt E. Incidence and recurrence rate of postpartum hemorrhage and manual removal of the placenta: A longitudinal linked national cohort study in The Netherlands. *Eur J Obstet Gynecol Reprod Biol.* 2019;238:114-119.

van den Akker T, Brobbel C, Dekkers OM, Bloemenkamp KW. Prevalence, indications, risk indicators, and outcomes of emergency peripartum hysterectomy worldwide: A systematic review and meta-analysis. *Obstet Gynecol.* 2016;128(6):1281-1294.

CASE 2 Cardiac Arrest on the Labor and Delivery Floor

Michael A. Frölich, MD, MS, and Mark Powell, MD

You have been emergently called to evaluate a patient in the labor and delivery suite. She is an otherwise healthy 29-year-old G3P2002 at 40.0 weeks' gestation who was admitted 8 h prior for a scheduled induction. After an oxytocin infusion was begun and the membranes were ruptured electively, an epidural was placed at the L3–L4 interspace. For the last 6 h, there have been no complications to the labor and the epidural has provided adequate analgesia. The patient's nurse has now STAT paged you because the patient has become acutely agitated and tachypneic. Vital signs upon entering the room are blood pressure 102/76 mm Hg, heart rate 118 beats/min, respiratory rate 32 breaths/min, and SpO₂ 84% on 6 L oxygen via nasal cannula. The nurse states she has stopped the oxytocin infusion. Noting the hypoxic respiratory distress, you call for help and elect to intubate the patient. Suddenly, the patient develops pulseless electrical activity (PEA) arrest, and Advanced Cardiac Life Support (ACLS) protocol is initiated.

1. While continuing ACLS, the next step is to:

   A. Have the nurse resume the oxytocin in an effort to deliver the fetus vaginally.
   B. Prepare the patient for a bedside cesarean delivery.
   C. Place a central venous line in an attempt to aspirate air, as this is most likely a venous air embolism.
   D. Discontinue and remove the epidural, as this is likely a high spinal.

The correct answer is B. For the best possible outcome for the baby, delivery should occur within 5 min of maternal cardiac arrest. Early delivery of the fetus will also relieve compression of the inferior vena cava (IVC), increase maternal preload and cardiac output, and allow for more effective resuscitation of the patient. During resuscitation of the pregnant patient, it is important to provide left uterine displacement to relieve pressure on the IVC to improve venous return to the heart. If return of spontaneous circulation is not achieved by minute 4, an incision should be made, so delivery of the baby can occur by minute 5. Transporting the patient to the operating room for STAT cesarean delivery wastes valuable time, and effective resuscitation may not be possible during transport; therefore, cesarean delivery should occur in the patient's room.

Option A is incorrect in that resumption of oxytocin will not allow an expedited vaginal delivery. Given the fact there are no venous sinuses open to the atmosphere, it is highly unlikely that the arrest is related to a venous air embolism (option C). If this was a cesarean delivery, then venous air embolism would be higher on the differential diagnosis list. A high or total spinal (option D) is unlikely as well. Initially, the patient experienced isolated hypoxia with associated agitation and no excessive weakness. Bradycardia from loss of cardiac accelerator fibers (T2–T4) was also not present. The epidural infusion had provided a stable level of analgesia for hours and there was no mention of manipulation of the catheter.

2. After delivery of the fetus, the obstetrician notes excessive uterine bleeding. You also note oozing around the patient's IV. Which of these lab values would you *least* expect to find in disseminated intravascular coagulation (DIC)?

   A. International normalized ratio (INR) 2.5.
   B. Partial thromboplastin time (PTT) 68 s.
   C. Platelets 89,000/μL.
   D. Fibrinogen 340 mg/dL.

The correct answer is D. DIC is a result of systemic activation of the coagulation system, with generalized clot formation, breakdown, and consumption of coagulation factors and platelets. DIC is not a primary disease, but results from another pathological process. The extrinsic pathway is activated when factor VII is exposed to tissue factor, leading to activation of thrombin, which cleaves fibrinogen to fibrin. Platelet activation and aggregation also occur. DIC is a consumptive process, which will cause depletion of factors and platelets. Thus elevation in PTT and INR along with a decrease in platelet count is expected. Fibrinogen levels are typically decreased in DIC.

3. Given this clinical scenario, the most likely diagnosis is:

   A. Local anesthetic toxicity.
   B. Amniotic fluid embolism (AFE).
   C. Venous air embolism (VAE).
   D. High spinal.

The correct answer is B. Amniotic fluid enters the maternal circulation via ruptured membranes and small tears in the maternal vasculature, most likely in the lower uterine and cervical vessels. As with VAE, a negative gradient must exist to drive amniotic fluid into the maternal circulation. There is a biphasic response to AFE. In phase 1, amniotic fluid causes the release of biochemical mediators—leukotrienes, thromboxane, bradykinin, prostaglandins, and arachidonic acid—which cause pulmonary artery spasm, leading to acute-onset pulmonary hypertension. Acute right-heart failure ensues and leads to hypoxemia via V/Q mismatch and hypotension. Phase 1 is acute and transient, lasting up to 30 min. Phase 2 occurs if patients survive the initial insult. Patients experience left ventricular failure, pulmonary edema, and DIC. All other options listed also can cause circulatory collapse but would not explain the overall clinical picture. The patient had an adequate level of analgesia with no adjustment to the epidural, so local anesthetic toxicity would be very low on the differential. There were no maternal vessels exposed to the atmosphere leading to VAE. A high spinal would likely cause bradycardia and hypotension with involvement of cardiac accelerator fibers. Respiratory compromise requiring intubation would occur with motor block of the phrenic nerve (C3–C5). DIC would not be seen with a high spinal.

4. The least common sign or symptom of AFE is:

A. Hypotension.
B. Chest pain.
C. Fetal distress.
D. Cardiopulmonary arrest.

The correct answer is B. Common signs and symptoms are listed in order of descending frequency: hypotension (100%), fetal distress (100%), pulmonary edema or adult respiratory distress syndrome (93%), cardiopulmonary arrest (87%), cyanosis (83%), coagulopathy (83%), dyspnea (49%), seizure (48%), uterine atony (23%), bronchospasm (15%), transient hypertension (11%), cough (7%), headache (7%), and chest pain (2%).

5. Treatment would include all of the following *except*:

A. Intubation and mechanical ventilation.
B. Fluid therapy.
C. Inotropic support.
D. Delayed delivery of the fetus.

The correct answer is D. Prompt recognition, resuscitation, and delivery of the fetus are vital in the management of AFE. As there is no way to prevent or reverse maternal absorption of amniotic fluid, management of AFE is primarily resuscitative. The airway should be controlled with intubation and mechanical ventilation. Hemodynamic stability should be provided with fluid resuscitation, inotropes, and vasopressors. Labs should be drawn and factors and platelets replaced as needed. Delivery of the fetus must be expedited in order to optimize both maternal and fetal outcomes.

DID YOU LEARN?

- The signs and symptoms of AFE.
- The importance of early recognition of AFE.
- Management of AFE.
- The importance of an expeditious delivery of the fetus during maternal cardiac arrest.

CHAPTER 34 Obstetric Anesthesia

Reference

Tamura N, Farhana M, Oda T, Itoh H, Kanayama N. Amniotic fluid embolism: Pathophysiology from the perspective of pathology. *J Obstet Gynaecol Res.* 2017;43(4):627-632.

CASE 3 — Parturient with Congenital Ventricular Septum Defect and Eisenmenger Syndrome

Madhumani Rupasinghe, MBBS, FRCA

A 20-year-old primiparous woman at 34 weeks' gestation was admitted to labor and delivery triage with a 1-week history of dizziness, fatigue, dyspnea, and lower-extremity edema. She was diagnosed with congenital heart disease 10 years ago but remained asymptomatic and without therapy until this time. There is no other significant past medical history. Vital signs are heart rate 84 beats/min, respiratory rate 20 breaths/min, blood pressure 125/80 mm Hg, and SpO$_2$ 88% on room air. She has cyanosis and clubbing of her fingers. Cardiac auscultation reveals a loud second heart sound and a grade 5/6 systolic murmur maximal along the left sternal border. There is moderate lower-extremity edema.

Laboratory results include hemoglobin 14.5 g/dL, hematocrit 45%, platelets 173,000/dL, and normal prothrombin time (PT) and activated PTT. Blood gases reveal pH 7.35, PaO$_2$ 61 mm Hg, PaCO$_2$ 34 mm Hg, bicarbonate 18.1 mmol/L, base excess (BE) −6.6, and SaO$_2$ 90%.

1. The most useful diagnostic test to order at this time is:

A. ECG.
B. Chest radiograph.
C. Bedside echocardiogram.
D. Chest computed tomography (CT).

The correct answer is C. The clinical findings in this case signify underlying right-heart pathology. Cardiac auscultation findings that should prompt further cardiovascular investigation during any pregnancy include grade 3/6 or more systolic

murmurs, diastolic murmurs, a fixed-split second heart sound, a loud fourth heart sound, and/or an opening snap.

ECG and chest radiograph do not provide the most useful information in this scenario and will delay diagnosis. During pregnancy, elevation of the diaphragm shifts the heart's position in the chest, resulting in the appearance of an enlarged heart on a chest radiograph and in left axis deviation and T-wave changes on the ECG.

Pulmonary embolism is a leading cause of death in pregnancy and may present with some of the clinical features exhibited by this patient. Chest CT is recommended only when bilateral leg Doppler ultrasound test is negative.

Transthoracic echocardiography and Doppler examination show a 15-mm ventricular septal defect (VSD) with bidirectional flow, pulmonary hypertension (pulmonary artery systolic pressure of 115 mm Hg), mild dilation of the right atrium, right ventricular hypertrophy, and an estimated left ventricular ejection fraction of 61%. Based upon the initial clinical presentation and subsequent investigations, a diagnosis of congenital ventricular septum defect with Eisenmenger physiology was made.

2. Which of the following is *not true* about Eisenmenger syndrome?

A. Central cyanosis with clubbing is a frequent feature of advanced disease.
B. Right-to-left shunting is present.
C. Paradoxical embolism is a possibility.
D. Red blood cell production is decreased.

The correct answer is D. The reduction in pulmonary oxygen transfer reduces blood oxygen saturation, leading to compensatory increase in red blood cell production as a mechanism to increase oxygen delivery. Hence, polycythemia is common.

VSD is a common congenital heart defect, accounting for 25% to 35% of congenital heart disease. Eisenmenger syndrome is defined as the development of pulmonary hypertension in response to a left-to-right cardiac shunt (ie, VSD) with consequent bidirectional or reversal (right-to-left) of shunt flow. With advanced disease, the pressures within the right heart may exceed those within the left heart, and such patients are chronically hypoxemic with cyanosis and digital clubbing. The presence of shunt flow between the right and left sides of the heart, regardless of the direction of blood flow, mandates meticulous exclusion of air bubbles and particulate material from intravenous fluids in order to minimize the risk of paradoxical embolism into the cerebral or coronary circulations.

The patient is admitted to the intensive care unit (ICU) for management by a multidisciplinary team of obstetricians, cardiologists, critical care specialists, and obstetric anesthesiologists. After observation and stabilization, a cesarean section is performed under combined spinal-epidural anesthesia.

3. Decreasing which of the following is *most* detrimental when considering regional anesthesia?

A. Hematocrit.
B. Systemic vascular resistance.
C. Pulmonary vascular resistance.
D. Preload.

The correct answer is B. Patients with congenital right-to-left or bidirectional shunts do not benefit from abrupt increases in pulmonary vascular resistance or decreases in systemic vascular resistance.

Reductions in venous return (preload) are also poorly tolerated. Hypovolemia can cause an increase in right-to-left shunting, reduced cardiac output, and refractory hypoxemia. Similarly, volume overload should also be avoided as it cannot be accommodated by the compromised pulmonary vascular bed and/or right ventricle and can result in heart failure and increasing right-to-left shunt. When considering major conduction blockade anesthesia, adequate fluid loading prior to placement of the regional technique is essential. On the other hand, one must be mindful that when the block wears off, the additional fluid load can lead to hypervolemia. These patients are better managed with a low-dose combined spinal-epidural technique, carefully titrated epidural anesthesia, or general anesthesia.

Patients develop secondary erythrocytosis with an increase in hematocrit due to increased erythropoietin production in response to long-standing hypoxemia. Therapeutic phlebotomy is indicated only if hemoglobin is greater than 20 g/dL and hematocrit >65%, or if erythrocytosis is associated with headache, progressively increasing fatigue, or other symptoms of hyperviscosity in the absence of dehydration or anemia.

After delivery, the patient was started on prophylactic low-molecular-weight heparin (LMWH).

4. Which of the following is true regarding postoperative thromboprophylaxis after cesarean section?

A. Anti-Xa level is predictive of the risk of bleeding.
B. If presence of blood is noticed during epidural needle and/or epidural catheter placement, initiation of LMWH therapy should be delayed for 12 h.
C. A twice-daily LMWH dosing regimen is not associated with an increased risk of spinal hematoma
D. Administration of LMWH prophylaxis should be delayed for 6 to 12 h following cesarean section.

The **correct answer is D.** Administration of LMWH prophylaxis should be delayed for 6 to 12 h after delivery (no sooner than 4 h after epidural catheter removal) as long as hemostasis is assured and there has not been a bloody or traumatic epidural.

Anti-Xa level is not predictive of the risk of bleeding following use of LMWH, and routine monitoring of anti-Xa levels is not recommended.

Patients on preoperative LMWH thromboprophylaxis can be assumed to have altered coagulation. In these patients, epidural or spinal needle placement should occur at least 10 to 12 h following the last LMWH dose. The presence of blood during needle and catheter placement does not necessitate postponement of surgery, but initiation of LMWH therapy in this setting should be delayed for 24 h postoperatively.

With once-daily LMWH dosing, the first postoperative dose should be administered 6 to 12 h postoperatively. The second postoperative dose should occur no sooner than 24 h after the first dose. Indwelling neuraxial catheters may be safely maintained; however, the catheter should be removed a minimum of 10 to 12 h after the last dose of LMWH. Subsequent LMWH dosing should occur at least 4 h after catheter removal.

A twice-daily LMWH dosage regimen is associated with an increased risk of spinal hematoma. With this regimen, the first dose of LMWH should be administered no earlier than 24 h postoperatively, regardless of anesthetic technique, and only in the presence of adequate (surgical) hemostasis. Indwelling catheters should be removed before initiation of twice-daily LMWH thromboprophylaxis. If a continuous neuraxial catheter technique is selected, the catheter may remain indwelling overnight but must be removed before the first dose of LMWH. Administration of LMWH should be delayed for 4 h following epidural catheter removal.

DID YOU LEARN?

- Significance of investigation of abnormal cardiovascular physical findings during pregnancy.
- Physiology, diagnosis, and management of Eisenmenger syndrome.
- Issues related to postoperative thromboprophylaxis and regional anesthesia.

References

Bates SM, Middeldorp S, Rodger M, James AH, Greer I. Guidance for the treatment and prevention of obstetric-associated venous thromboembolism. *J Thromb Thrombolysis.* 2016;41:92-128.

Bhatt AB, DeFaria Yeh D. Pregnancy and adult congenital heart disease. *Cardiol Clin.* 2015;33(4):611-623.

Canobbio MM, Warnes CA, Aboulhosn J, et al. Management of pregnancy in patients with complex congenital heart disease: A scientific statement for healthcare professionals from the American Heart Association. *Circulation.* 2017;135:e50-e87.

CASE 4   Umbilical Cord Prolapse

Madhumani Rupasinghe, MBBS, FRCA

A 29-year-old woman, G7P5, at 37 weeks' gestation is admitted in labor. Her only past medical history is five uncomplicated, spontaneous, vaginal deliveries. On palpation, the baby is noted to be small for gestational age and the fetal head is not engaged in the pelvis. The patient is now having contractions every 2 to 4 min, lasting 60 to 90 s. On vaginal exam, the patient was found to be 4 cm dilated, 90% effaced, with the fetal head at −2 station with bulging membranes. You have been called to the room because the patient requests an epidural for labor analgesia. You note that her vital signs are blood pressure 110/72 mm Hg, heart rate 90 beats/min, and SpO$_2$ 99% on room air. Continuous fetal monitoring has been initiated. After you obtain her history and consent, the nurse helps you to position the patient.

1. While you are setting up your epidural tray, what is *most* important to monitor?

   A. Continuous fetal monitoring.
   B. Maternal blood pressure.
   C. Maternal heart rate.
   D. Maternal oxygen saturation.

The correct answer is A. Intrauterine asphyxia during labor is the most common cause of neonatal depression. Fetal monitoring throughout labor is helpful in identifying which babies may be at risk, detecting fetal distress, and evaluating the effect of acute interventions.

As you are getting ready to place the epidural, the patient complains of a sudden gush of water. The fetal heart rate is heard decelerating down to 90 beats/min and the trace is as noted in the figure on the next page.

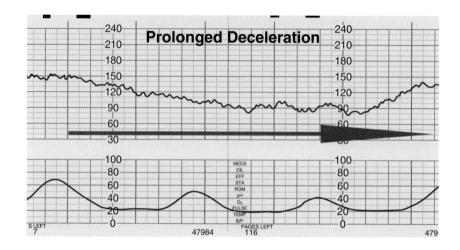

2. Given the mother's history and physical examination and the current clinical scenario, the next *best* step is to:

A. Put the patient in the left lateral position.
B. Provide supplemental oxygen.
C. Initiate IV hydration.
D. Ask the obstetrician to quickly perform a vaginal examination.

The correct answer is D. Prolapse of the umbilical cord complicates 0.2% to 0.6% of deliveries. Umbilical cord compression following prolapse can rapidly lead to fetal asphyxia. The diagnosis is suspected after sudden fetal bradycardia or profound decelerations and is confirmed by physical examination.

Although acute interventions—which include positioning to prevent aortocaval compression, correcting maternal hypotension with fluids and/or vasopressors, provision of supplemental oxygen, and decreasing uterine contractions by stopping oxytocin or administering tocolytics—are helpful, the next critical step is to confirm the diagnosis by vaginal exam.

There are two types of cord prolapse. In *overt prolapse*, the cord protrudes in advance of the fetal presenting part and is visible or palpable on examination. In *occult prolapse*, the cord descends alongside, but not past, the presenting part.

Predisposing factors for umbilical cord prolapse include excessive cord length, malpresentation, low birthweight, grand parity (more than five pregnancies), multiple gestations, and artificial rupture of membranes.

3. On vaginal examination, the obstetrician confirms umbilical cord prolapse. What is the next step in management?

A. Put the patient in left lateral position.
B. Put the patient in knee–chest position.
C. Administer nitroglycerin 50 to 100 μg IV.
D. Place an epidural in the lateral position.

The correct answer is B. Traditionally, umbilical cord prolapse has been managed by minimizing pressure on the cord while preparing for delivery. The steps involve manual pushing of the presenting fetal part back up into the pelvis, immediate steep Trendelenburg or knee–chest position, instillation of fluid in the bladder, and fundic reduction. Unless the cervix is fully dilated and an immediate spontaneous or instrumental delivery can be achieved, most obstetricians would opt for emergent delivery by cesarean section.

4. The patient is rushed to the operating room in knee–chest position for an emergency cesarean section, with the obstetric resident pushing the fetal head back into the pelvis. In anticipation of induction of general anesthesia in this patient:

   A. Mendelson syndrome can be prevented with 30 mL of particulate antacid.
   B. Cricoid pressure is useful in preventing active vomiting.
   C. Hemoglobin oxygen desaturation is likely to occur more rapidly following induction as compared to a nonpregnant patient.
   D. The incidence of difficult intubation is twice that of the general surgical population.

The correct answer is C. The combination of increased oxygen consumption and decreased functional residual capacity secondary to increased intraabdominal pressure promotes rapid desaturation in the term parturient.

Mendelson suggested criteria that increase the risk of aspiration during cesarean section: low pH (<2.5), gastric volume greater than 25 mL, and the presence of particulate material in the aspirated fluid. To prevent Mendelson, or aspiration, syndrome, a nonparticulate antacid such as sodium citrate is administered with metoclopramide and an H_2-receptor antagonist. Although controversial, cricoid pressure may be useful in preventing passive regurgitation. In active vomiting, cricoid pressure is contraindicated because the combination of vomiting and cricoid pressure may result in esophageal rupture.

Pulmonary aspiration of gastric contents and failed endotracheal intubation are the major causes of maternal morbidity and mortality associated with general anesthesia. The incidence of difficult intubation is many times greater in the obstetric patient compared to the general population, probably due to a combination of factors including anatomical changes such as weight gain and upper airway edema, which increase the Mallampati score and make intubation technically more difficult. Most experts now recognize that the advent of video laryngoscopy may reduce the likelihood of failed intubation. Difficult intubation remains more common in emergency situations due to lack of preparation.

DID YOU LEARN?

- The importance of fetal monitoring.
- The methods of identification of cord prolapse.

- The management of cord prolapse.
- The complications of general anesthesia in the obstetric patient.

Reference

Holbrook BD, Phelan ST. Umbilical cord prolapse. *Obstet Gynecol Clin North Am.* 2013;40(1):1-14.

CASE 5 — Parturient with Hypognathia, Large Tongue, and Repetitive Late Fetal Decelerations Without Epidural Analgesia

Michael A. Frölich, MD, MS, and Mark Powell, MD

Your partner is called to perform a preanesthetic evaluation on a 25-year-old primigravida admitted in term labor. Her medical history is unremarkable except for a prior laparoscopic inguinal hernia repair at age 21 in which the patient noted a sore throat and a chipped front tooth postoperatively. On airway exam, he notes hypognathia, a large tongue, and a chipped top left central incisor. The uvula is not visible. After discussing the risks and benefits of an epidural, the patient does not want epidural analgesia and wishes for a "natural birth."

Three hours later, the patient is taken to the operating room for an emergent cesarean delivery for recurrent late decelerations. Ten minutes later, you are called to the operating room STAT.

1. The risk of failed intubation in pregnancy is how many times more likely when compared to nonpregnant patients?

A. No difference.
B. Twice.
C. Four times.
D. More than four times.

The correct answer is D. Despite significant advancement in airway technology, there has been very little change in the reported overall incidence of failed intubation in the pregnant population since the 1980s. The rate of failed intubation in parturients is approximately 1:300, which is approximately eight times higher than the general population (1:2330). Nevertheless it is likely that the full impact of widespread availability video laryngoscopy and video fiberoptic bronchoscopy has not yet been reported. Several physiological changes of pregnancy, such as edema of the oropharynx and vocal cords, contribute to the difficult intubation.

Parturients often have large breasts, which may greatly increase the difficulty of inserting the laryngoscope blade in the patient's mouth.

2. Rapid desaturation occurs in term parturients due to an *increase* in:

A. Minute ventilation.
B. Functional residual capacity.
C. Oxygen consumption.
D. Closing capacity.

The correct answer is C. Minute ventilation is increased by approximately 50% in pregnancy. The majority of this increase is due to an increase in tidal volume with minimal contribution from an increase in respiratory rate. This hyperventilation above baseline will lead to a decrease in $PaCO_2$ and a mild respiratory alkalosis. However, an increase in minute ventilation is not the cause of rapid desaturation in pregnancy. Pregnancy has no effect on the closing capacity. Due to an increase in intraabdominal pressure, pregnancy will result in a *decrease* of the functional residual capacity by about 20%. Functional residual capacity will often be below the closing capacity, which promotes shunting of arterial blood and early desaturation. There is an approximately 20% *increase* in oxygen consumption above baseline in pregnancy, which will contribute to rapid desaturation.

3. Upon arrival to the operating room, your partner attempts direct laryngoscopy twice with a grade IV view, and you attempt once without success. The patient's SpO_2 is beginning to decrease and the obstetrician notes severe fetal distress on the fetal heart monitor. You are able to adequately mask ventilate. Your next action is to:

A. Wake up the patient and attempt a spinal anesthetic.
B. Wake up the patient and secure airway with awake fiberoptic intubation.
C. Place an intubating laryngeal mask airway (LMA), hold cricoid pressure, and proceed with cesarean delivery.
D. Perform an emergent tracheostomy.

The correct answer is C. A difficult airway should have been anticipated given the patient's history and physical examination, and the risk of a difficult airway and failed intubation should have been part of the initial discussion with the patient during the preanesthetic evaluation. Video laryngoscopy should likely have been the first choice for this patient. Placement of a labor epidural that could have been converted to a surgical block would have avoided the need for general anesthesia for an emergent cesarean delivery. If time allowed, spinal anesthesia would also have been an appropriate first choice. However, your partner has induced general anesthesia and is unable to intubate the patient. The obstetric patient adds more complexity to the difficult airway algorithm in that the status of the fetus has to be considered. In this scenario, the fetus is in severe distress, and delivery needs

Obstetric Anesthesia

to occur immediately for the best possible outcome. This would eliminate options A and B. If no fetal distress was present, then it would be appropriate to awaken the patient and attempt an alternate means of anesthesia. If you cannot intubate or ventilate with mask or LMA, then it would be appropriate to proceed with a surgical airway. However, you could mask-ventilate, so the best option would be to continue mask ventilation or place an LMA, hold cricoid pressure, and proceed with emergent cesarean delivery.

4. After successful placement of the intubating LMA and delivery of the baby, you call for the difficult airway cart for fiberoptic placement of an endotracheal tube. You easily secure the airway; however, you notice what appears to be gastric content in the trachea. Inspiratory pressure increases from 20 cm H_2O to 35 cm H_2O, and diffuse wheezing is heard during auscultation of bilateral lung fields. Which of the following would be an appropriate next step in treatment?

A. Bronchial lavage with sodium bicarbonate.
B. Suctioning of the gastric content from the airway.
C. Prophylactic administration of 1 g of ceftriaxone.
D. Prophylactic administration of 8 mg of dexamethasone.

The correct answer is B. Pregnancy causes a decrease in gastric motility and upward displacement of the stomach and esophagus by the gravid uterus, lessening the effectiveness of the gastroesophageal sphincter as a mechanical barrier. Due to these normal physiological changes of pregnancy, parturients are at greater risk for aspiration and should be considered as having a full stomach regardless of their NPO status. Prophylaxis with a nonparticulate antacid, H_2 blocker, and metoclopramide are given to increase the gastric pH and motility prior to any procedure. This patient was difficult to intubate and required prolonged ventilation with an unsecured airway, leading to further risk of aspiration. If gastric contents are noted in the oropharynx, the patient should be placed in Trendelenburg position, suctioned, and intubated if she is unable to protect her airway. After securing the airway, a bronchoscope can be inserted down the endotracheal tube and then suctioned if gastric content is present in the airway. In our case, the patient was already intubated and gastric content was noted in the airway, so the next step would be to suction the gastric content. Since acid pH-related tissue injury is an immediate event, neutralizing the pH would provide no benefit and the extra solution may worsen any existing hypoxemia. As the gastric solution is sterile, antibiotic administration is not indicated and may select for resistant strains of bacteria. Corticosteriod administration has no immediate benefit for acute lung injury secondary to gastric aspiration.

DID YOU LEARN?

- The incidence of failed intubation in the obstetric population.
- Causes of rapid desaturation in the obstetric patient.

- Modification of the difficult airway algorithm to account for fetal distress.
- Management of aspiration.

References

Practice guidelines for obstetric anesthesia: An updated report by the American Society of Anesthesiologists Task Force on Obstetric Anesthesia and the Society for Obstetric Anesthesia and Perinatology. *Anesthesiology.* 2016;124(2):270-300.

Lee AS, Ryu JH. Aspiration pneumonia and related syndromes. *Mayo Clin Proc.* 2018; 93(6):752-762.

Mushambi MC, Jaladi S. Airway management and training in obstetric anaesthesia. *Curr Opin Anaesthesiol.* 2016;29(3):261-267.

Scott-Brown S, Russell R. Video laryngoscopes and the obstetric airway. *Int J Obstet Anesth.* 2015;24(2):137-146.

CASE 6   Patient with History of Chronic Low Back Pain for Placement of a Cervical Cerclage

Michael A. Frölich, MD, MS, and Mark Powell, MD

You are being called to evaluate a 32-year-old G3P0020 at 14.0 weeks' gestation with a history of repeated pregnancy losses due to cervical incompetence. Her cervical exam is rapidly changing, and she is now scheduled for emergent cerclage placement. The patient has a history of gastroesophageal reflux disease (GERD), obesity (body mass index = 42 kg/m^2), borderline hypertension, and chronic low back pain that is currently managed with oral methadone 30 mg twice a day, but no other medications. She is also complaining of a productive cough over the past few days without other constitutional symptoms. She had undergone a lumbar laminectomy and discectomy for a herniated disk 1 year ago without information on whether instrumentation was used for spine stabilization. Upon examination of her back, there is a 3-inch midline scar extending from the T12 to L2 spinous processes. The airway exam reveals normal neck extension but a small mouth opening and a large tongue with only the hard palate visible. Her oral temperature is 99.2°F, blood pressure is 143/87 mm Hg, and SpO$_2$ is 97% on room air.

1. What is the most appropriate way to proceed with this patient?

   A. Proceed with cerclage placement using deep sedation/general anesthesia with propofol.

   B. Obtain both lumbar spine radiographs to ascertain the presence of surgical hardware and a chest radiograph to rule out pneumonia prior to surgery. Make anesthetic plan contingent on radiographic findings.

   C. Obtain a chest radiograph and white blood cell (WBC) count. Plan for a spinal anesthetic below the level of the lumbar surgery scar.

   D. Proceed with general anesthesia without any further evaluation.

The correct answer is C. A chest radiograph and WBC are indicated preoperative tests for a patient with a productive cough. The radiation exposure to the unborn child from a chest radiograph is minimal, but the radiation exposure from a lumbar spine radiograph is considerably greater. The mean radiation exposure from a lumbar spine x-ray is 1.7 millisievert (mSv) compared to 0.1 mSv for a standard chest radiograph. In addition, spinal anesthesia is feasible in a patient with limited back surgery and has even been reported in patients with spinal instrumentation. Hence, a spine film would be of no value with respect to formulating the anesthetic plan.

The patient's chest radiograph shows no acute changes, and her WBC count is 14,000/μL. A spinal anesthetic is performed, and 10 mg of hyperbaric bupivacaine is injected after withdrawal of clear cerebrospinal fluid at the level of the L4–L5 interspace. However, when the surgeon attempts to place the cervical suture 20 min later, the patient complains of excruciating right-sided pain. There appears to be one-sided anesthetic sparing. The patient requests general anesthesia and refuses any further attempt at regional anesthesia.

2. What is the most appropriate anesthetic choice in this situation?

   A. Mask anesthesia with sevoflurane.
   B. General anesthesia with awake fiber-optic intubation.
   C. General anesthesia with rapid-sequence induction.
   D. Deep sedation with ketamine and propofol.

The correct answer is B. Pregnant patients are at increased risk of pulmonary aspiration, and airway protection via a cuffed endotracheal tube is needed. Most experts agree that aspiration risk increases with the second trimester, due to hormonal effects relaxing lower esophageal sphincter pressure. The history of GERD, whether related to pregnancy or not, is a risk factor for pulmonary aspiration. With only the hard palate visible, the patient is classified as a Mallampati IV airway—a predictor of difficult visualization of the larynx with traditional laryngoscopy. The most appropriate choice is therefore use of an awake fiber-optic intubation.

The case proceeds well under general anesthesia. However, with 1.5 MAC sevoflurane and after having received 150 μg of fentanyl IV, the patient's blood pressure is 187/110 mm Hg with a heart rate of 123 beats/min. A repeated blood pressure reading is 186/112 mm Hg with a heart rate of 125 beats/min.

3. Given this clinical scenario, the most appropriate treatment is:

   A. Labetalol 20 mg IV in divided doses.
   B. Increase volatile anesthesia to 2 MAC.
   C. Hydralazine 10 mg IV.
   D. Esmolol 50 mg IV.

The correct answer is A. The patient appears to have an adequate level of anesthesia. Antihypertensive treatment is indicated in a patient with a sustained blood pressure in the severely hypertensive range. The typical times of onset of action of IV antihypertensive drugs are hydralazine, 10 to 20 min; labetalol, 5 to 10 min; sodium nitroprusside, 0.5 to 1 min; nitroglycerine, 1 to 2 min; and nicardipine, 5 to 15 min. Among those choices, only labetalol also reduces heart rate. Reports of fetal distress and neonatal bradycardia have discouraged the use of esmolol in pregnancy. Given the hemodynamic presentation, the best treatment choice is labetalol 20 mg IV in divided doses.

Immediately following the uneventful cerclage, the patient is extubated and transported to the postanesthesia care unit (PACU). Her blood pressure upon arrival is 142/87 mm Hg, heart rate is 118 beats/min, and room air SpO$_2$ is 98%. She complains of excruciating back pain (9 on a 10-point visual analog pain rating scale) and indicates that she did not take her last two doses of methadone. She does not have any drug allergies.

4. The most appropriate pain management plan is:

   A. Methadone 30 mg IV.
   B. Fentanyl 50 µg IV every 10 min, with maximum total dose of 250 µg IV in PACU. Discontinue methadone during pregnancy.
   C. Buprenorphine 300 µg IV. Resume oral methadone 30 mg twice a day when oral intake allowed.
   D. Morphine 4 mg IV every 15 min, maximum 30 mg IV in PACU. Resume oral methadone 30 mg twice a day when oral intake allowed.

The correct answer is D. This patient is likely opioid-tolerant, and a higher dose, given in the controlled setting of the PACU, is appropriate. The patient will also have to resume maintenance opioid therapy to prevent acute opioid withdrawal, which may produce harmful maternal and fetal effects. Buprenorphine is a mixed agonist–antagonist opioid receptor modulator that is not recommended for the treatment of acute pain. Switching from methadone to buprenorphine requires a long-term treatment plan. IV methadone is approximately two to eight times more potent relative to a chronically administered oral maintenance dose, and 30 mg IV would likely be too high a dose for a patient on 60 mg daily oral methadone maintenance therapy. In general, equianalgesic ratios are considered crude estimates at best, and therefore, it is imperative that careful consideration is given to individualizing the dose of the selected opioid. Dosage titration of a new opioid should be completed slowly and with frequent monitoring. However, 250 µg of IV fentanyl will likely be inadequate for the opioid-tolerant patient.

DID YOU LEARN?

- Management of the patient with history of back surgery.
- Considerations for radiation exposure during pregnancy.
- Antihypertensive treatment options in pregnancy.
- Therapeutic considerations in the opioid-tolerant pregnant patient.

References

Ballantyne JC. Opioids for the treatment of chronic pain: mistakes made, lessons learned, and future directions. *Anesth Analg.* 2017;125(5):1769-1778.

Hubbert CH. Epidural anesthesia in patients with spinal fusion. *Anesth Analg.* 1985;64:843.

Raymond BL, Kook BT, Richardson MG. The opioid epidemic and pregnancy: implications for anesthetic care. *Curr Opin Anaesthesiol.* 2018;31(3):243-250.

Sutter MB, Leeman L, Hsi A. Neonatal opioid withdrawal syndrome. *Obstet Gynecol Clin North Am.* 2014;41:317-334.

Too GT, Hill JB. Hypertensive crisis during pregnancy and postpartum period. *Semin Perinatol.* 2013;37:280-287.

CASE 7 — Severe Preeclampsia in an Obese Patient with Chronic Hypertension

Michael A. Frölich, MD, MS, and Mark Powell, MD

A 36-year-old G4P3 at 35.4 weeks' gestation is admitted to the labor and delivery floor from clinic for induction of labor due to accelerated hypertension and new-onset headache. She was diagnosed with preeclampsia at 23 weeks of pregnancy. Her past medical history is significant for essential hypertension, obesity, and a prior pregnancy complicated by preeclampsia. Home medications include labetalol 200 mg twice daily and a prenatal vitamin. Her blood pressure was 185/118 mm Hg in clinic today, and repeat blood pressure was 187/112 mm Hg. Admission laboratory studies have been drawn, and the results are pending.

1. All of the following are criteria for diagnosis of severe preeclampsia *except*:

    A. A blood pressure of 170/115 mm Hg with repeat of 165/108 mm Hg 4 h later.
    B. New-onset headache.
    C. Severe persistent right upper quadrant pain.
    D. Proteinuria of 5 g/d.

The correct answer is D. Traditionally, two criteria have to be met for the diagnosis of preeclampsia: (1) new-onset hypertension of 140/90 mm Hg or higher after 20 weeks of pregnancy; and (2) proteinuria of ≥ 300 mg/d. However, in the absence of proteinuria, the diagnosis of preeclampsia can be made with new-onset hypertension and any of the following: (1) thrombocytopenia with platelet count less than 100,000/μL; (2) acute kidney injury with serum creatinine >1.1 mg/dL, or doubling of serum creatinine in the absence of preexisting kidney disease; (3) impaired liver function, with elevated levels of hepatic transaminases to twice normal concentrations or greater; (4) pulmonary edema; or (5) cerebral or visual symptoms. Although preeclampsia patients have classically been divided into two categories, mild and severe, it should be noted that mild preeclampsia is associated with adverse outcomes, and the American College of Obstetricians and Gynecologists Task Force on Hypertension in Pregnancy suggests that the term "preeclampsia without severe features" be used instead. Findings that further increase the risks and place the patient into the severe preeclampsia category include a blood pressure of 160/110 mm Hg or higher on two occasions at least 4 h apart or a blood pressure of at least 140/90 mm Hg and any of the above-mentioned criteria, and severe, persistent right upper quadrant or epigastric pain. Since studies have shown minimal association between the quantity of protein in the urine and patient outcome, the amount of proteinuria, ie, >5 g/d, has been removed from the criteria for severe preeclampsia.

2. Which of the following would *not* be a risk factor for the development of preeclampsia?

A. Age >40 years.
B. Smoking.
C. Obesity.
D. Primiparity.

The correct answer is B. Risk factors for development of preeclampsia include personal history of preeclampsia, history of preeclampsia in a first-degree relative, multiple gestations, chronic hypertension, obesity, maternal age >40 years, first pregnancy, and/or diabetes. Smoking has been associated with reduced risk of developing preeclampsia.

The patient is given a labetalol 20-mg IV bolus, a Foley catheter is placed, and a magnesium sulfate 4-g IV bolus is administered over 20 min followed by a magnesium sulfate infusion of 2 g/h IV. Total urine output over 4 h is 80 mL. You are emergently called to the room because the patient has been found unresponsive. The nurse states that the patient began to complain of flushing and difficulty breathing and then became apneic. You secure the patient's airway, initiate mechanical ventilation, and order a STAT serum magnesium level.

3. What serum magnesium level would you expect in this patient?

A. 1 mEq/L.
B. 5 mEq/L.
C. 10 mEq/L.
D. >10 mEq/L.

The correct answer is D. A normal serum magnesium level is between 1.5 and 2.5 mEq/L. For seizure prophylaxis in preeclampsia, therapeutic levels are between 4 and 6 mEq/L. Loss of deep tendon reflexes occurs at a magnesium level of 10 mEq/L. At 15 mEq/L, the patient can experience respiratory arrest, and at levels of ≥20 mEq/L, the patient can develop asystole and cardiovascular collapse.

4. What is the likely cause of the supratheraputic levels of serum magnesium in this patient?

   A. Drug administration error.
   B. Acute liver failure.
   C. Acute kidney injury.
   D. Drug interaction with labetalol.
   E. A and/or C

The correct answer is E. Since magnesium is primarily excreted by the kidneys, caution should be exercised when administrating magnesium sulfate to patients with acute or chronic kidney insufficiency, as magnesium can accumulate to toxic levels. In this case, the patient has been diagnosed with severe preeclampsia and has diminished urine output. Although our patient does not have laboratory data to confirm the diagnosis at this time, oliguria in the setting of severe preeclampsia suggests acute kidney injury. Finally, those who investigate adverse outcomes in a health system appreciate that drug administration errors are much more common than we would like to admit.

5. Which of the following IV medications is the treatment for magnesium sulfate toxicity?

   A. Calcium.
   B. Atropine.
   C. Epinephrine.
   D. Isoproterenol.

The correct answer is A. Calcium (either 1 g of calcium gluconate or 300 mg of calcium chloride) IV is used as the reversal agent for magnesium sulfate toxicity. However, this does not eliminate the magnesium from circulation. In a patient with adequate kidney function, IV fluids and a loop diuretic can also be given. Renal replacement therapy should be considered in patients with kidney failure and severe side effects from magnesium toxicity. Until the patient is stabilized, mechanical ventilation and cardiovascular support may be required.

The patient's blood pressure is now 200/120 mm Hg, and recurrent late decelerations are noted on the fetal tracing. The patient is taken for emergent cesarean delivery under general anesthesia. Labetalol 20 mg IV, propofol 120 mg IV, rocuronium 50 mg IV, and 1.6% end-tidal sevoflurane with 100% FiO_2 are administered prior to incision. An uncomplicated cesarean delivery is performed. At the end of the 1-h procedure, the patient is noted to have very weak respiratory effort and zero twitches on a neuromuscular stimulator train-of-four.

6. What is the likely cause of the patient's failure to wean from the ventilator?

   A. Hemorrhagic stroke.
   B. Pseudocholinesterase deficiency.
   C. Magnesium.
   D. Hypoglycemia.

The correct answer is C. Although hemorrhagic stroke and hypoglycemia should be included in the differential diagnosis of delayed emergence, neither diagnosis in and of itself would produce zero twitches on a neuromuscular stimulator train-of-four. Magnesium will decrease both the release of acetylcholine from the nerve and the response of the motor end-plate to acetylcholine. The effects of both succinylcholine and nondepolarizing muscle relaxants are potentiated by magnesium sulfate. Even small doses of magnesium will markedly intensify neuromuscular blockade. The patient received rocuronium and not succinylcholine; therefore, pseudocholinesterase deficiency would be incorrect.

DID YOU LEARN?

- The diagnostic criteria for mild and severe preeclampsia and risk factors for the development of preeclampsia.
- Magnesium toxicity and treatment.
- The potentiation of muscle relaxants by magnesium.

References

Frawley P, Butterworth JF 4th. Do antiarrhythmic doses of magnesium potentiate vecuronium? *Nurse Anesth.* 1992;3(1):8-13.

Roberts JM, August PA, Gaiser RR, et al. Hypertension in pregnancy: Report of the American College of Obstetricians and Gynecologists' Task Force on Hypertension in Pregnancy. *Obstet Gynecol.* 2013;122:1122-1131.

CASE 8   Pregnant Patient with HIV

Michael A. Frölich, MD, MS, and Mark Powell, MD

A 26-year-old primigravida is to be evaluated in the high-risk obstetric anesthesia clinic for newly diagnosed human immunodeficiency virus (HIV) infection. The patient was diagnosed with HIV at her first prenatal visit. Her latest laboratory studies show a CD4 count of 680 cells/mm^3 and a viral load of 220 copies/mL. Her medications include a combination lamivudine-zidovudine tablet and lopinavir-ritonavir tablet that are taken daily. She is 32 weeks pregnant and is asymptomatic from her HIV.

1. She is concerned about the risk of HIV infection in her baby. Given her current clinical picture, you tell her the risk of HIV transmission is:

   A. 2%.
   B. 10%.
   C. 20%.
   D. 25%.

The correct answer is A. If the patient does not receive antiretroviral therapy during pregnancy and delivery, the risk of vertical transmission is approximately 25%. This risk is reduced to 5% to 8% if zidovudine is taken by the mother during pregnancy and delivery and given to the neonate for the first 6 weeks of life. In patients with a viral load of 1000 copies/mL or less at the time of delivery, the risk is further reduced to 2% or less.

2. The patient is concerned that her baby would be at a higher risk of infection if she delivered vaginally and requests a cesarean delivery. At what viral load should a patient be counseled on the benefits of a scheduled cesarean delivery?

   A. 250 copies/mL.
   B. 500 copies/mL.
   C. 1000 copies/mL.
   D. 1500 copies/mL.

The correct answer is C. The American College of Obstetricians and Gynecologists (ACOG) Committee on Obstetric Practice recommends counseling patients on the potential benefit of cesarean delivery to reduce the risk of vertical transmission of HIV to the newborn in patients with a viral load of 1000 copies/mL or higher. Although under most circumstances cesarean deliveries should not be scheduled before 39 weeks' gestational age, ACOG endorses early (38 weeks' gestational age) delivery in HIV-infected patients to reduce the likelihood of spontaneous labor and rupture of membranes. The fetus is at increased risk of infection during labor with maternal–fetal microtransfusions during uterine contractions, and during delivery via cervicovaginal secretions. The benefit of decreased fetal transmission should be weighed against the risk of increased morbidity of elective cesarean delivery, especially in patients with low CD4 cell counts.

3. The patient is also very anxious about experiencing pain during labor and delivery and desires to receive the most effective, yet safe, form of analgesia. Due to her HIV status, you suggest the patient receive:

   A. IV meperidine as needed.
   B. IV fentanyl patient-controlled analgesia (PCA).
   C. IV remifentanil PCA.
   D. Epidural bupivacaine-fentanyl.

The correct answer is D. Currently, there are limited data addressing the concern for neurological or infectious complications in HIV patients undergoing neuraxial anesthesia. Reports have shown the safe administration of neuraxial anesthesia in HIV-infected patients; however, all have looked at relatively healthy patients in early stages of HIV infection as opposed to patients with more advanced forms of the disease. A major challenge in HIV-infected patients is post-neuraxial anesthesia follow-up, as most neurologic symptoms will be unrelated to the anesthetic performed. Approximately 90% of HIV patients have pathological changes within the nervous system at autopsy. Neurological complications such as aseptic meningitis, chronic headaches, or polyneuropathy can often be erroneously associated with the epidural or spinal block. Also, some of the retroviral medications used can lead to neurotoxicity. After a detailed history and physical examination addressing any neurological derangements, it would be appropriate to discuss the risks and benefits of epidural placement for pain control during labor and delivery, as this will provide superior analgesia when compared to IV administration of opioid analgesic agents. All preexisting neurological symptoms and signs should be carefully documented so that baseline neurological function is established for postprocedure follow-up.

4. Laboratory studies were drawn at her 37th-week appointment and showed a viral load of 240 copies/mL and a CD4 count of 660 cells/mm^3. The patient was scheduled for induction of labor at 39 weeks' gestational age. She now presents to labor and delivery for induction. On placement of the IV, the nurse accidentally sticks herself with an 18-gauge IV contaminated with the patient's blood. The risk of seroconversion is:

   A. 0.2%.
   B. 2%.
   C. 12%.
   D. 20%.

The correct answer is A. The risk of seroconversion in practitioners who have a needlestick injury with HIV-infected blood is extremely rare, at approximately 0.2% to 0.3%. The risk is approximately 2% with hepatitis C and 20% with hepatitis B. Certain risk factors can increase the risk and include injury with a large-diameter needle, deep injury, visible blood on the device, a procedure involving a needle placed in the HIV-infected patient's artery or vein, emergency procedures, and exposure to blood of a patient who died within 2 months from acquired immunodeficiency syndrome. Although no prospective studies can confirm its efficacy, prophylactic use of zidovudine within 4 h of exposure appears to be protective.

5. After zidovudine administration, an oxytocin infusion is begun. Shortly thereafter, your colleague is called to place a labor epidural. While placing the epidural, your partner inadvertently accesses the subarachnoid space with free-flow of cerebrospinal fluid. The epidural catheter is threaded into the subarachnoid space and is used for labor analgesia. The labor and delivery is uncomplicated. Postpartum, the patient is diagnosed with a post-dural puncture headache (PDPH). After IV hydration, caffeine, and oral analgesics have failed by postpartum day 2, the patient desires definitive treatment. While discussing treatment options with the patient, you:

A. Suggest that she continue with conservative therapy, as the headache should resolve within 24 h.
B. Suggest no further therapy, as the headache should resolve within 24 h.
C. Tell her that a blood patch is contraindicated due to risk of HIV contamination within the central nervous system (CNS).
D. Offer her a blood patch.

The correct answer is D. As in this scenario, after 24 h of conservative therapy, a more invasive and definitive treatment of an epidural blood patch can be discussed with the patient. Inoculating the CNS with HIV should be of no concern, as involvement of the CNS occurs within the first several months of the infection. Although data are lacking for HIV-infected patients treated with a blood patch for PDPH, one small study following nine patients anywhere from 6 months to 2 years after the procedure showed no complications attributed to the blood patch. Therefore, in a patient with a debilitating PDPH in whom conservative therapy has failed, a blood patch would be an appropriate treatment option after risks and benefits of the procedure have been discussed.

DID YOU LEARN?

- The risk of vertical transmission of HIV from mother to newborn during labor and delivery and treatments to reduce this risk.
- The risk of neuraxial procedures in HIV-infected patients.
- The risk of seroconversion in practitioners involved in needlesticks with HIV-contaminated blood.

References

ACOG Committee Opinion No. 751 Summary: Labor and delivery management of women with human immunodeficiency virus infection. *Obstet Gynecol*. 2018;132(3):803-804.

Gronwald C, Vowinkel T, Hahnenkamp K. Regional anesthetic procedures in immunosuppressed patients: Risk of infection. *Curr Opin Anaesthesiol*. 2011;24(6):698-704.

Lima YA, Cardoso LP, Reis MN, Stefani MM. Incident and long-term HIV-1 infection among pregnant women in Brazil: Transmitted drug resistance and mother-to-child transmission. *J Med Virol*. 2016;88(11):1936-1943.

Nwaiwu CA, Egro FM, Smith S, et al. Seroconversion rate among health care workers exposed to HIV-contaminated body fluids: The University of Pittsburgh 13-year experience. *Am J Infect Control*. 2017;45(8):896-900.

CASE 9 · Obese Patient Without IV Access for Urgent Cesarean Section

Michael A. Frölich, MD, MS, and Mark Powell, MD

You are called to evaluate a 32-year-old G4P3 undergoing urgent repeat cesarean delivery for recurrent late decelerations. She presented 30 min earlier with painful contractions. Her past medical history includes two prior cesarean deliveries, morbid obesity, essential hypertension, obstructive sleep apnea (OSA), and a right femoral vein thrombosis for which she is currently taking enoxaparin. Her last enoxaparin injection was 4 h ago. She is 64″ tall and weighs 165 kg and has a body mass index of 62. Vital signs include blood pressure 165/102 mm Hg, pulse 106 beats/min, respiratory rate 22 breaths/min, and SpO_2 93% on room air. On airway exam, she has a large neck, poor oral opening, full dentition, and a Mallampati class IV airway. The nursing staff is unable to obtain a peripheral IV or perform phlebotomy for routine laboratory evaluation.

1. Your most appropriate next action is to:

   A. Proceed to the operating room (OR) and perform an inhalational induction.

   B. Administer supplemental O_2, position the patient in left lateral tilt, and place a right internal jugular vein central venous line (CVL) under ultrasound guidance.

   C. Administer supplemental O_2 and position the patient supine for placement of a left femoral vein CVL.

   D. Allow for oral hydration in an effort to facilitate peripheral IV placement.

The correct answer is B. IV access must be obtained prior to proceeding with cesarean delivery to allow blood withdrawal for laboratory studies, provide an IV route for medication administration, and because urgent massive resuscitation may be required during or after procedure. Although this is an urgent case, proceeding to the OR for an inhalational induction could prove disastrous. The patient has multiple risk factors for a difficult intubation and mask ventilation, including pregnancy, a small mouth opening, and morbid obesity. The parturient is also at high risk for aspiration despite her NPO status. Inhalational induction without IV access would place the patient at great risk for an anesthetic-related complication, including death. The appropriate action is to attempt restoration of the normal arterial O_2 tension to the fetus by administering supplemental O_2 to the mother and also by placing her in left lateral tilt position, which will alleviate aortocaval compression. Relief of vena cava compression will increase venous return and potentially correct maternal hypotension, and improved flow through the aorta will improve uterine perfusion. There are multiple reasons that a femoral CVL would not be the first choice for central venous access in this patient: supine positioning for this procedure would likely promote aortocaval compression, and the patient's body habitus may make placement difficult and unsterile. The subclavian approach would also be reasonable for placement of a CVL. It also might be possible to place a large-bore IV in a peripheral site with ultrasound guidance. Oral hydration will not acutely facilitate peripheral IV placement and will further increase aspiration risk.

2. After performing the above procedures, the recurrent late fetal decelerations improve; however, the patient remains in active labor, and the obstetrician requests to proceed with cesarean delivery. Blood is sent for routine laboratory analysis. Your choice of anesthetic will be:

A. Epidural.
B. Spinal.
C. Combined spinal-epidural.
D. General anesthesia with awake fiber-optic intubation.

The correct answer is D. Due to the risk of spinal hematoma, the American Society of Regional Anesthesia and Pain Medicine recommends against the placement of an epidural or spinal needle or catheter for 12 h after receiving a prophylactic dose of enoxaparin and for 24 h after receiving a full-dose of enoxaparin. General anesthesia is indicated if the case cannot be delayed for at least 24 h from the patient's last enoxaparin injection. Awake fiber-optic intubation is an appropriate airway technique in this case because of the patient's risks for difficult mask ventilation, failed intubation, rapid blood O_2 desaturation, and aspiration.

3. After adequate application of topical anesthesia to the airway, you are able to intubate the trachea with the fiber-optic bronchoscope. Which of the following nerves provides sensory innervation to the arytenoids?

A. Recurrent laryngeal nerve.
B. Superior laryngeal nerve, internal branch.
C. Superior laryngeal nerve, external branch.
D. Glossopharyngeal nerve.

The correct answer is B. The internal branch of the superior laryngeal nerve provides sensory innervation to the posterior surface of the epiglottis and to the structures between the epiglottis and vocal cords, including the arytenoids. The recurrent laryngeal nerve provides sensory innervation to airway below the level of the vocal cords and motor nerve innervation to all intrinsic laryngeal muscles except the cricothyroid muscle, which is supplied by the external branch of the superior laryngeal nerve. The external branch of the superior laryngeal nerve only has motor function. The glossopharyngeal nerve provides sensory innervation to the anterior surface of the epiglottis and to structures above the epiglottis, including the vallecula, walls of the pharynx, tonsils, and posterior third of the tongue.

After the procedure, the patient was extubated and taken to the recovery room. Twenty minutes later, you get called to evaluate the patient for postoperative pain control. The patient is somnolent but readily and appropriately responsive to verbal communication. She reports moderate incisional pain. The patient's vital signs are blood pressure 158/90 mm Hg, pulse 106 beats/min, respirations 16 breaths/min, and SpO_2 90% on 2 L O_2 via nasal cannula.

4. The most appropriate IV pain control at this time is:

A. None until her O_2 saturation improves.
B. Morphine 2 mg.
C. Fentanyl 100 μg.
D. Ketorolac 30 mg.

The correct answer is D. Although the patient is somnolent, she is verbally responsive and is reporting moderate pain at her incision site. Postoperative pain control should be a priority. However, she does have a history of OSA and currently exhibits low O_2 saturation with supplemental O_2. Patients with OSA are at increased risk for adverse respiratory events, and opioid analgesics should be utilized with caution. If no contraindication exists, nonsteroidal anti-inflammatory drugs (NSAIDs), such as ketorolac, are a first-line treatment for postprocedure acute pain control, as they are not associated with respiratory depression or somnolence. IV acetaminophen is another excellent analgesic option in this situation for the same reason. Regional anesthesia (such as a transverse abdominis plane block) would be an ideal option for OSA patients at high risk for adverse respiratory events in the postoperative period.

DID YOU LEARN?

- The implications of aortocaval compression and importance of left lateral tilt.
- Guidelines for neuraxial anesthesia and enoxaparin administration.
- Sensory innervation of the airway.
- Pain control in patients with OSA.

Recommended Reading

Frölich MA. Obstetric anesthesia. In: Butterworth IV JF, Mackey DC, Wasnick JD, eds. *Morgan & Mikhail's Clinical Anesthesiology,* 6th ed. New York, NY: McGraw-Hill Education; 2018:861-896.

References

Chung F, Memtsoudis SG, Ramachandran SK, et al. Society of Anesthesia and Sleep Medicine guidelines on preoperative screening and assessment of adult patients with obstructive sleep apnea. *Anesth Analg.* 2016;123(2):452-473.

Leffert LR, Dubois HM, Butwick AJ, et al. Neuraxial anesthesia in obstetric patients receiving thromboprophylaxis with unfractionated or low-molecular-weight heparin: A systematic review of spinal epidural hematoma. *Anesth Analg.* 2017;125(1):223-231.

Netter FH. *Atlas of Human Anatomy,* 3rd ed. Teterboro: Icon Learning Systems; 2003:58.

CHAPTER 35

Pediatric Anesthesia

CASE 1 — Inhalation Induction in Two Siblings

Jason Noble, MD

Two siblings present for surgery on the same day. The younger one is a 1-year-old girl who is scheduled for myringotomy tubes for recurrent otitis media. She has a remote history of esophageal reflux, but she has had no signs or symptoms from this for 3 months. Her vital signs on admission are blood pressure 83/52 mm Hg, heart rate 116 beats/min, respiratory rate 27 breaths/min, SaO_2 97%, and weight 10 kg. The older sibling is a 12-year-old boy who is scheduled for adenoidectomy for chronic sinusitis. His vital signs on admission are blood pressure 94/62 mm Hg, heart rate 85 beats/min, respiratory rate 22 breaths/min, SaO_2 98%, and weight 44 kg. Both children were born at term. Neither one has any evidence of sleep-disordered breathing or other respiratory abnormalities. Both were given water to drink this morning shortly after waking, which was 4 h ago.

Both children are induced by inhalation technique with a mixture of sevoflurane in oxygen at similar inhaled concentrations. Both inductions proceed without complication.

1. Which of the following is the best explanation for the 1-year-old losing consciousness more quickly than the 12-year-old?

    A. The infant has a smaller mass and requires a smaller amount of sevoflurane.
    B. On a per-kilogram basis, the infant has less anatomical dead space.
    C. The infant has a smaller functional residual capacity (FRC).
    D. The blood/gas coefficient of sevoflurane is increased in the infant.
    E. A, B, and C.

The correct answer is C. Infants and neonates have faster induction times with inhaled anesthetic agents than adults and older children due to a number of physiological and anatomical differences. Infants and neonates have relatively smaller FRC and greater minute ventilations. This results in a more rapid turnover of alveolar gas and more rapid increase in alveolar concentration of volatile anesthetic. A higher percentage of an infant's cardiac output is directed toward vessel-rich organs, resulting in a more rapid delivery of agent to the central nervous system. The blood/gas solubility coefficients of anesthetic agents are reduced, not increased, in very young pediatric patients. This means less agent will dissolve in the blood, and partial pressure of the agent in the alveoli will increase more quickly. All of these qualities result in a more rapid rise of the concentration of agent in brain tissue.

Volatile anesthetic agents exert their effects when they achieve sufficient concentrations in the brain. The speed of onset of this effect is determined by the rate that concentrations increase in alveolar gas, not the speed at which a total anesthetic dose is administered. Anatomic pulmonary dead space on a per-kilogram basis is similar in all age groups.

Both children show a decrease in blood pressure after induction. Despite identical end-tidal concentrations of sevoflurane, the change from baseline value is more pronounced in the 1-year-old.

2. The most likely explanation for this difference is that:

A. The infant's heart is more sensitive to the depressant effects of sevoflurane.
B. Greater sevoflurane-induced decreases in sympathetic tone in the infant.
C. Greater reductions of heart rate in the infant.
D. Greater anesthetic depth despite similar alveolar concentrations of sevoflurane in the infant.

The correct answer is A. The blood pressure of neonates and infants is especially sensitive to volatile anesthetics for several reasons. The immature myocardium itself is more sensitive to the direct depressant effects of anesthetic agents. The sympathetic nervous system and baroreceptor reflexes are not yet well developed in infants and children. Therefore, compensatory mechanisms dependent on the sympathetic nervous system, such as tachycardia and systemic vasoconstriction, will be less effective in infants. The parasympathetic system is relatively unopposed in infants, and thus bradycardia is a bigger problem than tachycardia in this population, and bradycardia can lead to cardiac arrest.

The immature heart is also relatively noncompliant, meaning it has only a limited ability to increase stroke volume when needed to increase cardiac output. Changes in cardiac output are thus almost completely dependent on heart rate (in the absence of hypovolemia) to accommodate changing requirements. In infants and neonates, changes in ventricular filling time (from heart rate changes) do not usually influence cardiac output.

Halogenated agents have an increased MAC in infants and children compared to adults. Sevoflurane is unique among them in that it does not also have a greater MAC in infants when compared to neonates.

Both patients are allowed to breathe spontaneously for the duration of their respective procedures. Prior to the start of surgery, the infant has a greater end-tidal carbon dioxide tension than her older sibling.

3. Which explanation for this is most likely correct?

   A. The increased lung compliance of the infant results in more extensive atelectasis.
   B. The older child's larger tidal volume breaths result in greater alveolar ventilation.
   C. Weaker diaphragmatic and accessory muscles in the infant produce less efficient ventilation.
   D. Infants have a greater baseline carbon dioxide tension.
   E. Both A and B

The correct answer is C. Neonates and infants have several characteristics that may result in problems with oxygenation and ventilation during general anesthesia. The lungs do not mature fully until late childhood. In infants and neonates, the lungs have fewer and smaller alveoli as well as smaller airways. Aside from directly affecting gas exchange and decreasing FRC, this decreases lung compliance and increases airway resistance. All of these factors increase the work of breathing.

Work of breathing is of greater importance to infants and neonates than to older children and adults. Infants and neonates have respiratory muscles with a relatively reduced concentration of type I fibers, and therefore, these muscles fatigue more easily. The framework these muscles work against is also less mechanically efficient than in an adult. Very young children have ribs that are more horizontally oriented, which means the muscles less efficiently expand the volume of the thoracic cavity when they contract. The ribs also contain more cartilage, making the chest wall more compliant. As a result, the chest wall collapses inwardly during inspiration, further reducing the ability of the muscles to expand the chest cavity.

It is these combined factors, not increased lung compliance, which cause greater atelectasis in infants during anesthesia. Tidal volumes, like anatomic dead space, remain similar throughout life on a per-kilogram basis. In neonates and infants, both hypoxic and hypercapnic respiratory drives are poorly developed; either hypoxia or hypercapnia may cause respiratory depression instead of stimulation in this patient population.

DID YOU LEARN?

- Age differences in FRC.
- Age differences in susceptibility to left ventricular depression from volatile anesthetics.

- Age differences in work of breathing and susceptibility to respiratory muscle fatigue.

References

Cote CJ, Lerman J, Anderson B. *A Practice of Anesthesia for Infants and Children*. 6th ed. Philadelphia, PA: Elsevier; 2018.

Davis PJ, Cladis FP. *Smith's Anesthesia for Infants and Children*. 9th ed. Philadelphia, PA: Elsevier; 2016.

CASE 2 Sudden Bradycardia During Strabismus Surgery

Linh T. Nguyen, MD

You are assigned to anesthetize a healthy 10-year-old, 32-kg boy scheduled for strabismus surgery. His preoperative vital signs are blood pressure 110/65 mm Hg, pulse 90 beats/min, respiratory rate 20 breaths/min, and room air SpO_2 99%. Standard ASA monitors are placed. He has an uneventful induction and intubation with propofol 100 mg intravenously (IV), rocuronium 20 mg IV, and fentanyl 150 µg IV. General anesthesia is maintained with sevoflurane, using a mixture of 50% air and 50% oxygen. Fifteen minutes after initiation of the surgical procedure, when the surgeon retracts the medial rectus muscle, you note that the heart rate abruptly decreases to 40 beats/min, with a concomitant decrease in blood pressure.

1. What is the most likely cause of the vital signs change?

A. Bezold-Jarisch reflex.
B. Oculocardiac reflex.
C. Bainbridge reflex.
D. Cushing reflex.

The correct answer is B. The *oculocardiac reflex* (OCR) was first described in 1908 by Bernard Aschner and Giuseppe Dagnini in separate publications. It is activated by traction on the extraocular muscles and/or by pressure applied to the globe, and its most common manifestation is sudden-onset bradycardia. However, this reflex may also produce asystole or cardiac arrhythmias such as nodal rhythm or ventricular fibrillation. The incidence of the OCR during strabismus surgery is reported to be between 32% and 90%.

The afferent pathway of this reflex consists of ciliary nerves, which travel from the ciliary ganglion via the ophthalmic branch of the trigeminal nerve (cranial nerve V) to the trigeminal (Gasserian) ganglion. The fibers then synapse with fibers that travel to the main sensory nucleus of the trigeminal nerve in the medulla. Short *internuncial fibers* connect the main sensory nucleus of the trigeminal nerve to the motor nucleus of the vagus nerve (cranial nerve X). The efferent pathway of the reflex consists of nerve fibers from the motor nucleus of the vagus nerve innervating the sinoatrial node in the heart.

Stimulation of the maxillary or mandibular divisions of the trigeminal nerve can also elicit reflex bradycardia, cardiac arrhythmias, or asystole. This phenomenon has been reported to occur during skull-base surgeries, including resection of tumors at the cerebellopontine angle, and during maxillofacial procedures on the temporomandibular joint or repair of facial fractures. This reflex is referred to as the *trigeminocardiac reflex*.

The *Bezold-Jarisch reflex* refers to the triad of bradycardia, hypotension, and peripheral vasodilation in response to the activation of mechanosensitive receptors in the walls of the ventricles by a rapid fall in cardiac preload. It is postulated that this reflex may be responsible for the sudden bradycardia or asystole that may be observed with spinal anesthesia, rapid blood loss, high gravitational force aerobatic maneuvers, and rarely after administration of nitroglycerin.

The *Bainbridge reflex*, also called the *atrial reflex*, is characterized by an increase in heart rate in response to increased central venous volume and is initiated by activation of atrial stretch receptors.

The *Cushing reflex* consists of bradycardia, hypertension, and irregular respiration initiated by excessively elevated intracranial pressure (ICP) and may herald impending brain herniation.

2. At this point, what should you do immediately?

   A. Administer ephedrine IV.
   B. Administer atropine IV.
   C. Ask the surgeon to stop surgical manipulation.
   D. Do nothing and continue to observe.

The correct answer is C. The first step in the management of the OCR during strabismus surgery is to ask the surgeon to immediately halt ophthalmic stimulation—in this case, to release the traction on the extraocular muscle. The bradycardia or cardiac dysrhythmias will usually resolve simply by removing the inciting stimulus. Inaction and observation are not an option, as continued stimulation may provoke lethal arrhythmias and/or asystole.

The incidence of asystole during strabismus surgery under general anesthesia was reported to be 0.1% (4 out of 3628 consecutive cases) in a recent study. Of the four cases of asystole, the heart rate recovered to the pretraction heart rate in each case with release of the traction. IV atropine was given after heart rate recovery in each of these four cases, and each case proceeded uneventfully (Min and Hwang, 2009).

In this case, the physiological mechanism of the bradycardia and resulting hypotension involves the stimulation of the vagus nerve. Therefore, a vagolytic agent is used in the treatment of the oculocardiac reflex. Ephedrine is commonly used to treat hypotension under anesthesia. However, it does not have anticholinergic properties and is not the drug of choice for treatment of the OCR.

3. What factor(s) will increase the likelihood of the OCR?

  A. Hypoxemia.
  B. Opioids.
  C. Hypercarbia.
  D. All of the above.

The correct answer is D. Hypoxemia, hypercarbia, and the use of opioids increase the likelihood of the OCR. Dexdemetomidine, a selective α_2-adrenergic receptor agonist frequently used in pediatric strabismus surgery to prevent emergence agitation, also potentiates the OCR when given as an IV bolus (Arnold et al., 2018). Rapidly acting IV opioids have a greater augmenting effect upon the OCR than slower-acting opioids. Remifentanil has the greatest effect compared to sufentanil or fentanyl (Arnold et al., 2004).

4. Which of the following statements is true?

  A. Retrobulbar block is nearly always effective in preventing the OCR.
  B. IV anticholinergic medication should not routinely be used in strabismus surgery to prevent the OCR.
  C. The OCR fatigues after repeated activation.
  D. IV atropine is preferable to IV glycopyrrolate to prevent the bradycardia from the OCR.

The correct answer is C. The oculocardiac reflex fatigues after repeated stimulation. Retrobulbar block is ineffective in preventing the OCR, and sinus arrest has been reported in patients who have received, or are undergoing administration of, a retrobulbar block. Prophylactic anticholinergic administration has been reported to decrease the frequency of the OCR in children undergoing strabismus surgery from up to 90% to less than 50%. Although both atropine and glycopyrrolate are equally effective in the prevention of the OCR, glycopyrrolate causes less tachycardia. The IV route is more effective than the intramuscular route (Mirakhur et al., 1982, 1986).

DID YOU LEARN?

- The afferent and efferent limbs of the OCR.
- Management of the bradycardia caused by the OCR.
- Predisposing or potentiating risk factors for the activation of the OCR.
- The effectiveness of the retrobulbar block and IV anticholinergics in preventing the activation of the OCR.

Recommended Reading

Butterworth IV JF, Mackey DC, Wasnick JD, eds. Anesthesia for ophthalmic surgery. In: *Morgan & Mikhail's Clinical Anesthesiology.* 6th ed. New York, NY: McGraw-Hill Education; 2018:773-786.

References

Arnold RW, Biggs RE, Beerle BJ. Intravenous dexmedetomidine augments the oculocardiac reflex. *J AAPOS.* 2018:22(3):211-213.e1.

Arnold RW, Jensen PA, Kovtoun TA, Maurer SA, Schultz JA. The profound augmentation of the oculocardiac reflex by fast acting opioids. *Binocul Vis Strabismus Q.* 2004;19:215-222.

Campagna JA, Carter C. Clinical relevance of the Bezold-Jarisch reflex. *Anesthesiology.* 2003;98:1250-1260.

Crystal GJ, Salem RM. The Bainbridge and the "reverse" Bainbridge reflexes: History, physiology, and clinical relevance. *Anesth Analg.* 2012;114:520-532.

Lubbers HT, Zweifel D, Gratz KW, Kruse A. Classification of potential risk factors for trigeminocardiac reflex in craniomaxillofacial surgery. *J Oral Maxillofac Surg.* 2010;68:1317.

Min SW, Hwang JM. The incidence of asystole in patients undergoing strabismus surgery. *Eye.* 2009;23:864-866.

Mirakhur RK, Jones CJ, Dundee JW, Archer DB. IM or IV atropine or glycopyrrolate for the prevention of oculocardiac reflex in children undergoing squint surgery. *Br J Anaesth.* 1982;54:1059-1063.

Mirakhur RK, Shepherd WFI, Jones CJ. Ventilation and the oculocardiac reflex. Prevention of oculocardiac reflex during surgery for squint: Role of controlled ventilation and anticholinergic drugs. *Anaesthesia.* 1986;41:825-828.

Schaller B, Cornelius JF, Prabhakar H, et al. The trigeminocardiac reflex: An update of the current knowledge. *J Neurosurg Anesthesiol.* 2009;21:187.

Waldschmidt B, Gordon N. Anesthesia for pediatric ophthalmologic surgery. *J AAPOS.* 2019;23(3):127-131.

CASE 3   Hemorrhage in the PACU Following Tonsillectomy

Nischal K. Gautam, MD

You are called to the postanesthesia care unit (PACU) to evaluate a 10-year-old, 74-kg male patient with trisomy 21 who has undergone adenotonsillectomy. The patient is now restless, agitated, and has pulled out his IV catheter. Pulse oximetry has a poor waveform and intermittently indicates a heart rate of 65 beats/min and SpO$_2$ of 90% on room air. The blood pressure cuff indicates a mean pressure of 45 mm Hg. The preoperative assessment notes that this patient had a successful repair of complete atrioventricular canal defect and placement of a pacemaker generator for complete heart block in the past. Preoperatively, the pacemaker was reprogrammed to an asynchronous mode. The intraoperative anesthesia record documents laryngospasm during inhalational induction, which resolved with IV administration of propofol and rocuronium. Subsequent endotracheal intubation was atraumatic and easy. Sevoflurane anesthesia was used for the 40-min surgical procedure, during which 300 mL of IV lactated Ringer's was administered. At the conclusion of the surgery, 3 mg IV morphine was given before a "deep" extubation.

1. At this time, all the following are appropriate measures *except*:

   A. Administer oxygen.
   B. Examine the oropharynx.
   C. Deeply sedate the patient with weight-appropriate doses of IV propofol or intramuscular ketamine to facilitate examination and management.
   D. Establish IV or intraosseous access.

The correct answer is C. The child recovering from an adenotonsillectomy has a variety of reasons to be restless and agitated. Emergence delirium observed within 30 min of emergence from general anesthesia is associated with wild or poorly controlled motor activity, disorientation, and abnormal response to comfort measures, caregivers, and stimuli. However, before diagnosing postoperative disorientation as emergence delirium, a rapid initial examination to seek other common causes of restlessness and agitation—such as pain, hypoxemia, and hypovolemia—is warranted. Each of the above may act alone or in combinations to confound the clinical picture. In this child who appears restless and agitated with hypoxemia and hypotension, the clinical signs point toward hypovolemia from inadequate fluid replenishment, hemorrhage, and/or cardiopulmonary compromise. Deep sedation without a diagnosis and without securing the airway may hasten cardiovascular collapse.

Once the patient is gently restrained, copious blood is noted during examination of the oropharynx, and the surgical team decides to examine the naso-oropharynx under anesthesia. The patient is immediately returned to the operating room, where he is now noted to be lethargic with a respiratory rate of 46 breaths/min. The ECG reveals a regular rate of 65 beats/min, and pulse oximetry indicates SaO_2 of 90% on 6 L/min oxygen by simple face mask.

2. The following are appropriate next steps for this patient *except*:

   A. Rapid-sequence induction/intubation with cricoid pressure.
   B. Check hematocrit and send blood sample for type and crossmatch.
   C. Apply a magnet to the pacemaker.
   D. Alert the angiography suite.

The correct answer is C. Major hemorrhage occurring immediately after tonsillectomy (<24 h) is rare (<1% incidence) but may have devastating consequences.

The concerns for anesthetic management of any child with primary bleeding after adenotonsillectomy include anemia, hypovolemia, and a large volume of sequestered intragastric blood. Care in this instance is compounded by trisomy 21 (with possible atlantoaxial instability), obesity, and a pacemaker with suboptimal performance. Securing and protecting the airway is paramount in case of a primary tonsillar hemorrhage. Resuscitation with blood products may be required. Preoperatively, this child's pacemaker may have been placed in an asynchronous rate with no rate modulation in order to minimize effects of electrocautery, and the child is now unable to compensate for hypovolemia with appropriate heart rate responsiveness. Application of a magnet does nothing to change this asynchronous mode. The child needs reprogramming of the pacemaker device with the asynchronous rate closer to the intrinsic atrial rate and the asynchronous mode reverted to a synchronous mode as soon possible after use of electrocautery. Primary bleeding after adenoidectomy alone is extremely rare and occurs immediately after curettage. Arteriography should be considered when immediate bleeding in the adenoid bed is suggestive of aberrant courses of greater arteries.

3. During direct laryngoscopy, laryngeal visualization is obscured by the presence of clots and brisk bleeding. Oxygen saturation progressively drops to the low 80s. What constitutes the best subsequent course of action?

   A. Awaken the patient.
   B. Ventilate via laryngeal mask airway.
   C. Attempt flexible bronchoscopy.
   D. Proceed directly to rigid bronchoscopy and preparation for possible tracheostomy.

The correct answer is D. Difficult tracheal intubation with rapid-sequence induction may be encountered in a child with posttonsillectomy hemorrhage despite having no difficulties during initial intubation for the surgical procedure. Laryngeal views may be significantly hampered due to bleeding and obstruction from edematous tissues and clots during rapid-sequence reintubation. One or two rigid suction instruments may help facilitate laryngeal visualization while performing direct line-of-sight laryngoscopy, and rigid endoscopes should be available for this difficult intubation scenario that ensues with progressive hypoxemia. Tracheostomy may rarely be needed, and the trachea may be partially blocked with blood clots.

After achieving hemostasis, the patient is extubated when fully awake, but he continues to be tachypneic with an SpO_2 of 88% on 50% high-flow oxygen by simple face mask. Crackles are noted bilaterally in the lower lung fields. A chest radiograph shows intact pacemaker wires and bilateral patchy infiltrates in the lower lobes. Arterial blood gas reveals pH 7.30, $PaCO_2$ 37 mm Hg, PaO_2 52 mm Hg, and BE −4. Electrolytes are Na 145 mEq/L, K 2.8 mEq/L, chloride 115 mEq/L, and HCO_3 19 mEq/L.

4. What is true about the above scenario?

A. Arterial blood gases demonstrate anion gap metabolic acidosis and a shunt physiology.
B. Symptoms typically present late (24–48 h) after an aspiration episode.
C. Mechanical ventilation and flexible bronchoscopy may be indicated to evaluate worsening lung injury.
D. Antibiotics are the first line of therapy.

The correct answer is C. The arterial blood gas is consistent with a hyperchloremic metabolic acidosis with respiratory compensation and with hypoxemia due to ventilation–perfusion mismatch. Clinical signs point toward aspiration pneumonitis, although other confounders such as atelectasis and pulmonary edema need to be ruled out. In children, most of the blood from the tonsillar area is usually swallowed, which may subsequently result in hematemesis. Aspiration of this acidified blood or blood clots into the lungs during rapid-sequence intubation or emergence typically presents as hypoxemia and respiratory distress within 2 h of aspiration. The chest radiograph may reveal patchy opacities. The aspirated blood may act as a nidus for subsequent infection and may progress to pneumonia. Treatment is usually supportive with oxygen, and some cases may require mechanical ventilation, bronchoscopy, and therapeutic lavage.

DID YOU LEARN?

- Differential diagnosis of posttonsillectomy agitation.
- Types of bleeding after adenotonsillectomy.
- Management of primary hemorrhage after adenotonsillectomy.
- Approach to pulmonary aspiration.

References

Fields RG, Gencorelli FJ, Litman RS. Anesthetic management of the pediatric bleeding tonsil. *Paediatr Anaesth.* 2010;20:982-986.

Mitchell RB, Archer SM, Ishman SL, et al. Clinical practice guideline: Tonsillectomy in children (update). *Otolaryngol Head Neck Surg.* 2019;160(1 suppl):S1-S42.

Windfuhr JP, Schloendorff G, Sesterhenn AM, Prescher A, Kremer B. A devastating outcome after adenoidectomy and tonsillectomy: Ideas for improved prevention and management. *Otolaryngology.* 2009;140:191-196.

CASE 4 — Precipitous Delivery with Thick Meconium and No Neonatologist

Michael A. Frölich, MD, MS, and Mark Powell, MD

You are called STAT to the emergency department to care for a mother following precipitous delivery of a postterm fetus. Upon arrival, you see that the mother is currently stable; however, you note the fetus to be unresponsive and covered in thick meconium. The nurses are drying and stimulating the newborn and providing oxygen and oropharyngeal suctioning. Nevertheless, the neonate continues to have minimal respiratory effort. The neonatologist has been called from home but is 20 min away.

1. Your initial step is to:

   A. Continue to care for the mother, as you were called to evaluate her and not the newborn.
   B. Provide supplemental oxygen via face mask to the newborn.
   C. Provide positive-pressure ventilation via face mask to the newborn.
   D. Intubate the newborn and suction the airway.

The correct answer is D. Although you were called to care for the postpartum mother, she is stable at this moment, and care should be immediately directed toward the distressed newborn. Since this newborn exhibits depressed respirations, lax muscle tone, and a heart rate of less than 100 beats/min, the first step in resuscitation is tracheal intubation and suctioning. The goal of early intubation and suctioning is to minimize the risk of meconium aspiration. However, if a neonate is vigorous, tracheal suctioning is *not* recommended even in the presence of thick meconium. Supplemental oxygen alone will not improve the status of an unresponsive newborn. Positive-pressure ventilation via face mask may exacerbate the meconium aspiration.

2. Despite complete suctioning of the meconium from the airway, endotracheal intubation, and positive-pressure ventilation, the newborn is still lethargic, with a heart rate of 58 beats/min. Your next step is to:

   A. Transfer to ICU for mechanical ventilation.
   B. Administer epinephrine.
   C. Begin chest compressions.
   D. Continue to stimulate.

The correct answer is C. The first step of the neonatal resuscitation algorithm is to dry, stimulate, and (if necessary) clear the airway of the newborn. If the newborn is apneic and has a heart rate of less than 100 beats/min, then positive-pressure ventilation either by mask (if meconium is not present) or endotracheal tube is required. If, after 30 s of positive-pressure ventilation, the baby is still unresponsive or the heart rate remains less than 60 beats/min, chest compressions should be initiated. Epinephrine should be administered if the baby continues to be unresponsive or the heart rate remains less than 60 beats/min after at least 30 s of positive-pressure ventilation and chest compressions.

3. After continued resuscitation, you decide to administer epinephrine via the endotracheal tube. The correct dose is:

A. 0.1 mL/kg of 1:1000 solution.
B. 1 mL/kg of 1:1000 solution.
C. 0.1 mL/kg of 1:10,000 solution.
D. 1 mL/kg of 1:10,000 solution.

The correct answer is D. It is recommended to give a dilute (1:10,000) concentration of epinephrine. The standard dose for IV administration is 0.1 to 0.3 mL/kg. The endotracheal dose is approximately three times higher at 0.3 to 1 mL/kg.

4. After 5 min of resuscitation, the newborn has weak respiratory efforts, has some flexion, will grimace to stimulation, exhibits a pink torso with blue extremities, and has a heart rate of 110 beats/min. What is the Apgar score?

A. 2.
B. 4.
C. 6.
D. 8.

The correct answer is C. The Apgar score is composed of five criteria (see chart below), with each criterion scored from 0 to 2. Although the Apgar score is not a good predictor of neonatal outcome, it can provide insight into the newborn's response to resuscitation. Apgar scores are typically assessed at 1 and 5 min following delivery. If the 5-min score is less than 7, then subsequent scores should continue to be assessed at each 5-min interval for up to 20 min. From the chart below, the newborn in our scenario would be assigned a score of 6.

Category	0	1	2
Appearance (skin color)	Pale/blue	Pink body, blue extremities	All pink
Pulse	Absent	<100 beats/min	>100 beats/min
Grimace (reflex irritability)	Absent	Grimace	Cry
Activity (muscle tone)	Absent	Some flexion	Active motion
Respirations	Absent	Weak, irregular	Cry

Adapted with permission from Butterworth JF, Mackey DC, Wasnick JD: *Morgan and Mikhail's Clinical Anesthesiology*, 6th ed. New York, NY: McGraw-Hill Education; 2018.

5. After your resuscitation efforts, the newborn is stable. However, the nurse notes that the mother continues to have significant vaginal bleeding despite bimanual compression and oxytocin administration. Upon examination, she now appears pale and lethargic and has vital signs of blood pressure, 90/68 mm Hg; pulse, 120 beats/min; respiratory rate, 18 breaths/min; and SpO_2, 97%. You diagnose acute hypovolemia secondary to hemorrhage and order an emergent transfusion of packed red blood cells (RBCs). The patient's blood type is unknown. The most appropriate RBC type for emergent transfusion in this patient is:

A. O positive.
B. O negative.
C. AB positive.
D. AB negative.

The correct answer is B. Transfusion of ABO-incompatible blood leads to a severe hemolytic transfusion reaction. When blood is needed emergently and the patient's blood type is unknown, type O blood may be used. ABO blood group typing is determined by the antigens present (or absent) on the patient's RBC surfaces (see chart below). IgM antibodies are produced in reaction to surface antigens of common bacteria that closely resemble missing A- and/or B-type antigens, so anti-A and/or anti-B antibodies are present in the serum despite the patient having never been exposed to foreign RBCs. Therefore, when a patient's blood type is unknown, type O blood should be transfused, as those RBCs lack the A- and/or B-antigens that IgM antibodies in the recipient's serum would recognize as foreign and cause a hemolytic reaction.

Another common antigen on the RBC surface is the D Rhesus (Rh) antigen. Patients with this antigen are *Rh positive*, and those without are *Rh negative*. Rh-negative patients will only develop Rh antibodies after exposure to foreign RBCs (from blood transfusion or pregnancy) that have the Rh antigen present. Therefore, a hemolytic reaction will not occur with the first exposure of an Rh-negative patient to Rh-positive blood, but will occur in such patients with subsequent exposures to Rh-positive blood. Exposure to Rh-positive blood in an Rh-negative female of childbearing age may be detrimental to future pregnancies. If the fetus is Rh positive, then the antibodies developed by an Rh-negative mother from a previous Rh-positive blood exposure can cross the placenta and cause a hemolytic reaction in the fetus. This is why it is important to transfuse women of childbearing age with O-negative blood if type-specific blood is unavailable.

Type	A	B	AB	O
Surface antigen	A	B	A and B	None
Antibodies produced	B	A	None	A and B

6. Upon questioning, you note the mother has a past medical history significant for asthma. In an effort to improve uterine tone, you administer:

A. Terbutaline.
B. Methylergonovine.
C. Carboprost.
D. Magnesium sulfate.

The correct answer is B. First-line treatment for uterine atony is oxytocin. If oxytocin fails, second-line therapies include methylergonovine, an ergot derivative, or carboprost, a synthetic analogue of prostaglandin $F_{2\alpha}$. As carboprost can exacerbate bronchospasm, this drug should be avoided in asthmatics whenever possible. Terbutaline and magnesium sulfate cause uterine relaxation and are not used as uterotonics.

DID YOU LEARN?

- The goals of resuscitation of the depressed neonate with meconium aspiration.
- Emergency transfusion of un-crossmatched blood in a female of child-bearing age.
- Medications utilized for the treatment of uterine atony.

Recommended Readings

Butterworth IV JF, Mackey DC, Wasnick JD, eds. Pediatric anesthesia. In: *Morgan & Mikhail's Clinical Anesthesiology.* 6th ed. New York, NY: McGraw-Hill Education; 2018:897-928.

Frölich MA. Obstetric anesthesia. In: Butterworth IV JF, Mackey DC, Wasnick JD, eds. *Morgan & Mikhail's Clinical Anesthesiology.* 6th ed. New York, NY: McGraw-Hill Education; 2018:861-896.

References

Wyckoff MH, Aziz K, Escobedo MB, et al. Part 13: Neonatal resuscitation: 2015 American Heart Association guidelines update for cardiopulmonary resuscitation and emergency cardiovascular care. *Circulation.* 2015;132(18 Suppl 2):S543-S560.

Wyllie J, Perlman JM, Kattwinkel J, et al. Part 7: Neonatal resuscitation: 2015 International consensus on cardiopulmonary resuscitation and emergency cardiovascular care science with treatment recommendations. *Resuscitation.* 2015;95:e169-e201.

CHAPTER 36

Geriatric Anesthesia

| CASE 1 | Competing Priorities in a Patient with an Advanced Directive |

John F. Butterworth IV, MD

A 92-year-old woman presents with a pathological fracture of her right femur for an open reduction and internal fixation (ORIF). She is awake and alert, and conversing with her family. A chest radiograph and magnetic resonance imaging (MRI) of her chest reveal that she has (probable pathological) fractures of her sixth and seventh ribs on right side, masses in both breasts, and a mass in the right axilla. There is an infiltrate in the right lung suggestive of pneumonia. There is a left ventricular aneurysm and calcification of the aortic valve and mitral valve annulus. She finds coughing, deep breathing, or any repositioning in the bed very painful. Physical examination reveals symmetrical breath sounds and a soft systolic murmur. The ECG shows an old myocardial infarction. She has an advanced directive on the hospital chart stating that she does not want intubation, resuscitation, drugs, or any other artificial means of life support if her likelihood of at least 1 month of meaningful survival is less than 5%.

1. *If* you desired further cardiac evaluation, which of the following tests would be most likely to yield useful new information that might guide the choice of her anesthesia?

   A. Exercise ECG.
   B. Transthoracic echocardiogram.
   C. Pulmonary artery catheterization before induction of anesthesia.
   D. Radionuclide scintigraphy of left ventricle.
   E. Needle biopsy of axillary or breast mass.

The correct answer is B. Elderly patients with hip fractures either undergo ORIF or die of medical complications. This patient requires surgery, ideally within a day of injury. Given the age and condition of the patient, it would be reasonable to proceed to the operating room without further investigation. It would also be reasonable to perform a transthoracic echocardiogram to determine whether the valvular abnormalities identified on the MRI scan are associated with physiologically important valvular heart disease. Aortic stenosis would be the most important diagnosis that might be made.

An exercise ECG would be impossible in a patient with hip fracture. Pulmonary artery catheterization has never been shown to improve outcomes in surgical patients. Radionuclide scintigraphy of the left ventricle might identify coronary artery disease. However, the diagnosis has already been made by the presence of the left ventricular aneurysm. If the surgical specimen from the ORIF was not diagnostic for the form of cancer, postoperative needle biopsy of the axillary mass would be useful for prognosis and for treatment planning if the patient wishes to have radiation or drug treatment of her presumed stage IV breast cancer. Preoperative biopsy would have no relevance to the anesthetic.

The anesthesiologist in this case elected to obtain a transthoracic echocardiogram that showed mild-to-moderate aortic stenosis with a gradient of 30 mm Hg. The anesthesiologist performed a combined spinal/epidural anesthetic (CSE) after sedating the patient with 20 mg of ketamine intravenously (IV) prior to positioning the patient for needle puncture. After injecting 2 mL of 0.5% bupivacaine with 25 µg of fentanyl and 0.1 mg of morphine, she positions the patient on the fracture table. The patient appears to be comfortable. Unfortunately, the patient's blood pressure is now 50/25 mm Hg by arterial line with a heart rate of 82 beats/min.

2. Which of the following is the best choice?

A. Ephedrine 2.5 mg IV.
B. Phenylephrine 25 µg IV.
C. Phenylephrine 0.1 µg/kg/min.
D. Norepinephrine 0.1 µg/kg/min.
E. Epinephrine 2 mg IV.

The correct answer is D. This is a medical emergency, and the patient needs to have coronary perfusion pressure restored immediately. The first three choices represent inadequate doses of weaker drugs. This patient does not need an increase in inotropy or heart rate (and is not in cardiac arrest—at least not yet). Therefore, norepinephrine (D) is the best choice. Even though the patient has an advanced directive, it does not preclude the use of vasoactive drugs to counteract temporary side effects of procedures (eg, hypotension with a spinal anesthetic). The clinical practice of anesthesiology requires drug treatment of anesthetic-induced vasodilation. This would not constitute resuscitation per se.

Norepinephrine infusion restores the blood pressure and surgery proceeds uneventfully.

After 90 min, the ORIF is completed. The patient is brought to the postanesthesia care unit (PACU) where she is awake and stable for 25 min. The patient suddenly becomes tachycardic and tachypneic. Arterial saturation declines from 100% to 82% despite addition of nasal oxygen at a flow of 10 L/min. The ECG shows a new right bundle branch block. The patient begins coughing.

3. Which of the following is the *least* worrisome possibility?

  A. Myocardial infarction.
  B. Pulmonary embolism.
  C. Aspiration.
  D. Delirium.

The correct answer is D. Delirium is the diagnosis of least consequence at the immediate time, even though delirium can lead to a variety of adverse events. In this setting, exactly what should be done with a positive diagnosis of pulmonary embolism or myocardial infarction is problematic. Anticoagulation is not feasible until the risk of surgical bleeding is low. Percutaneous transluminal coronary intervention (PTCI) without the ability to anticoagulate has reduced likelihood of success. Even the diagnosis of aspiration could prove difficult to manage in a patient with an advanced directive proscribing tracheal intubation.

Of the choices, pulmonary embolism appears most likely. Aspiration would be unlikely to occur in an awake, stable patient, and if it had occurred during the surgery, it would be unlikely to present so abruptly in the PACU. Diagnosis of acute myocardial infarction could be made with cardiac enzymes (given an inconclusive finding on ECG).

4. Which of the following tests would most definitively confirm a diagnosis of pulmonary embolism?

  A. D-Dimer
  B. Troponin level.
  C. Spiral computed tomography (CT).
  D. Bedside echocardiogram.

The correct answer is C. The most definitive finding would be from a spiral CT where the diagnosis could be confirmed. A normal D-dimer would be inconsistent with pulmonary embolism, but an elevated D-dimer is not diagnostic. A normal troponin level is inconsistent with myocardial infarction. A major pulmonary embolism would be likely to show right ventricular dysfunction on a transthoracic echocardiogram, but this would not be diagnostic.

In this case, the spiral CT demonstrates a pulmonary embolus. Her arterial saturation improved to 92% while she inhaled 40% oxygen delivered by a face shield.

The situation was discussed with the patient and her family. They consented to placement of a vena cava filter to prevent further embolization, knowing that anticoagulation and thrombolysis could not be performed in this patient who had undergone ORIF only a few hours earlier.

DID YOU LEARN?

- Appropriate selection of diagnostic tests in patients requiring urgent surgery.
- Evaluation and management of suspected pulmonary embolism.
- Importance of differentiating between drugs used for resuscitation after an unexpected cardiac event versus similar drugs used to counteract a temporary side effect of an anesthetic (eg, hypotension during spinal anesthesia).

References

Colquhoun AD, Zuelzer W, Butterworth JF 4th. Improving the management of hip fractures in the elderly: a role for the perioperative surgical home? *Anesthesiology*. 2014;121(6):1144-1146.
Soffin EM, Gibbons MM, Wick EC, et al. Evidence review conducted for the agency for healthcare research and quality safety program for improving surgical care and recovery: focus on anesthesiology for hip fracture surgery. *Anesth Analg*. 2019;128(6):1107-1117.

CASE 2 — Patient with Disorientation

Kallol Chaudhuri, MD, PhD, and Angelo Riccione, DO

1. A 76-year-old woman with a history of breast cancer, with bony metastases to the spine, presents for a full-body MRI requiring general anesthesia. She denies alcohol use, lives independently, and does not smoke. The case proceeds uneventfully. Shortly after emerging from general anesthesia and extubation, the patient starts taking off her gown and fighting with members of the anesthesia staff. She is completely disoriented and is incoherent. This behavior lasts for about 30 min, after which she is completely alert and oriented and back to her baseline mental status. What is the most likely diagnosis?

   A. Stroke.
   B. Postoperative delirium.
   C. Delirium tremens.
   D. Normal pressure hydrocephalus.

Anesthetic Management — SECTION III

The correct answer is B. Given how quickly this episode resolved and that there is no mention of any motor deficits or neurological imaging/tests, stroke is unlikely. Delirium tremens is a condition associated with alcohol withdrawal, which typically manifests 2 to 5 days after an alcoholic's last drink of alcohol. This life-threatening condition includes hallucinosis, confusion, seizures, and possible cardiovascular collapse. It is typically treated acutely with benzodiazepines. This patient does not drink alcohol, so this diagnosis is impossible. Normal pressure hydrocephalus is a condition where an excess of cerebrospinal fluid is produced, resulting in enlarged ventricles and pressure on brain parenchyma. It manifests as gait disturbances, dementia, and urinary incontinence. The hallmark of this diagnosis, along with the clinical symptoms, is enlarged ventricles on brain imaging. In the absence of any imaging of this patient and lack of persistence of symptoms, this diagnosis is also unlikely.

Postoperative delirium is defined as a disturbance of consciousness with possible change in cognition, which develops up to 1 week after surgery and tends to fluctuate throughout the day.

2. Which of the following factors can predispose a patient to these types of actions postoperatively?

A. Diabetes.
B. Advanced age.
C. Impaired functional status preoperatively.
D. Benzodiazepine use.
E. All of the above.

The correct answer is E. Factors that predispose a patient to postoperative delirium include advanced age, diabetes, benzodiazepine use, and impaired functional status preoperatively. Other factors include the type of operation and length of surgery, atherosclerosis, and preexisting depression.

3. Which type of procedure requiring an anesthetic is notorious for being associated with postoperative delirium and postoperative cognitive dysfunction?

A. Colonoscopy.
B. Hip surgery.
C. Radical prostatectomy.
D. Mastectomy.

The correct answer is B. The most common procedures associated with postoperative delirium are hip surgery, cardiac surgery, and vascular surgery.

4. Which of the following is an effective method of postoperative intervention to prevent delirium after surgery?

A. Midazolam.
B. Leaving the patient in a dark room throughout the day.
C. Early mobilization.
D. Keeping the patient NPO.

The correct answer is C. Effective measures of preventing or moderating postoperative delirium include avoiding benzodiazepines; keeping lights on during the day and off at night to promote day–night awareness and a normal sleep cycle; getting patients out of bed and moving, as tolerated; and resuming oral intake as soon as possible.

DID YOU LEARN

- Potential causes of postoperative disorientation.
- Measures to reduce the incidence of postoperative delirium.
- Contributing factors leading to postoperative delirium.

Recommended Reading

Butterworth IV JF, Mackey DC, Wasnick JD, eds. Geriatric anesthesia. In: *Morgan & Mikhail's Clinical Anesthesiology.* 6th ed. New York, NY: McGraw-Hill Education; 2018:929-942.

References

Viramontes O, Luan Erfe BM, Erfe JM, et al. Cognitive impairment and postoperative outcomes in patients undergoing primary total hip arthroplasty: a systematic review. *J Clin Anesth.* 2019;56:65-76.
Vlisides P, Avidan M. Recent advances in preventing and managing postoperative delirium. *F1000Res.* 2019;8:pii: F1000.

SECTION IV

Regional Anesthesia & Pain Management

CHAPTER 37

Peripheral Nerve Blocks

CASE 1 — Upper Extremity Peripheral Nerve Blocks

Joel Feinstein, MD, and Brian M. Ilfeld, MD, MS

A 78-year-old man fractured his left distal radius during a fall and is now scheduled for open reduction and internal fixation of the fracture. He suffered no other significant injuries. During preoperative evaluation, the patient is noted to be in no distress and to be oriented to person, place, and time. His medical history includes stable coronary artery disease, and he is status post right circumflex coronary artery drug-eluting stent placement 2 years ago. Additional past medical history includes obstructive sleep apnea (OSA) with home continuous positive airway pressure therapy, chronic obstructive pulmonary disease (COPD), hypertension, and chronic kidney disease. Medications include lisinopril, tiotropium, carvedilol, adult low-dose aspirin, and clopidogrel, but the patient has not taken any medications for the past 2 days. The patient's height is 175 cm (5′9″), weight 98 kg, and body mass index 32. Vital signs include blood pressure 168/96 mm Hg and heart rate 73 beats/min. He is afebrile. Room air SpO_2 is 94%. Twelve-lead ECG shows normal sinus rhythm with Q waves in leads II, III, and aVF. Recent transthoracic echocardiography revealed left-ventricular ejection fraction of 35%, pulmonary artery pressure of 40 to 50 mm Hg, and no significant valvular dysfunction. After reviewing the chart and interviewing the patient, you recommend a regional anesthetic.

1. Which regional anesthetic block is the *best* option for both intraoperative anesthesia and postoperative analgesia for this patient?

   A. Interscalene.
   B. Supraclavicular.
   C. Axillary.
   D. Infraclavicular.
   E. Intravenous regional (Bier) block.

The best answer is D. A regional block will obviate the need for general anesthesia and minimize risk of anesthesia-related complications related to the patient's medical comorbidities. Updated guidelines from the ASA Task Force on Perioperative Management of Patients with Obstructive Sleep Apnea recommend that "regional analgesic techniques should be considered to reduce or eliminate the requirement for systemic opioids in patients at increased risk from obstructive sleep apnea." While several blocks could provide adequate anesthesia and postoperative analgesia for the surgical procedure, an *infraclavicular* block provides the best combination of safety, reliable surgical anesthesia, and superior perineural catheter function for continuous postoperative analgesia.

The *interscalene* approach blocks the C5 to C7 roots and is indicated for procedures on the shoulder and proximal humerus. Interscalene blocks reliably spare C8 and T1, making this block inappropriate for surgeries distal to the elbow.

The *supraclavicular* block is performed at the divisions level of the brachial plexus and can provide surgical anesthesia at, or distal to, the elbow. Ultrasound guidance has significantly enhanced the safety of this block, but there is still a small risk of a pneumothorax. Furthermore, while the risk of phrenic nerve palsy is less than with an interscalene block, the incidence of ipsilateral diaphragmatic paralysis is still reported to be as high as 50%, posing a risk of respiratory compromise in patients with significant preexisting pulmonary disease. In addition, continuous postoperative analgesia with supraclavicular perineural catheters is less easy to maintain than with infraclavicular catheters because supraclavicular catheters may be more easily dislodged.

Axillary block is performed at the terminal branches of the brachial plexus and will anesthetize the median, ulnar, and radial nerves. The musculocutaneous nerve emerges proximally to the axilla and terminates as the lateral antebrachial cutaneous nerve. It must be blocked separately where it travels through the coracobrachialis muscle for complete anesthesia of the forearm and wrist. Axillary perineural catheters provide inferior analgesia when compared to infraclavicular perineural catheters and also may have an increased risk of catheter dislodgement.

Bier block, or intravenous regional anesthesia, provides surgical anesthesia for soft tissue surgeries of limited duration but can be unreliable for coverage of osteal stimulation. Bier blocks provide no postoperative analgesia. For these reasons, brachial plexus blocks have widely supplanted Bier blocks as anesthesia for fracture fixation.

The patient refuses placement of a perineural catheter, so you elect to do a single-shot block with 45 mL of 0.5% bupivacaine. Within 5 min of block placement, the patient begins to show signs of altered mental status. His heart rate drops from 73 to 37 beats/min, and his systolic blood pressure drops to 70 mm Hg. ECG progresses from sinus rhythm to first-degree block and then to wide-complex ventricular tachycardia. The patient begins to seize.

2. Your treatment should include all of the following *except*:

A. Seizure suppression with an intravenous (IV) benzodiazepine.
B. Intralipid 20% 1.5 mL/kg IV over 1 min.

C. Epinephrine bolus 10 mcg/kg IV.
D. Initiation of advanced cardiac life support adjusted for local anesthetic toxicity.
E. Alert nearest facility with cardiopulmonary bypass.

The correct answer is C. Local anesthetic systemic toxicity can be caused by excessive total dose, rapid systemic absorption, or direct intravascular injection. Certain comorbidities increase the risk of developing local anesthetic toxicity. This patient's advanced age, ischemic heart disease, and heart failure all increase the risk of developing toxicity. Additional risk factors for local anesthetic toxicity can include conduction abnormalities, metabolic (eg, mitochondrial) disease, liver disease, low plasma protein concentration, metabolic acidosis, and medications that inhibit sodium channels.

Neurological symptoms are typically the initial presentation and may be subtle or overt. These symptoms can include manifestations of central nervous system excitation or depression or may be nonspecific. Significant toxicity often terminates with neurological involvement only, but severe cases may also include the cardiovascular system. Cardiovascular signs often include an initial hyperdynamic state that can progress to marked hypotension with cardiac conduction block or ventricular arrhythmia.

In vivo studies have shown that high dose (1 mg or 10 mcg/kg) IV epinephrine administration hinders the effectiveness of lipid rescue and overall resuscitation efforts. Reduced dosing of epinephrine at 1 mcg/kg IV is recommended during resuscitation. It is also recommended that vasopressin, calcium channel blockers, β-blockers, and additional local anesthetics be avoided.

Treatment of toxicity should begin immediately with basic and advanced cardiac life support measures adjusted for the anesthetic etiology. IV bolus delivery of lipid followed by an infusion is fundamental to management. An infusion of 0.25 mL/kg/min is recommended during resuscitation and should be continued for at least 10 min after the return of cardiovascular stability. The infusion can be doubled for persistent hypotension, and two additional boluses of 1.5 mL/kg may also be delivered. Prolonged cardiopulmonary resuscitation and cardiopulmonary bypass have resulted in successful resuscitation.

In an alternative scenario, 1 h into the case after uncomplicated infraclavicular blockade with 30 mL of 1.5% mepivacaine with 1:400,000 epinephrine, the patient's blood pressure begins to rise and he complains of pain. A small dose of fentanyl is administered IV with temporary relief, but shortly thereafter, the patient's complaints return and intensify.

3. What is the most likely source of the patient's pain?

A. Block resolution.
B. Surgical incision extension into lateral antebrachial distribution.
C. Tourniquet pain.
D. Inadequate sedation.

The correct answer is C. Tourniquets are commonly used for surgery of the extremity in order to reduce blood loss and to maintain a surgical field visually unobstructed by shed blood. The majority of awake or lightly sedated patients will complain of tourniquet pain within 30 to 60 min of tourniquet inflation. While the exact mechanism is complex, tourniquet pain is likely caused by neuronal ischemia. Forearm tourniquets have a longer time to onset of pain when compared to upper arm tourniquets and may be especially useful in selective surgeries.

Mepivacaine, an intermediate-duration local anesthetic, will provide surgical anesthesia for approximately 3 h.

A successful infraclavicular or supraclavicular block will provide complete anesthesia and analgesia at and below the elbow, including soft tissue and bone. These blocks will also anesthetize the lateral, posterior, and anterior portion of the upper arm, but will spare the medial portion of the upper arm. The intercostobrachial nerve innervates the cutaneous portion of the medial upper arm. Although evidence is lacking to support the practice, blockade of the intercostobrachial nerve is often added to brachial plexus blocks in an attempt to delay the onset of tourniquet pain. Infiltration of the superficial plane at the medial upper arm is used to block the intercostobrachial nerve.

If an axillary block was utilized for this procedure, a separate block of the musculocutaneous nerve would often be performed within the body of the coracobrachialis muscle. The lateral antebrachial cutaneous nerve is the terminal branch of the musculocutaneous nerve and is reliably blocked at the both the infraclavicular and supraclavicular locations.

Recommended Readings

Hadzic A. Section five: Upper extremity nerve blocks. *Textbook of Regional Anesthesia and Acute Pain Management*, 2nd ed. New York: McGraw-Hill; 2017:558-585.
Halaszynski TM. Ultrasound brachial plexus anesthesia and analgesia for upper extremity surgery: Essentials of our current understanding, 2011. *Curr Opin Anaesthesiol.* 2011;24(5):581-591.

References

American Society of Anesthesiologists: Practice guidelines for the perioperative management of patients with obstructive sleep apnea. *Anesthesiology.* 2014;120(2):268-286.
Hiller DB, Gregorio GD, Ripper R, et al. Epinephrine impairs lipid resuscitation from bupivacaine overdose: A threshold effect. *Anesthesiology.* 2009;111(3):498-505.
Horlocker TT, Hebl JR, Gali B, et al. Anesthetic, patient and surgical risk factors for neurologic complications after prolonged total knee arthroplasty. *Anesth Analg.* 2006;102: 950-955.
Mak PH, Irwin MG, Ooi CG, Chow BF. Incidence of diaphragmatic paralysis following supraclavicular brachial plexus block and its effect on pulmonary function. *Anaesthesia.* 2001;56:352-356.
Neal JM, Bernards CM, Butterworth JF, et al. ASRA practice advisory on local anesthetic systemic toxicity. *Reg Anesth Pain Med.* 2010;35:152-161.

CASE 2 — Peripheral Nerve Block for Mastectomy

Bahareh Khatibi, MD, and Brian M. Ilfeld, MD, MS

A 43-year-old, 50-kg woman with newly diagnosed intraductal breast cancer is scheduled for left mastectomy with tissue expander placement, sentinel node biopsy, and possible axillary dissection. Past medical history is significant for gastroesophageal reflux and tension headaches. She does not take any medications regularly. She reports a history of difficulty tolerating oral opioids secondary to severe vomiting and requests pain-management techniques minimizing the need for emetic-inducing medications. Laboratory values are within normal limits and include hemoglobin level of 11.5 g/dL, platelet count of 165,000/mcL, and international normalized ratio (INR) of 0.9.

1. You plan to offer a regional nerve block as part of the patient's pain management regimen. Which of the following nerve blocks would provide the *least* postoperative analgesia?

    A. Quadratus lumborum block.
    B. Erector spinae block.
    C. Intercostobrachial nerve block.
    D. Paravertebral nerve block.
    E. Thoracic epidural.

The correct answer is C. Intercostal, paravertebral, erector spinae, quadratus lumborum, and epidural blockade can all decrease postoperative pain associated with breast surgery. For intercostal blocks, analgesia is limited to the chest and upper abdomen at the specific thoracic dermatome levels related to where the block is performed. Epidural and paravertebral blockade can provide surgical anesthesia and postoperative analgesia for not only thoracic and upper abdominal procedures, but also lower abdominal procedures such as inguinal or abdominal hernia repair. Pectoralis and serratus plane blocks, quadratus lumborum, and erector spinae blocks are also effective for postoperative analgesia.

The intercostobrachial nerve provides cutaneous innervation to the medial aspect of the proximal arm and a portion of the axilla. The nerve is a branch of the T2 nerve root and thus is not anesthetized with a brachial plexus block. The intercostobrachial nerve block is performed with the patient in the supine position with the arm abducted and externally rotated. Local anesthetic is injected just distal to the axilla from the anterior deltoid prominence to the medial aspect of the arm and can be done with infiltration only or with ultrasound guidance. An intercostobrachial nerve block would not provide complete analgesia for the axillary dissection and would not cover any chest wall pain.

2. The patient decides that she would like a nerve block for postoperative pain in addition to a general anesthetic for the surgery. Your plan is to perform thoracic paravertebral nerve blocks. Which of the following is *false* regarding paravertebral blocks?

A. Paravertebral blocks can allow for targeted unilateral blockade.
B. Long-acting local anesthetics used for paravertebral blocks can have a duration of 16 to 24 h.
C. Paravertebral blocks are an alternative for patients who are poor candidates for epidural block secondary to prior spine surgery.
D. Paravertebral blocks are a good alternative for patients who are not candidates for epidural placement secondary to anticoagulation.

The correct answer is D. Paravertebral blocks have several advantages compared to intercostal blocks. Local anesthetics injected in the paravertebral space at one level may spread to multiple levels to anesthetize multiple spinal roots, whereas separate injections are necessary to anesthetize specific dermatomes for intercostal blocks. In addition, the intercostal region has high vascular flow, resulting in more rapid absorption into the blood. This can lead to an increased risk of local anesthetic systemic toxicity as well as decreased block duration compared to paravertebral blocks. Further, insertion of a perineural catheter is more feasible at the paravertebral space than an intercostal space.

When compared to epidural blocks, paravertebral nerve blocks can be performed to reliably provide unilateral blockade. However, in rare instances, paravertebral block can result in inadvertent epidural spread, which may lead to bilateral anesthesia or analgesia. Paravertebral blocks are an alternative to epidurals for patients who are not ideal candidates for neuraxial procedures, such as those with a history of multiple spine surgeries where placement may be difficult or epidural spread may be unpredictable. However, paravertebral blocks would not be a good alternative to epidurals for patients taking anticoagulants. The most recent American Society of Regional Anesthesia (ASRA) guidelines for performing regional blocks and managing perineural catheters recommend that similar parameters be followed for neuraxial blockade and more peripheral blocks, such as paravertebral blocks, in such circumstances.

3. The patient is concerned about possible risks from the nerve block. Which of the following is the *least* likely after a paravertebral nerve block performed by a proficient regional anesthetist?

A. Hypotension.
B. Pneumothorax.
C. Horner syndrome.
D. Pleural puncture.
E. Vascular puncture.

The correct answer is B. Several prospective studies have investigated the complication rates of paravertebral blocks. In one study, among the 367 patients who had received a thoracic or lumbar paravertebral block, the most frequent complication was hypotension (4.6%). Hypotension typically occurs secondary to blockade of sympathetic fibers and can be more pronounced if the paravertebral blocks are performed at multiple levels or bilaterally. Similarly, blockade of the sympathetic fibers at the C8 to T2 level or above can result in Horner syndrome, which is characterized by ptosis, miosis, and anhydrosis of the face on the ipsilateral side. Other complications found in the study were vascular puncture (3.8%), pleural puncture (1.1%), and pneumothorax (0.5%). In another study, which included 662 patients who underwent thoracic and lumbar paravertebral blocks, the complications recorded were inadvertent vascular puncture (6.8%), hypotension (4.0%), hematoma (2.4%), pain at site of skin puncture (1.3%), signs of epidural or intrathecal spread (1.0%), pleural puncture (0.8%), and pneumothorax (0.5%).

In preparation for the nerve block, the patient is placed in the sitting position and standard ASA monitors are placed. Oxygen is provided via face mask, and midazolam 1 mg and fentanyl 50 μg are administered IV. You perform a left-sided paravertebral block with ultrasound guidance at T2 and T4 and deposit 10 mL of 0.5% ropivacaine with 1:400,000 of epinephrine at each level. The patient tolerates the procedure well, with stable vital signs. Approximately 10 min later, the patient is taken to the operating room. After preoxygenation, general anesthesia is induced with fentanyl 200 μg, lidocaine 100 mg, and propofol 180 mg, and muscle relaxation is provided with succinylcholine 70 mg IV. After intubation and initiation of mechanical ventilation with sevoflurane, her blood pressure decreases from 129/85 to 79/58 mm Hg.

4. Which of the following is *least likely* to be a contributing factor to the patient's hypotension?

    A. Inappropriate anesthetic depth.
    B. Local anesthetic toxicity.
    C. Sympathectomy from paravertebral block.
    D. Total spinal.
    E. Pneumothorax.

The correct answer is D. Hypotension can be a common occurrence after the induction of general anesthesia. One of the most common causes of postinduction hypotension is the decrease in systemic vascular resistance that results as a side effect of many induction agents. However, it is important to rule out other etiologies of hypotension and to treat reversible causes.

The cause of hypotension in this patient is likely multifactorial. In addition, in patients who have blocks that significantly reduce the level of nociceptive stimulus, doses for anesthetic maintenance may need to be adjusted downward to match the decreased level of stimulation. Specific nerve blocks that reduce sympathetic tone and block cardiac accelerator nerve fibers, such as thoracic paravertebral blocks, can also exacerbate hypotension because patient are not able to fully compensate for hypotension by increasing heart rate and contractility. A pneumothorax is also a possible cause of hypotension if it is large enough to induce tension physiology. It is possible for a pneumothorax to remain relatively small and undetected during spontaneous tidal breathing, but then manifest itself after positive-pressure ventilation increases the pneumothorax volume. Finally, one must also consider local anesthetic systemic toxicity in any patient receiving local anesthetics. This is especially possible for this patient, who received ropivacaine 2 mg/kg for the paravertbral blocks and an additional 2 mg/kg lidocaine IV at the time of general anesthesia induction. The hypotension that can occur with systemic ropivacaine or bupivacaine toxicity is typically associated with cardiac arrhythmias, including conduction block, bradycardia, ventricular arrhythmias, or asystole.

In this patient with hypotension after induction, initial management includes checking endotracheal tube depth, verifying end-tidal carbon dioxide, and listening to breath sounds to confirm tracheal intubation and assess for endobronchial intubation, mucous plugging, bronchospasm, or pneumothorax/hemothorax. Anesthetic depth and intravascular volume status must be assessed, and all medications administered must be verified. Anaphylactic/anaphylactoid reactions should be considered. Temporizing maneuvers, such as reducing anesthetic depth and administering additional IV fluids and vasoactive medications, should be instituted, and any identified underlying cause of the hypotension should be corrected.

Although intrathecal injection of local anesthetic is a potential complication of performing a paravertebral block, the onset of the spinal blockade would likely occur more rapidly following the block and is not consistent with the delayed onset of hypotension in this patient.

DID YOU LEARN?

- Alternative nerve block techniques for postoperative pain management after mastectomy.
- The advantages and disadvantages of paravertebral block compared to epidural and intercostal block.
- Complication profile for paravertebral blockade.
- Potential contributing causes and management of intraoperative hypotension in a patient with a paravertebral block under general anesthesia.

References

Abrahams M, Derby R, Horn JL. Update on ultrasound for truncal blocks: A review of the evidence. *Reg Anesth Pain Med*. 2016;41(2):275-288.

Horlocker TT, Vandermeuelen E, Kopp SL, et al. Regional anesthesia in the patient receiving antithrombotic or thrombolytic therapy: American Society of Regional Anesthesia and Pain Medicine Evidence-Based Guidelines (Fourth Edition). *Reg Anesth Pain Med*. 2018;43(3):263-309.

CASE 3 Infraclavicular Block for Hand Surgery

Matthew T. Charous, MD, and Brian M. Ilfeld, MD, MS

ER 37 Peripheral Nerve Blocks

You are scheduled to care for a 78-year-old man who is undergoing left first meta-carpalphalangeal (MCP) arthroplasty for osteoarthritis. The patient has hypertension and coronary artery disease (CAD) and underwent angioplasty and insertion of a drug-eluting stent (DES) 6 months prior. He has a remote history of smoking (1 pack per day for 10 years, quit >30 years ago). Home medications include metoprolol, simvastatin, aspirin, and clopidogrel. The clopidogrel was discontinued by the patient's cardiologist 7 days ago, but the patient has continued his aspirin therapy (81 mg, once per day). The patient is to be discharged following surgery. The surgeon asks that the procedure be performed under peripheral nerve block and monitored anesthesia care. The benefits and risks of peripheral nerve blocks are outlined to the patient, and he agrees to undergo a brachial plexus block.

1. At this point, your next action is to:

A. Cancel the surgery and insist that the patient discontinue all antiplatelet medications, including the aspirin, prior to surgery.
B. Perform a general anesthetic.
C. Proceed with brachial plexus block as planned.
D. Perform a median nerve block.

The correct answer is C. The patient has already discontinued his clopidrogel, which is acceptable given that his DES placement was 6 months ago. Since a DES had been placed recently, discontinuation of dual antiplatelet therapy (both aspirin and a thienopyridine, the most popular of which is clopidogrel) within 30 days and also prior to 6 months would place the patient at a significantly increased risk of stent thrombosis and perioperative myocardial infarction. Stent thrombosis in patients with DES undergoing noncardiac surgery is of highest risk in surgeries that take place closer to the timing of stent placement. Prior studies suggested that dual antiplatelet therapy be continued at least 12 months following deployment of a DES. However, as stent design continues to evolve, more recent investigations suggest that 6 months of dual antiplatelet therapy achieves the same benefit as a longer duration, while minimizing hemorrhagic complications such as gastrointestinal bleeding. Many sources advocate discontinuation of clopidogrel 7 to 10 days prior to a surgical procedure, or 5 days prior to a surgical procedure for high-risk patients (eg, prior myocardial infarction, history of percutaneous coronary intervention). Aspirin and nonsteroidal anti-inflammatory drugs (NSAIDs) are not contraindicated with spinal or epidural anesthesia; so by extension, a patient on aspirin therapy would be a suitable candidate for brachial plexus block.

There is no compelling reason to perform a general anesthetic for this patient. Both induction and intubation are associated with hemodynamic changes

333

(hypotension, hypertension, tachycardia), all of which place additional stress on the patient's cardiovascular system. An isolated median nerve block for first MCP arthroplasty would not provide the necessary anesthetic coverage for the surgical procedure.

The patient's vital signs prior to the block are noninvasive blood pressure, 136/79 mm Hg; heart rate, 68 beats/min; unlabored respiratory rate, 12 breaths/min; and SpO$_2$ 99% on 2 L/min oxygen by nasal cannula. The patient is placed in the supine position. His operative arm (left) is bent approximately 90 degrees at the elbow and is positioned in abduction and external rotation so that you can use the infraclavicular approach to the brachial plexus. The patient states that he is comfortable. The infraclavicular fossa is prepped and draped in sterile fashion. After local infiltration with lidocaine, a 17 G Tuohy needle is passed utilizing ultrasound guidance, and 25 mL of mepivacaine 2.0% with epinephrine 1:300,000 is injected. An epidural catheter is then passed through the Tuohy needle, with the needle tip location between the posterior cord and the subclavian/axillary artery. The patient is then placed in a semi-recumbent position.

Ten minutes following completion of the nerve block, the patient begins to complain of left chest discomfort. His vital signs include blood pressure, 143/84 mm Hg; heart rate, 70 beats/min; respiratory rate, 16 breaths/min; and SpO$_2$, 97% on 2 L/min nasal cannula oxygen. His breathing is unlabored. He does note that taking large breaths produces a modest increase in pain over his left chest. Auscultation of right and left chest reveals similar breath sounds.

2. The most appropriate immediate action would be to first:

A. Cancel the surgery and discharge the patient home.
B. Immediately obtain an ECG and chest radiograph.
C. Reassure the patient and proceed with surgery as planned.
D. Administer morphine.

The correct answer is B. Canceling the surgery before determining the etiology of the patient's chest pain is premature. Moreover, a patient suffering from chest pain should be thoroughly evaluated before either discharge from medical care or proceeding with a scheduled surgery. Administration of morphine may make the patient feel better but does little to establish a cause of the patient's chest pain. Obtaining an ECG, especially in a patient with known coronary artery disease, can be helpful to identify changes that indicate new ischemia.

This patient has a remote history of smoking but does not have any history of chronic obstructive pulmonary disease (COPD) and has never needed any pulmonary treatments in the past. Given that the patient quit so long ago (>30 years) and is able to exercise vigorously multiple times per week, it is unlikely that the patient is experiencing any respiratory event due to either asthma or COPD exacerbation.

Given the close proximity to the thoracic cavity, infraclavicular nerve blocks carry a risk of iatrogenic pneumothorax. This risk is theoretically reduced, but not eliminated, when the block is performed with ultrasound guidance. Positive-pressure ventilation in a patient with a small, physiologically tolerable pneumothorax may convert it into a rapidly deteriorating tension pneumothorax.

Brachial plexus blockade may produce hemidiaphragmatic paresis, commonly referred to as phrenic nerve paresis. The diaphragm is innervated by the phrenic nerve, which receives contributions from cervical nerves C3 to C5. These nerve roots may be anesthetized before joining to form the phrenic nerve due to cephalad spread of local anesthetic; the phrenic nerve may also be reversibly paralyzed due to migration of local anesthetic across the anterior scalene muscle. Hemidiaphragmatic paresis results in 20% to 40% decrease in both forced expiratory volume in 1 s (FEV_1) and forced vital capacity (FVC). Clearly, the risk of hemidiaphragmatic paresis is greater for blocks performed above the clavicle, where the administered local anesthetic is closest to the contributing cervical nerve roots and to the phrenic nerve. However, blocks of the brachial plexus below the level of the clavicle—but still close to the clavicle (eg, infraclavicular blocks)—may still cause phrenic nerve paresis. In this regard, dosing the catheter with additional local anesthetic volume may either cause phrenic nerve paresis or extend the duration of the paresis if it has already occurred. Obtaining a chest radiograph in this patient is a high-yield and minimally invasive test: One may ascertain the presence of either hemidiaphragmatic paresis or a clinically large pneumothorax. One can also use bedside ultrasound to assess hemidiaphragmatic paresis.

The ECG is unremarkable. A telephone call to the patient's cardiologist reveals that the patient has been adherent to his medication regimen and that his last exercise echocardiogram 6 months ago showed no evidence of ischemia. Moreover, the patient has been active and swims multiple times per week.

The chest radiograph shows no evidence of either a pneumothorax or hemidiaphragmatic paresis. The patient's condition is still unchanged. His shortness of breath has not worsened, and the rest of his vital signs are stable. He continues to complain of pain over his left chest. At this point, the patient's gown is taken down to allow for a thorough physical examination. His left pectoral muscle is decidedly enlarged compared the right side. In fact, the left chest area involving his pectoralis muscle is now nearly three times the size of the same area on the right. The presumptive diagnosis is hemorrhage, and a prompt ultrasound scan reveals extensive fluid throughout the left pectoralis muscle.

3. Which of the following is the best course of action at this point?

   A. Type and crossmatch the patient and administer 2 units of packed red blood cells.
   B. Obtain central venous access and admit the patient to the intensive care unit.
   C. Discharge the patient home with instructions to return if bleeding increases.
   D. Apply compression to the left chest, consult a vascular surgeon, and obtain a hemoglobin/hematocrit level.

The correct answer is D. At this point, the patient is hemodynamically stable, and administration of blood products or placement of a central venous catheter is unjustified. In addition, given that the patient's condition continues to evolve, it is prudent to admit the patient for ongoing observation and monitoring. Since the bleeding appears to continue, external compression of the area may slow or stop it. Though a preliminary ultrasound was performed, a dedicated vascular ultrasound examination and consultation with a vascular surgeon would better delineate any source of hemorrhage and whether an intervention is needed. Lastly, obtaining a hemoglobin/hematocrit would help establish the degree of blood loss. This test should be repeated several hours later, since in the acute setting it may not accurately reflect the true extent of blood loss.

A vascular surgeon is consulted and a vascular ultrasound examination is conducted. The patient's condition has now stabilized, expansion of the chest wall hematoma has ceased, and no site of active bleeding is seen on the ultrasound examination, though a significant hematoma is observed within the substance of the pectoralis major. The decision is made to admit the patient to a monitored telemetry inpatient ward, with repeat hemoglobin/hematocrit level the following morning. If the level is acceptable, the patient is to be discharged and an alternate date for the original surgery will be set.

4. What is the most likely etiology of the patient's source of bleeding?

   A. Intercostal vein.
   B. Subcutaneous vein.
   C. Axillary artery.
   D. Arterial branch to the pectoralis muscle.

The correct answer is D. The intercostal veins lie deep to both the pectoralis major and minor muscles, as well as to the brachial plexus at this level. A subcutaneous vein would be extremely unlikely to cause such a significant hematoma, even with a patient on an antiplatelet medication. In addition, a subcutaneous vein puncture would have been easily compressible through external compression. The subclavian/axillary artery is always at risk for accidental puncture, despite ultrasound guidance, as the cords of the brachial plexus are immediately dorsal to this vessel. However, puncture of the subclavian/axillary artery in this case scenario would not account for the hematoma observed in the substance of the pectoralis major muscle.

The most likely source of this patient's bleeding would be an arterial branch to the pectoralis muscle. The main arterial supply to the pectoralis major is the thoracoacromial trunk (TAT), or artery, which is a take-off from the first or second segment of the axillary artery. The TAT gives rise to a number of branches that feed the pectoralis major: clavicular, deltoid, and pectoral. In addition, the pectoralis major receives contributions from perforating vessels from the superior thoracic artery, the internal thoracic artery, and the anterior intercostal arteries.

5. What are the American Society of Regional Anesthesia and Pain Medicine (ASRA) guidelines for performance of a peripheral nerve block on a patient taking an antiplatelet medication?

    A. No contraindication.
    B. Absolute contraindication.
    C. Relative contraindication.
    D. All antiplatelet medications must be stopped 1 week prior to surgery.

The correct answer is C. The risk of hemorrhagic complication is dependent on type of peripheral nerve block and type of antiplatelet medication. The most recent edition of the ASRA guidelines state that the "risk after plexus and peripheral techniques remains undefined . . . in a series of 4,879 patients undergoing cardiac catheterization and/or coronary angioplasty, the frequency of vascular complications was 0.39%." In addition, the ASRA guidelines also note 13 hemorrhagic complications in patients on antiplatelet/antithrombotic medications following peripheral or plexus block. The main complication in these patients was blood loss, not nerve injury. Thus, one must distinguish the relative risks associated with certain blocks. Some areas are anatomically amenable to compression should bleeding occur. Other areas, however, such as the paravertebral space, are impossible to compress, and their close proximity to critical structures (eg, the spinal cord) carry unacceptable risk. With regard to neuraxial and deep plexus/peripheral block procedures, ASRA guidelines are as follows for antiplatelet medications:

NSAIDs: no risk.
NSAIDs + heparin/low-molecular-weight heparin or oral anticoagulant: Recommend against block.
Thienopyridine therapy
   Ticlopidine: 14 days.
   Clopidogrel: 7 days.
Glycoprotein IIb/IIIa inhibitors
   Abciximab: 24–48 h.
   Eptifibatide/tirofiban: 4–8 h.

DID YOU LEARN?

- Various side effects and complications associated with infraclavicular nerve block.
- Methods for investigating chest pain following an infraclavicular nerve block.
- Blood supply to the pectoralis muscle.
- Approach to performing nerve blocks on a patient taking antiplatelet medication.

Recommended Readings

Elazab EEB, Nabil NM. Pectoralis major muscle: Anatomical features of its arterial supply. *Eur J Plast Surg.* 2012;35(1):9-18.

Flannery L, Liu R, Elmariah S. Dual antiplatelet therapy: How long is long enough? *Curr Treat Options Cardiovasc Med.* 2019;21(4):17.

Gopalakrishnan M, Lotfi AS. Stent thrombosis. *Semin Thromb Hemost.* 2018;44(1):46-51.

Horlocker TT, Wedel DJ, Rowlingson JC, et al. Regional anesthesia in the patient receiving antithrombotic or thrombolytic therapy: American Society of Regional Anesthesia and Pain Medicine Evidence-Based Guidelines (third edition). *Reg Anesth Pain Med.* 2010;35:64-101.

Urmey WF. Chapter 16: Pulmonary complications. In: Neal JM, Rathmell JP, eds. *Complications in Regional Anesthesia and Pain Medicine*, 2nd ed. Philadelphia, PA: Wolters Kluwer;2013.

CASE 4 Upper Extremity Peripheral Nerve Blocks

Arpita D. Badami, MD, and Brian M. Ilfeld, MD, MS

A 56-year-old woman presents for carpal tunnel release. She has a history of coronary artery disease (CAD) and severe chronic obstructive pulmonary disease (COPD), but denies any chest pain or shortness of breath with activity, although her activity is limited. She also denies any recent infections or hospitalization. She uses inhalers on a daily basis. Her height is 152 cm (5′4″), and her weight is 106 kg. She is afebrile and has a heart rate of 63 beats/min, blood pressure of 130/65 mm Hg, and respiratory rate of 16 breaths/min. Her room air SpO_2 is 96%.

1. What is your anesthetic management of choice for this patient?

   A. General anesthesia.
   B. Intravenous regional (Bier) block.
   C. Median and ulnar nerve block.
   D. Supraclavicular nerve block.
   E. Either B or C.

The correct answer is E. In a patient with morbid obesity and severe COPD, it would be advantageous to avoid a general anesthetic or deep sedation and the potential for associated pulmonary complications.

A Bier block, also referred to as intravenous regional anesthesia, can provide surgical anesthesia to the distal upper extremity and would be appropriate for this procedure. Bier blocks are ideal for short surgical procedures (45–60 min). Tourniquet pain can develop after 20 to 30 min, and is typically poorly tolerated with durations exceeding 60 min regardless of technique or patient selection. For upper extremity procedures, a catheter is inserted into a vein on the dorsum of the hand of the operative extremity. A single tourniquet may be used for short procedures (~20 min duration), or double tourniquet for longer procedures. The extremity is elevated and exsanguinated using an Esmarch bandage, wrapping from distal to proximal, and the proximal tourniquet is then inflated. Local anesthetic, typically 25 to 50 mL of 0.5% lidocaine, is slowly injected through the IV in the hand. Surgical anesthesia is established after 5 to 10 min. For procedures lasting longer than 30 min, the distal tourniquet can be inflated over the already anesthetized area and the proximal tourniquet released if the patient complains of tourniquet pain. Disadvantages of a Bier block include not providing analgesia beyond complete release of the tourniquet and difficulty in completely exsanguinating the extremity when there is a traumatic injury involved. These factors should be taken into consideration for patient selection.

A median and ulnar nerve block (see figure below) would also be appropriate for this surgical procedure. The combination of these two blocks provides targeted surgical anesthesia and can provide postoperative analgesia if a long-acting local anesthetic is used. Alternatively, local anesthesia by the surgeon works quite well if no tourniquet is required.

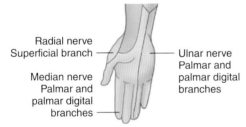

Radial nerve
Superficial branch

Ulnar nerve
Palmar and
palmar digital
branches

Median nerve
Palmar and
palmar digital
branches

Sensory blockade provided by median and ulnar nerve block. (Adapted with permission from Butterworth JF, Mackey DC, Wasnick JD: *Morgan and Mikhail's Clinical Anesthesiology*, 6th ed. New York, NY: McGraw-Hill Education; 2018.)

A supraclavicular nerve block is performed at the division level of the brachial plexus and offers dense anesthesia for procedures at or distal to the elbow. It would certainly provide sensory blockade in the desired operative area. However, there are several reasons why it is not the best choice for this patient. A supraclavicular block results in sensory and motor blockade extending well beyond the surgical site, and a completely insensate and immobile arm/hand could prove to be more bothersome than beneficial to the patient. Relatively uncommon complications of a supraclavicular block include pneumothorax, due to the proximity of pleura to the brachial plexus at this location (see the next figure), and phrenic nerve blockade. In a patient with significant pulmonary disease, these complications could be devastating. Thus, given other regional anesthetic options, it is better to avoid a supraclavicular block in this patient.

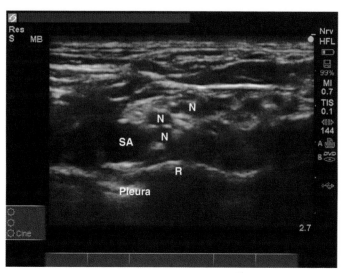

Ultrasound image of the brachial plexus in the supraclavicular fossa. Note proximity of pleura to brachial plexus. (SA, subclavian artery; R, ribs; N, brachial plexus in cross-section.) (Reproduced with permission from Butterworth JF, Mackey DC, Wasnick JD: *Morgan and Mikhail's Clinical Anesthesiology*, 6th ed. New York, NY: McGraw-Hill Education; 2018.)

You decide to proceed with a Bier block. The patient tolerates the procedure well. The surgeon is finished with the procedure in 8 min. The tourniquet is released, and the patient is readied for transport to the postanesthesia care unit (PACU). Suddenly, the patient becomes agitated and appears confused.

2. Your next course of action is to:

   A. Reassure the patient.
   B. Give the patient propofol.
   C. Ensure adequate oxygenation and ventilation, and monitor the patient.
   D. Get the code cart.

The correct answer is C. The patient has likely developed local anesthetic systemic toxicity (LAST) to lidocaine. When performing a Bier block, it is recommended to leave the tourniquet inflated at least 15 to 20 min to allow tissue absorption of the local anesthetic and to subsequently deflate gradually. In this case, the tourniquet was only inflated for 8 min. The anesthesia provider should be vigilant for signs and symptoms of LAST and should act promptly.

The classic symptoms of LAST include symptoms of central nervous system (CNS) excitation such as auditory changes, circumoral numbness, and metallic taste, and signs may include slurred speech and agitation that may progress to seizures and/or CNS depression. In classic descriptions, cardiac toxicity follows CNS toxicity: initial signs of hypertension, tachycardia, or ventricular arrhythmia progressing to cardiac depression (bradycardia, conduction block, asystole, and decreased contractility). There is marked variation in the presentation of LAST, including time from local anesthetic administration to onset, initial manifestations, and duration; however, with Bier blocks, onset of symptoms is usually immediately after release of the tourniquet, and indeed, CNS side effects can be expected when the tourniquet has been inflated for only a short time. Cardiac symptoms can present without any initial CNS symptoms with long-acting local anesthetics such as ropivacaine or bupivacaine, but this has not been reported with lidocaine.

Focusing on prevention can decrease the frequency and severity of LAST, although there is no single method that can completely eliminate risk. The overarching goal is to reduce the plasma concentration of local anesthetic. Recommendations for LAST prevention include:

- Using the lowest effective dose of local anesthetic.
- Incremental injection, and aspiration prior to each injection.
- Use of an intravascular indicator such as epinephrine. Intravascular injection of epinephrine 10 to 15 μg produces an increase in heart rate of at least 10 beats/min or an increase in systolic blood pressure of at least 15 mm Hg. However, epinephrine as an intravascular indicator may not be reliable in patients who are taking a β-blocker, in active labor, elderly, or under general/neuraxial anesthesia. In pediatric patients, an intravascular injection of epinephrine 0.5 mcg/kg produces an increase in systolic blood pressure of at least 15 mm Hg. However, epinephrine is never used in Bier blocks.

Treating LAST begins with early recognition and effective airway management to avoid hypoxia and acidosis, which can worsen LAST. After airway management, administration of lipid emulsion therapy should be considered at the first signs of LAST with long-acting local anesthetics, which can prevent further progression to seizure or cardiac arrhythmia. Initial IV dosing of 20% lipid emulsion is 1.5 mL/kg followed by 0.25 mL/kg/min infusion. If no improvement is seen, a re-bolus of intralipid emulsion may be given. The upper limit of dosing for intralipid emulsion is 10 mL/kg over 30 min. It would be inappropriate to administer intralipid to this patient inasmuch as the response to lidocaine will be short lived and will almost never produce any cardiac side effects.

Propofol should not be used as a substitute for intralipid. It has a low content of lipid, and thus a large volume of propofol would be required to deliver a sufficient amount of lipid to combat LAST, resulting in myocardial depression. If seizures occur, a benzodiazepine is the drug of choice for termination. If a benzodiazepine is not readily available, small doses of propofol may be used.

If cardiac arrest occurs after ropivacaine or bupivacaine, standard advanced cardiac life support (ACLS) is recommended, with reduced doses of epinephrine (10–100 μg bolus). Vasopressin is not recommended. Calcium channel blockers and β-blockers should be avoided. Amiodarone is the medication of choice for ventricular arrhythmias. Failure to respond to lipid emulsion, vasopressor therapy, and ACLS should prompt institution of cardiopulmonary bypass.

Fortunately, in this case, reassurance and monitoring sufficed. The patient returned to baseline over about a 5-min interval and was taken to the PACU after receiving only an additional 1 mg of midazolam.

Your next patient is a 65-year-old woman who presents for fixation of a distal radius fracture. She has a history of CAD with drug-eluting stents placed 1 year ago (currently taking aspirin), chronic back pain (consuming a significant amount of opiate analgesics), and a long history of smoking. The surgeon is concerned about pain control for this patient and asks your advice on intraoperative and postoperative management.

3. After careful consideration, you decide the *optimal* anesthetic plan is an enhanced recovery program with preoperative and postoperative multimodal systemic analgesia and:

   A. Single-injection supraclavicular nerve block.
   B. General anesthesia.
   C. Continuous interscalene peripheral nerve block.
   D. Continuous infraclavicular peripheral nerve block.

The correct answer is D. It can be challenging to provide adequate postoperative pain control for the patient who is already taking opioids for chronic pain, and the best approach in this case is an enhanced recovery program with multimodal analgesia. The scientific rationale for multimodal analgesia is to combine different classes of medications, having different (multimodal) pharmacological mechanisms of action and additive or synergistic effects, in order to control multiple perioperative pathophysiological factors that lead to postoperative pain and its sequelae. Regional anesthesia, nonsteroidal anti-inflammatory drugs (NSAIDs), acetaminophen, gabapentin or pregabalin, and opioids are some of the multimodal component options available. Regional anesthesia may provide potent analgesia, reducing systemic opioid analgesic requirements and thereby opioid-related side effects.

Patients with chronic pain and opioid tolerance benefit from a continuous peripheral nerve block administered in the hospital or ambulatory setting. An ambulatory infraclavicular brachial plexus perineural infusion with ropivicaine using a portable infusion pump, combined with multimodal analgesia, decreases pain, sleep disturbance, opioid use and opioid-related side effects, and improves overall satisfaction for moderately painful orthopedic surgery of the upper extremity at, or distal to, the elbow. It would be ideal for this patient.

A single-injection supraclavicular block (answer A) is not necessarily the wrong answer; however, it is not the *best* option for this patient. It would provide surgical anesthesia, as well as prolonged analgesia if a long-acting anesthetic is used. However, the maximum duration of a single-injection peripheral nerve block is 8 to 24 h, and the patient may have significant pain if there is no analgesic regimen in place following resolution of the block's sensory component. A continuous peripheral nerve block provides an alternative option when prolonged analgesia is desired.

General anesthesia (answer B) is an acceptable approach in treating this patient; however, a regional anesthetic technique should be considered when trying to utilize a multimodal analgesic approach, unless there is a contraindication. Aspirin therapy is not a contraindication to regional anesthesia and may be continued in the perioperative period. It is important to review anticoagulant medication and coagulation status of a patient prior to proceeding with regional anesthesia.

An interscalene brachial plexus block (answer C) is indicated for procedures involving the shoulder and upper arm. Cervical roots 5 to 7 are the most densely blocked with this approach, and the ulnar nerve may be spared. Interscalene blocks are not appropriate for surgery at or distal to the elbow, since they do not reliably produce surgical-quality sensory or motor blockade in the hand and distal arm.

DID YOU LEARN?

- Indications for intravenous regional anesthesia.
- Various sites of brachial plexus blockade and appropriate selection of regional anesthetic based on patient and surgical consideration.
- Recognition, prevention, and treatment of local anesthetic systemic toxicity.
- Role of regional anesthesia in perioperative pain management.

Recommended Readings

Baldini G, Miller T. Enhanced recovery protocols & optimization of perioperative outcomes. In: Butterworth IV JF, Mackey DC, Wasnick JD, eds. *Morgan and Mikhail's Clinical Anesthesiology*, 6th ed. New York, NY: McGraw-Hill; 2018:1111-1132.

Mariano ER. Anesthesia for orthopedic surgery. In: Butterworth IV JF, Mackey DC, Wasnick JD, eds. *Morgan and Mikhail's Clinical Anesthesiology*, 6th ed. New York, NY: McGraw-Hill; 2018:803-818.

References

Blackburn EW, Shafritz AB. Why do Bier blocks work for hand surgery…most of the time? *J Hand Surg*. 2010;35(6):1022-1024.

Madison SJ, Ilfeld BM. Chapter 46: Peripheral nerve blocks. In: Butterworth JF, Mackey DC, Wasnick JD, eds. *Morgan and Mikhail's Clinical Anesthesiology*, 5th ed. New York, NY: McGraw-Hill; 2013.

Mulroy MF, Hejtmanek MR. Prevention of local anesthetic toxicity. *Reg Anesth Pain Med*. 2010;35:175-178.

Neal JM, Bernards CM, Butterworth JF, et al. ASRA Practice Advisory on Local Anesthetic Systemic Toxicity. *Reg Anesth Pain Med*. 2010;35:152-161.

Weinberg GL. Treatment of local anesthetic systemic toxicity. *Reg Anesth Pain Med*. 2010;35:186-191.

CASE 5   Peripheral Nerve Block for Arteriovenous Fistula Placement

Bahareh Khatibi, MD, and Brian M. Ilfeld, MD, MS

A 67-year-old man with worsening kidney function is scheduled for arteriovenous fistula (AVF) placement in the left forearm. Past medical history is significant for diabetes mellitus, chronic obstructive lung disease, and coronary artery disease. He has a right coronary artery drug-eluting stent that was placed 1 year ago. He stopped taking clopidogrel 10 days ago, but has continued prophylactic aspirin. ECG reveals normal sinus rhythm with Q waves in the inferior leads. Laboratory values include hemoglobin, 13 g/dL; platelet count, 180,000/μL; creatinine, 1.5 mg/dL; fingerstick blood glucose, 114 mg/dL; and an international normalized ratio (INR) of 1.1.

1. Which of the following can you tell the patient about the role of anesthetic type in surgical patients?

A. Regional anesthesia reduces mortality compared to general anesthesia.
B. Regional anesthesia may reduce the stress response and the development of chronic pain.
C. Regional anesthesia has no benefits over local anesthesia for AVF placement.
D. Regional anesthesia has been shown to decrease the risk of postoperative delirium when compared to general anesthesia.

The correct answer is B. Regional anesthesia may lead to reductions in the stress response, postoperative analgesic requirements, opioid-related side effects, general anesthesia requirements, and the development of chronic pain.

Studies focused on specific outcomes of regional anesthesia have shown benefits related to its use in surgery and postoperative analgesia. For peripheral nerve blocks, perioperative opioid consumption may be reduced or avoided entirely, particularly with perineural catheter techniques. For total knee replacement, patients with continuous femoral or adductor canal nerve blockade have been shown to have less pain on movement and to achieve earlier or improved mobilization when compared to those receiving IV patient-controlled analgesia or placebo. Studies of epidural analgesia for major abdominal surgery and abdominal aortic surgery have revealed superior analgesia when compared to intravenous opioid-based analgesia. The use of epidural analgesia in those studies resulted in reduced need for postoperative mechanical ventilation, reduced rate of postoperative myocardial infarction, and reduced gastric and renal complications. However, these benefits have not been shown to result in a reduction in mortality.

Postoperative cognitive complications have been associated with poor short- and long-term outcomes. The role of anesthesia in cognitive dysfunction, particularly general anesthesia versus regional anesthesia, remains unclear. Although it appears that general anesthesia may increase the risk of developing postoperative cognitive dysfunction when compared to spinal, epidural, or intravenous block, the same benefit has not been shown for postoperative delirium.

When compared to local anesthesia, brachial plexus blockade for AVF placement is associated with sympathectomy-induced peripheral arteriovenous dilation, resulting in reduced peripheral resistance and increased local blood flow, thus offering an ideal background for fistula creation and short-term patency.

The patient would like to avoid general anesthesia if possible. The surgeon does not want to use local infiltration with monitored anesthetic care (MAC) and suggests a peripheral nerve block.

2. According to current guidelines on anticoagulation and regional anesthesia, which of the following is true?

A. A peripheral nerve block is not recommended because the patient has taken aspirin within the past 7 days.
B. A peripheral nerve block may be offered because the patient stopped taking clopidogrel over 7 days ago.
C. A peripheral nerve block may be offered because aspirin use is not a consideration in bleeding risk for nerve blocks.
D. A peripheral nerve block is not recommended because he has taken concurrent antiplatelet medications in the past 14 days.

The correct answer is B. The hemorrhagic risks after peripheral nerve block technique are not well defined. However, the latest American Society of Regional Anesthesia and Pain Medicine (ASRA) guidelines recommend that their consensus statements regarding neuraxial techniques in anticoagulated patients be applied to patients undergoing peripheral nerve blocks.

The guidelines do not specify concerns as to the timing of nerve block techniques in patients taking NSAIDs, including aspirin, alone. However, the performance of blocks is discouraged in patients taking aspirin with concurrent or expected use of other medications affecting clotting mechanisms such as oral anticoagulants, unfractionated heparin, and low-molecular-weight heparin.

For the thienopyridine derivatives ticlopidine and clopidogrel, the guidelines recommend that the time intervals between discontinuation of therapy and nerve blockade are 14 days and 7 days, respectively. For clopidogrel, if a block is indicated between 5 and 7 days, it is recommended that normalization of platelet function should be documented.

The ASRA guidelines represent the collective experience of experts in neuraxial anesthesia and anticoagulation. As with any medical procedure, the risks, benefits, and alternatives of regional techniques must be assessed on a patient-specific basis.

You choose to proceed with a peripheral nerve block with MAC for surgical anesthesia for the AVF placement.

3. Which of the following is true about peripheral nerve blocks for this patient?

A. An interscalene nerve block will provide the most complete coverage of all upper extremity nerve blocks.

B. An axillary nerve block will provide sufficient coverage of the forearm as long as the musculocutaneous nerve is also blocked.

C. A supraclavicular block will provide nearly complete and consistent coverage of the arm.

D. An infraclavicular nerve block is associated with a greater risk of pneumothorax than a supraclavicular nerve block.

The correct answer is C. An infraclavicular nerve block provides excellent anesthesia for procedures at or distal to the elbow. Supraclavicular nerve blocks provide anesthesia to a similar distribution, but may be associated with sparing of the ulnar nerve. Interscalene blocks provide better coverage of the shoulder and upper arm, but may have ulnar sparing. Other potential drawbacks to the infraclavicular and supraclavicular blocks are the slight risk of pneumothorax and potential for hemidiaphragmatic paralysis.

An axillary block ultrasound view includes the median, ulnar, and radial nerves in the proximal upper arm. The axillary, musculocutaneous, and medial brachial cutaneous nerves branch from the brachial plexus proximal to the location of an axillary block and are usually spared. The musculocutaneous nerve, a branch of the lateral cord, can sometimes be seen and blocked in the axillary block ultrasound view. This nerve terminates as the lateral antebrachial cutaneous nerve and provides cutaneous innervation of the lateral aspect of the forearm and wrist. The medial forearm receives innervation from the medial antebrachial cutaneous nerve, which is not visualized and cannot be blocked in the axillary block view. Unfortunately, nearly all initial arteriovenous fistulas for dialysis access are at least partly in the medial forearm.

The patient has decreased sensation in the appropriate distribution after supraclavicular nerve block with 12 mL ropivacaine 0.5% and is taken to the operating room for surgery. A propofol infusion is started at 100 mcg/kg/min for sedation, and surgery is started. Approximately 15 min after the start of surgery, the patient starts to move, appears agitated, and does not follow commands appropriately.

4. Your first choice of action is:

A. Increase the propofol dose to decrease patient agitation.

B. Administer fentanyl for pain control.

C. Administer lipid emulsion therapy for local anesthetic systemic toxicity.

D. None of the above.

The correct answer is D. Agitation is a nonspecific symptom resulting from any one or all of pain, anxiety, medication effects, and cerebral or metabolic derangements. It is important to quickly rule out common, reversible causes of agitation and altered mental status, including hypoxia and hypercarbia. Immediately provide 100% oxygen by mask and ensure the patient is ventilating appropriately. In this case, consider decreasing the dose of propofol, since it may be causing hypoventilation and/or cerebral disinhibition. Meanwhile, other patient-specific causes of altered sensorium should be sought and treated if found. In this diabetic patient, hypoglycemia may be a cause. Since the patient had a nerve block, local anesthetic systemic toxicity (LAST) must also be considered, even with the small dose used in this case.

The management of LAST begins with risk reduction during performance of the block. Use the least dose of local anesthetic needed to achieve the desired block. Consider using a pharmacologic indicator for intravascular injection, such as epinephrine 5 mcg/mL, in the local anesthetic solution. Aspirate prior to each local anesthetic injection, and inject incrementally while simultaneously monitoring for signs and/or symptoms of LAST.

Since signs and symptoms of LAST may be delayed for up to 30 min following injection, monitor the patient with standard ASA monitors during and after the block. Consider LAST in any patient with altered mental status, neurological symptoms, and/or cardiovascular instability. Neurological symptoms and signs include metallic taste, circumoral numbness or tingling, diplopia, tinnitus, dizziness, agitation, confusion, muscle twitching, seizure activity, drowsiness, slurred speech, obtundation, coma, or apnea. Cardiovascular signs may only manifest in severe cases, but include hyperdynamic circulation initially, followed by progressive hypotension with cardiac conduction block, bradycardia, or asystole. Ventricular arrhythmias, including ventricular tachycardia, torsades de pointes, and ventricular fibrillation, may be seen.

If LAST is suspected, immediately summon assistance and provide airway management with 100% oxygen. Benzodiazepines can be administered if the patient is experiencing seizures. Alert the nearest facility with cardiopulmonary bypass capability because this will take time to initiate and coordinate if needed. If LAST is the result of longer acting agents such as ropivacaine or bupivacaine, provide advanced cardiac life support, but reduce epinephrine doses to less than 1 mcg/kg and avoid administration of vasopressin, calcium channel blockers, β-blockers, and local anesthetics. Implement lipid therapy on the basis of LAST severity and rate of progression. Evidence for efficacy of lipid therapy is strongest for ropivacaine and bupivacaine, and much less convincing for lidocaine or mepivcaine. Administer IV lipid emulsion (20%) bolus of 1.5 mL/kg of lean body mass over 1 min, and then initiate IV infusion at a rate of 0.25 mL/kg/min. The upper total limit for lipid emulsion dose is approximately 10 mL/kg over the first 30 min. Since cardiovascular depression can recur after treatment, prolonged monitoring of patients with LAST is warranted.

DID YOU LEARN?

- The role of different anesthetic modalities in the outcome of surgical patients.
- Recommendations for the use of regional anesthesia in patients taking anticoagulants.
- The distribution of upper extremity nerve blocks, including potential advantages and disadvantages.
- Management of altered mental status and local anesthetic systemic toxicity in a surgical patient.

Recommended Reading

Madison SJ, Ilfeld B. Peripheral nerve blocks. In: Butterworth IV JF, Mackey DC, Wasnick JD, eds. *Morgan and Mikhail's Clinical Anesthesiology*, 6th ed. New York, NY: McGraw-Hill; 2018:997-1046.

References

Gitman M, Barrington MJ. Local anesthetic systemic toxicity: A review of recent case reports and registries. *Reg Anesth Pain Med.* 2018;43(2):124-130.

Horlocker TT, Wedel DJ, Rowlingson JC, et al. Regional anesthesia in the patient receiving antithrombotic or thrombolytic therapy: American Society of Regional Anesthesia and Pain Medicine Evidence-Based Guidelines (third edition). *Reg Anesth Pain Med.* 2010;35(1):64-101.

Lo Monte A, Damiano G, Mularo A, et al. Comparison between local and regional anesthesia in arteriovenous fistula creation. *J Vasc Access.* 2011;12(4):331-335.

Neal JM, Barrington MJ, Fettiplace MR, et al. The Third American Society of Regional Anesthesia and Pain Medicine Practice Advisory on local anesthetic systemic toxicity: Executive summary 2017. *Reg Anesth Pain Med.* 2018;43(2):113-123.

CHAPTER 38

Chronic Pain Management

CASE 1 | Painful Foot Numbness Before Scheduled Colorectal Surgery

Carrie Johnson, MD, and Larry C. Driver, MD

A 67-year-old man with newly diagnosed colorectal cancer presents to the preoperative anesthesia assessment clinic for evaluation 1 day prior to a scheduled low anterior resection. He has worked as a farmer in a rural community with limited medical care. A diagnosis of type 2 diabetes was made 10 years ago, but he states he does not regularly check his glucose levels and he has not taken the prescribed medicine because it did not "sit well" with him. Besides feeling unsettled by the cancer diagnosis, his primary complaint is a painfully numb, pins-and-needles sensation in both feet that has become progressively worse over the past 2 years. After taking his medical history and performing a physical examination, you determine that he has painful diabetic neuropathy.

1. What is the most common form of diabetic neuropathy?

   A. Mononeuropathy multiplex.
   B. Compression mononeuropathy.
   C. Distal symmetric polyneuropathy.
   D. Proximal motor neuropathy.

The correct answer is C. Diabetic neuropathy is most commonly a sensory disturbance with a bilateral pattern of distal small-fiber nerve involvement. Standard presentation includes a gradual onset of paresthesias (abnormal, but not painful, sensations, either spontaneous or evoked) and pain in the feet and legs. Symptoms typically begin in the toes and gradually ascend over months to years in a stocking distribution. Fingertips and hands can also be involved, although this is usually later in the disease course. Common features include burning pain, often worse at night, and allodynia (sensations of pain in response to a nonnoxious stimulus, such as light touch). Physical examination reveals distal sensory loss primarily affecting vibratory sense and proprioception. Of note, severe sensory loss leads to unnoticed microtrauma, placing patients at risk for foot ulcers and neuropathic arthropathy (Charcot joints).

2. Which of the following factors, if present in this patient, would have been most likely to prevent the development of his painful diabetic neuropathy?

  A. Chronic alcohol use.
  B. Chemotherapy treatment for his colorectal cancer.
  C. History of chronic back pain.
  D. Tight glycemic control.

The correct answer is D. The importance of glycemic control cannot be over-emphasized in diabetic patients who have, or are at risk for, neuropathy. This is supported by scientific evidence showing a 60% reduction in the incidence of neuropathy over a 5-year period with tight glycemic control. Conversely, alcohol use and history of chronic pain are known to place diabetic patients at increased risk for the development of neuropathic pain. Many chemotherapeutic agents cause peripheral neuropathies, and recent data suggest cancer patients may manifest a subclinical neuropathic syndrome prior to administration of chemotherapy.

You mention this case to one of your colleagues who suggests that you initiate pharmacotherapy with a medication that is both a first-line agent for treatment of diabetic neuropathy and beneficial for management of perioperative pain.

3. What is the described medication?

  A. Celecoxib.
  B. Pregabalin.
  C. Fluoxetine.
  D. Meperidine.

The correct answer is B. The anticonvulsants pregabalin and gabapentin are considered first-line agents in the treatment of numerous neuropathic pain syndromes, including diabetic neuropathy. These agents are structural analogs to γ-aminobutyric acid (GABA), but their activity is thought to be primarily through calcium channel modulation. Common side effects include sedation, dizziness, and edema. Moreover, several studies demonstrate that even a single 150-mg oral dose of pregabalin administered preoperatively reduces postoperative pain and decreases opioid consumption. This offers a unique opportunity to the anesthesiologist evaluating patients in the preoperative setting. Starting an anticonvulsant could prove not only beneficial for postoperative pain management, but also provide additional benefit for long-term management of a patient's chronic neuropathic pain.

Antidepressant medications including tricyclic antidepressants (TCAs) and serotonin-norepinephrine reuptake inhibitors (SNRIs) have also been well-studied and are routinely utilized in treating neuropathic pain states such as diabetic neuropathy. TCAs are considered most efficacious and can work synergistically with gabapentinoids, but their use is limited by anticholinergic side effects. Selective serotonin reuptake inhibitors (SSRIs), such as fluoxetine, are less effective for neuropathic pain and are not considered first-line agents.

Opioids are sometimes used for difficult-to-treat neuropathic pain states. However, their use is controversial and must be considered in the context of risk of misuse and/or abuse. The opioid meperidine would not be an appropriate choice for treatment of diabetic neuropathy. Nonsteroidal anti-inflammatory drugs (NSAIDs), like celecoxib, are excellent adjuvant medications for management of perioperative pain. These medications are not, however, efficacious in treating neuropathic pain states.

4. Given what you know about this patient, in planning for his anesthetic, you would be concerned about all of the following *except*:

A. Inaccurate pulse oximetry.
B. Risk of aspiration.
C. Impaired heart rate control.
D. Postural hypotension.

The correct answer is A. The potential presence of autonomic neuropathy should be considered in any patient with history of diabetes, but especially in patients with known diabetes-related neuropathy. Autonomic dysfunction occurs in up to 40% of diabetics and in greater than 50% of diabetic patients with coexisting hypertension. It is a serious and common complication of diabetes, which significantly influences perioperative management.

Characteristic abnormalities include orthostatic hypotension, lack of heart rate variability (including the presence of resting tachycardia), gastroparesis, esophageal dysmotility, and erectile dysfunction. Many anesthesiologists will treat diabetics as if having a "full stomach," with nonparticulate antacid premedication and rapid-sequence induction and intubation. Of note, patients with diabetic autonomic neuropathy are at increased cardiac risk due to postinduction hypotension, limited ability of the heart to adapt to changes in intravascular volume, and potential for silent postoperative myocardial ischemia. Preoperative awareness and associated anesthetic planning are critical for optimizing the care of these patients in the perioperative setting.

Conversely, based on history of diabetes and presence of peripheral neuropathy, there is no particular reason to expect inaccurate pulse oximetry. Conditions that may affect reliability of pulse oximetry include carboxyhemoglobinemia, methemoglobinemia, poor pulsation (eg, left-ventricular assist device patients), pulsatile veins (eg, tricuspid regurgitation), and cold extremities.

DID YOU LEARN?

- Characteristics and presentation of diabetic neuropathy.
- The importance of glycemic control in prevention of diabetic neuropathy.
- Optimal treatment of diabetic neuropathic pain.
- Perioperative considerations of a patient with autonomic neuropathy.

Recommended Reading

Benzon H, Raja SN, Liu S, Fishman SM, Cohen SP, eds. *Essentials of Pain Medicine*, 4th ed. Philadelphia, PA: Elsevier; 2017.

References

Agarwal A, Gautam S, Gupta D, et al. Evaluation of a single preoperative dose of pregabalin for attenuation of postoperative pain after laparoscopic cholecystectomy. *Br J Anaesth*. 2008;101(5):700-704.

Boyette-Davis JA, Eng C, Wang XS, et al. Subclinical peripheral neuropathy is a common finding in colorectal cancer patients prior to chemotherapy. *Clin Cancer Res*. 2012;18(11):3180-3187.

Diabetes Control and Complications Trial Research Group. The effect of intensive treatment of diabetes on the development and progression of long-term complications in insulin-dependent diabetes mellitus. *N Engl J Med*. 2003;329:977-986.

Vinik AI, Maser RE, Mitchell BD, Freeman R. Diabetic autonomic neuropathy. *Diabetes Care*. 2003;26:1553-1579.

CASE 2	Chronic Muscle Pain and Fatigue

Erik Hustak, MD, and Larry C. Driver, MD

A 55-year-old female ultrasound technician presents with chronic fatigue and chronic, progressive, right-sided, posterior neck and shoulder pain. Her medical history is significant for obesity (body mass index 35 kg/m^2), hypertension, and diabetes mellitus. After conservative treatment with NSAIDs and acetaminophen, the primary care physician ordered a shoulder radiograph and cervical spine magnetic resonance imaging studies that were both unremarkable. A diagnosis of nonspecific musculoskeletal pain is made, and referral to a pain management specialist for further evaluation and management is entertained.

1. What is the most appropriate next step?

   A. Order a urine drug screen.
   B. Order a complete blood count, erythrocyte sedimentation rate, and C-reactive protein level.
   C. Order an EMG/NCS.
   D. Perform a focused history and physical exam of the neck and shoulder.

The correct answer is D. Soft tissue disorders are a common primary care complaint. The differential diagnosis is broad for nonspecific "musculoskeletal pain" with no clear etiology from a radiological standpoint. One must understand that the afferent nociceptive input is complex and often arises from soft tissue structures not easily assessed with a simple blood test or radiograph. A focused history and physical exam is of paramount importance when evaluating a regional pain complaint. Nociceptive afferent input from bones, muscles, and tendons along with their attachment points and concomitant fascial planes can all explain regional pain syndromes.

Myofascial pain syndrome (MPS) is a clinical diagnosis based on a focused history and physical exam. Universally accepted diagnostic criteria are lacking. In general, MPS is characterized by the presence of "trigger points" located within "taut bands" in muscle or fascia that can trigger the presenting pain. Applying compression to these specific points can "trigger" a referred pain pattern to what is known as the "target zone." In addition to this local "twitch response," palpation of a trigger point can also be associated with autonomic phenomena. MPS is more prevalent in women than men (65% vs 35% of middle-aged patients, respectively), and it seems to be more common with age (85% of all such complaints are from the population older than 65 years). The underlying mechanism is thought to arise from repetitive muscle trauma or overuse promoting pathological development of regional dysfunctional trigger points.

2. A differential diagnosis of MPS versus fibromyalgia is considered. Which of the following statements is *most* accurate?

   A. Fibromyalgia is confirmed by the presence of at least 11/18 tender points on physical exam.
   B. Trigger points of MPS are identical to tender points of fibromyalgia.
   C. Patients with fibromyalgia by definition have tender points in a specific distribution and cannot have trigger points.
   D. Palpation of MPS "trigger points" gives rise to pain at a distant site, whereas palpation of fibromyalgia "tender points" typically causes pain at the site of palpation.

The correct answer is D. Fibromyalgia is a clinical diagnosis of diffuse musculoskeletal pain, which typically presents with other associated medical conditions including fatigue and psychiatric problems. Although the American College of

CHAPTER 38 · Chronic Pain Management

Rheumatology (ACR) classification of 1990 includes 11/18 tender points of widespread pain, the 2010 ACR preliminary diagnostic criteria are based on at least 3 months of symptoms that exceed various thresholds based on a widespread pain index (WPI) and a symptom severity scale (SS) in the absence of a disorder that would otherwise explain the patient's pain.

Fibromyalgia often coexists with other medical disorders, and the "trigger points" of MPS can be present in addition to the "tender points" of fibromyalgia. Although debatable in the literature, palpation of trigger points of MPS may "trigger" pain elsewhere. The "tender points" of fibromyalgia often follow the 1990 ACR pattern and are not associated with taut bands, and typically cause pain at the site of palpation. Although the underlying mechanism of fibromyalgia is unknown, it is not thought to represent an inflammatory condition or a motor end-plate dysfunction.

3. Which of the following statements most accurately portrays the underlying mechanism surrounding the development of MPS?

   A. MPS is psychogenic in origin, which often necessitates antidepressant pharmacotherapy.
   B. Although the exact etiology is unknown, an environment conducive to hyperpolarization of the motor end-plate would explain MPS.
   C. Excessive acetylcholine production and release is thought to play a role in the development of MPS.
   D. Repetitive trauma *alone* explains the genesis of a taut band with its corresponding trigger point.

The correct answer is C. The underlying mechanism of MPS is thought to arise from repetitive muscle trauma and/or overuse that promotes pathological development of dysfunctional motor nerve terminal end-plates caught in a state of increased acetylcholine production and release. Muscle fiber activation and sarcomere shortening facilitate the creation of a hypoxic local environment, prompting the release of inflammatory mediators and nociceptor activation. This is known as the *integrated hypothesis*. In addition, the development of trigger points in areas not exposed to a provocative traumatic event can also occur. This has been theorized as a *neurogenic expression of central sensitization*, perhaps in response to a primary medical condition or visceral event located within the corresponding myotomal segment, leading to trigger point creation.

4. A diagnosis of MPS is made based on clinical evaluation. What is the most appropriate treatment plan?

   A. Weak opioid agonist trial with upward titration as necessary.
   B. Muscle relaxant therapy.
   C. Trigger point injections with local anesthetic or "dry needling" techniques.
   D. Physical therapy with strengthening exercises.

The correct answer is C. Since MPS is thought to occur secondary to end-plate dysfunction and/or is possibly related to a central sensitization phenomenon, as discussed earlier, the therapeutic approach needs to be focused accordingly. After a taut band is identified on physical exam, the first-line treatment is often trigger point injections in order to break the cycle of end-plate dysfunction. Many different techniques have been advocated, including injection of local anesthetics, dry needling, and the injection of botulinum toxin. The injection of botulinum toxin can be costly, and its effectiveness has been questioned. Acupuncture and therapeutic ultrasound have also been utilized. From a pharmacological standpoint, opioid agonist therapy would not be first-line therapy. One could consider NSAIDs along with a centrally acting α_2-agonist in order to combat the central sensitization phenomenon discussed earlier. However, this should be considered as an addition to trigger point injection, not as an alternative. Finally, identifying clues of repetitive trauma or overuse in the clinical history is key in developing a strategy to prevent the formation of trigger points. In this particular case, a careful work history may point to an occupational ergonomic hazard that needs to be addressed.

DID YOU LEARN?

- The initial diagnostic approach for MPS.
- What distinguishes MPS from fibromyalgia.
- The pathophysiology of "trigger point" development in MPS versus the "tender points" of fibromyalgia.

Recommended Readings

Giamberardino MA, Affaitati G, Fabrizio A, Costantini R. Myofascial pain syndromes and their evaluation. *Best Pract Res Clin Rheumatol.* 2011;25(2):185-198.

Häuser W, Sarzi-Puttini P, Fitzcharles MA. Fibromyalgia syndrome: Under-, over- and misdiagnosis. *Clin Exp Rheumatol.* 2019;37:90-97.

Kamanli A, Kaya A, Ardicoglu O, Ozgocmen S, Zengin FO, Bayik Y. Comparison of lidocaine injection, botulinum toxin injection, and dry needling to triggerpoints in myofascial pain syndrome. *Rheumatol Int.* 2005;25(8):604-611.

Katz RS, Wolfe F, Michaud K. Fibromyalgia diagnosis: A comparison of clinical, survey, and American College of Rheumatology criteria. *Arthritis Rheumatol.* 2006;54(1):169-176.

Malanga GA, Gwynn MW, Smith R, Miller D. Tizanidine is effective in the treatment of myofascial pain syndrome. *Pain Physician.* 2002;5(4):422-432.

Mense S, Simons DG, Russell IJ. *Muscle Pain: Understanding Its Nature, Diagnosis, and Treatment.* Philadelphia, PA: Lippincott Williams and Wilkins; 2001:385.

Money S. Pathophysiology of trigger points in myofascial pain syndrome. *J Pain Palliat Care Pharmacother.* 2017;31(2):158-159.

Wolfe F, Clauw DJ, Fitzcharles MA, et al. The American College of Rheumatology preliminary diagnostic criteria for fibromyalgia and measurement of symptom severity. *Arthritis Care Res (Hoboken).* 2010;62(5):600-610.

CASE 3   Persistent Chest Wall Pain Following an Episode of Shingles

Shiraz Yazdani, MD, and Larry C. Driver, MD

An 81-year-old woman presents to the pain medicine clinic with a complaint of left-sided chest wall pain. Her past medical history includes type 2 diabetes mellitus, hypertension, and varicella infection at age 6. Three months ago, she developed a vesicular rash consistent with herpes zoster in a T7 and T8 distribution on her left side. Her primary care physician prescribed a course of acyclovir, with subsequent resolution of her rash. Since then, she has had burning pain in the same distribution. She describes significant allodynia and limitation of activities of daily living due to the pain. She has failed a trial of acetaminophen with codeine. She has tried no other treatments for her pain. On physical examination, her temperature is 37.1°C; heart rate, 91 beats/min; blood pressure, 147/88 mm Hg; and respiratory rate, 22 breaths/min. She is visibly uncomfortable. Examination of her chest wall reveals evidence of well-healed scars from her previous vesicular rash in the aforementioned T7 and T8 distributions.

1. What is the next appropriate action in the treatment of this patient's pain?

   A. Perform paravertebral local anesthetic injections.
   B. Prescribe 5% topical lidocaine patch.
   C. Prescribe immediate-release morphine.
   D. Prescribe amitriptyline.

The correct answer is B. The incidences of herpes zoster and postherpetic neuralgia both increase with age, and the incidence of herpes zoster in patients older than 85 years of age approaches 50%. Postherpetic neuralgia is often refractory to many analgesic modalities. First-line treatment includes topical lidocaine and capsaicin. Geriatric patients are susceptible to the adverse effects of many medications, including opioids, membrane stabilizers, and antidepressants. Topical preparations are advantageous because there is minimal systemic absorption of the medication and they have been shown to be effective in providing analgesia to those with postherpetic neuralgia with allodynia. The next step, if needed, is to begin a trial of membrane stabilizers such as gabapentin or pregabalin, followed by antidepressants. Amitriptyline has been shown to be effective, but is often not as well tolerated as nortriptyline due to its higher incidence of anticholinergic side effects. Opioids are typically not effective for neuropathic pain states and are often poorly tolerated by elderly patients. Should a patient fail these measures, treatment can progress to interventional procedures such as neural blockade with local anesthetics perhaps combined with steroids. More invasive modalities such as spinal cord stimulation can also be effective for refractory postherpetic neuralgia pain.

2. Which of the following pathophysiological mechanisms explains the pain associated with postherpetic neuralgia?

   A. Type IV hypersensitivity reaction to the latent virus.
   B. IL-2–mediated autoimmune destruction of dorsal root ganglia cells.
   C. Sensory neuronal inflammation caused by viral replication.
   D. Cytotoxic sensitivity reaction to viral antigens.

The correct answer is C. Varicella-zoster is the primary viral infection that causes chickenpox. Once the primary infection is resolved, the virus is kept dormant by cell-mediated immunity. These dormant viral particles are present in sensory nerve ganglia, most commonly in the trigeminal and thoracic regions. Reactivation of the virus can occur due to reduced immune function, which can be due to age-related decreases in immunity, immunosuppressive medications, and/or physical or psychological stress. During this reactivation process, the virus travels along the affected sensory nerves, leading to the pathognomonic unilateral rash in a dermatomal distribution. Replication of the virus leads to inflammation in these sensory neurons, leading to pain. Ultimately, this may lead to loss of cells, myelin, axons, fibrosis of the ganglion, and dorsal horn atrophy.

Following this neural insult, sensitization and deafferentation can occur. Nociceptors in the peripheral and central nervous systems develop a reduced threshold for action potential firing, leading to allodynia. Loss of afferent neurons can lead to spontaneous firing centrally, leading to further pain in the area of sensory damage. Neuronal sprouting may also play a role in the development of the allodynia and hyperalgesia present in postherpetic neuralgia.

3. The patient completes a trial of topical lidocaine without relief. She next tries various membrane stabilizers and antidepressants, but they have intolerable side effects. She asks about high-dose capsaicin therapy. What is one of the mechanisms of action of high-dose (8% w/v) capsaicin therapy in the treatment of postherpetic neuralgia?

   A. Depletion of neuropeptides from peripheral cells.
   B. Destruction of replicating viral cells.
   C. Downregulation of nociceptors at the site of application.
   D. Stabilization of neuronal membranes.

The correct answer is A. Capsaicin is a noxious compound found in chili peppers that is often utilized in the treatment of postherpetic neuralgia. It can be purchased in low concentration (0.025% to 0.075%) over-the-counter topical creams, and 8% w/v topical capsaicin is available by prescription. Since it is a topical treatment, systemic toxicity is unlikely. Capsaicin stimulates free nerve endings of C-fibers in the area where it is applied, leading to depolarization and release of neuropeptides. This is interpreted as a painful, burning sensation. Due to this, topical lidocaine is used prior to capsaicin treatment. Repeated capsaicin application causes depletion of neuropeptides such as substance P from the painful areas, leading to pain relief.

4. What is the most effective way to prevent herpes zoster and subsequent post-herpetic neuralgia in the geriatric population?
   A. Administration of the varicella vaccine.
   B. Increasing vitamin C intake to 2000 mg per day.
   C. Neuraxial injection of valacyclovir.
   D. Administration of the zoster vaccine.

The correct answer is D. Administration of the zoster vaccine, which contains attenuated varicella virus particles, has been shown to dramatically decrease the incidence of both herpes zoster and postherpetic neuralgia. This vaccine is typically given to patients older than 60 years. In contrast, the varicella vaccine, which contains a lower concentration of attenuated varicella virus particles and which is widely used for younger patients in order to prevent primary varicella infection, may not be as effective in preventing herpes zoster in elderly patients.

Adjusting vitamin C intake has not been recommended as a means to reduce the incidence of postherpetic neuralgia. If reactivation does occur and a patient has active herpes zoster, oral or intravenous antivirals such as valacyclovir are recommended. However, neuraxial injection of valacyclovir is not recommended.

DID YOU LEARN?

- Appropriate management of postherpetic neuralgia.
- Pathophysiology of herpes zoster and the mechanism of pain from postherpetic neuralgia.
- Mechanisms of commonly used topical agents in the treatment of postherpetic neuralgia.
- Effective mechanisms to decrease the incidence of postherpetic neuralgia.

References

Arvin A. Aging, immunity, and the varicella-zoster virus. *N Engl J Med*. 2005;352:2266-2267.

Benzon HT. *Practical Management of Pain*. Philadelphia, PA: Elsevier/Mosby; 2014.

Harke H, Gretenkort P, Ladleif HU, et al. Spinal cord stimulation in postherpetic neuralgia and in acute herpes zoster pain. *Anesth Analg*. 2002;94:694-700.

Johnson R, McElhaney J, Pedalino B, et al. Prevention of herpes zoster and its painful and debilitating complications. *Int J Infect Dis*. 2007;11(suppl 2):S43-S48.

Saguil A, Kane S, Mercado M, Lauters R. Postherpetic neuralgia and trigeminal neuralgia. *Am Fam Physician*. 2017;96(10):656-663.

Watson CP, Vernich L, Chipman M, et al. Nortriptyline versus amitriptyline in postherpetic neuralgia: A randomized trial. *Neurology*. 1998;51:1166-1171.

CASE 4   Lumbar Sympathetic Block

Shiraz Yazdani, MD, and Salahadin Abdi, MD, PhD

A 44-year-old, 65-kg woman comes to your office complaining of right lower leg pain. The pain began 7 weeks after she suffered a stress fracture in her right foot, which was treated with casting. She states that putting socks on her foot causes extreme pain. Light touch of the foot on examination confirms allodynia. The skin appears normal, although hair in the affected area is noticeably thinner than on the contralateral extremity. Your medical student asks if this represents a case of complex regional pain syndrome, and if so, what can be done to treat it.

1. Your next action is to:

  A. Order a computed tomography (CT) scan of the right lower extremity with intravenous (IV) contrast.
  B. Obtain a peroneal nerve biopsy.
  C. Perform quantitative sensory testing.
  D. Complete a thorough history and physical examination.

The correct answer is D. Complex regional pain syndrome (CRPS) type I (previously referred to as *reflex sympathetic dystrophy*) and type II (previously referred to as *causalgia*) are diagnoses principally made by history and physical examination. The chief difference between CRPS type II and CRPS type I is that type II is associated with a defined nerve injury. Although tests are useful in confirming the diagnosis, there is currently no one tool that is considered 100% reliable for confirming CRPS. Primary physical changes include sensory, motor, trophic, sudomotor, and autonomic neuropathies. If there is an inciting event, it should be identified, with or without recognized nerve injury. Useful tests include quantitative sensory testing. Thermoregulatory sweat tests can measure changes in temperature typical of those seen in patients with CRPS. Sudomotor changes can be tested via quantitative sudomotor axon reflex tests. Three-phase bone scintigraphy may detect joint and bone changes. CT imaging has not been shown to be useful in the diagnosis of CRPS, although magnetic resonance imaging has high sensitivity and can be helpful. A peroneal nerve biopsy would not necessarily show any changes and could lead to nerve injury, complicating the clinical picture.

After diagnosing the patient with CRPS I, you elect to perform a fluoroscopically guided lumbar sympathetic block. Once the 22-gauge needle is placed in appropriate position and confirmed with injection of contrast, you begin injection of 10 mL of 0.25% bupivacaine. After completion of the injection, the patient complains of nausea. Her mean arterial pressure has decreased from a preoperative measurement of 75 mm Hg to 50 mm Hg.

2. Which of the following is the most likely explanation?

   A. Accidental intravascular injection of local anesthetic.
   B. Accidental subarachnoid block.
   C. Sympatholysis leading to venous pooling and arterial vasodilation.
   D. Acute blood loss from aorta injury.

The correct answer is C. Image-guided lumbar sympathetic block is a relatively safe procedure with rare complications, which can be largely avoided with careful needle positioning and with fluoroscopic confirmation of appropriate contrast spread. Peripheral vasodilation from sympathectomy is to be expected, and in a volume-depleted patient, can lead to hypotension from venous pooling of blood and hypovolemia. Intravascular injection would be less likely, given verification of appropriate contrast spread. Additionally, even if the full amount of the injectate were intravascular, 25 mg of systemic bupivacaine is well below the toxic dose of 2.5 mg/kg for this 65-kg patient and most likely would not cause local anesthetic toxicity. Inadvertent subarachnoid block is a known complication, but unlikely because of the aforementioned verification of contrast spread. Acute blood loss from needle injury to the aorta can certainly cause hypotension, but would be low on the differential diagnosis given the relatively small gauge of the needle. The aorta has a thick wall, and the smooth muscle in the tunica media is sufficient to halt bleeding from a 22-gauge puncture.

Your patient responds well and reports 80% relief of her lower extremity pain. Your medical student is interested in learning more about the procedure and is curious about which types of patients could benefit from this intervention.

3. Which of the following is another indication for lumbar sympathetic block?

   A. Ischemic pain from peripheral vascular insufficiency.
   B. Postoperative pain from repair of a tibial plateau fracture.
   C. Perirectal pain from squamous cell carcinoma.
   D. Acute pain from epididymitis.

The correct answer is A. Lumbar sympathetic block indications include vascular insufficiency in the lower extremity, including Raynaud phenomenon, Buerger disease (thromboangitis obliterans), peripheral vascular disease, and frostbite. Sympathetically mediated pain, such as that of CRPS, can be treated with this intervention as well. Hyperhidrosis and phantom limb syndrome have also been successfully treated. Lumbar sympathetic block is not an appropriate intervention for postoperative pain. A patient with perirectal pain would be better served by a ganglion impar block. Acute pain from epididymitis should not be treated with a lumbar sympathetic block.

DID YOU LEARN?

- The different types of CRPS.
- Diagnostic tools useful in CRPS.
- Indications, techniques, and complications of lumbar sympathetic block.

Recommended Readings

Benzon H, Rathmell J, Wu C, Turk D, Argoff C, Hurley W. *Practical Management of Pain*, 5th ed. Philadelphia, PA: Mosby; 2014.

Birklein F, Ajit SK, Goebel A, Perez RSGM, Sommer C. Complex regional pain syndrome-phenotypic characteristics and potential biomarkers. *Nat Rev Neurol*. 2018;14(5): 272-284.

Fishman S, Ballantyne J, Rathmell J, eds. *Bonica's Management of Pain*, 4th ed. Philadelphia, PA: Wolters Kluwer/Lippincott, Williams and Wilkins; 2010.

Longmire DR. An electrophysiological approach to the evaluation of regional sympathetic dysfunction: A proposed classification. *Pain Physician*. 200;9:69-82.

Raj P, Lou L, Erdine S, et al. *Interventional Pain Management: Image-Guided Procedures*, 2nd ed. Philadelphia, PA: Saunders Elsevier; 2008.

Urits I, Shen AH, Jones MR, Viswanath O, Kaye AD. Complex regional pain syndrome, current concepts and treatment options. *Curr Pain Headache Rep*. 2018;22(2):10.

CASE 5 | Superior Hypogastric Block in a Patient with Pelvic Pain

Shiraz Yazdani, MD, and Salahadin Abdi, MD, PhD

A 59-year-old woman with a history of locally invasive cervical squamous cell carcinoma presents with a chief complaint of pelvic pain. She describes the pain as a deep ache that has been unrelieved by a variety of oral medications, including opioid analgesics and adjuvant medications. She asks if there are any interventional procedures that could help alleviate her pain.

1. Which of the following is the most appropriate interventional procedure for this patient?

   A. Pudendal nerve block.
   B. Transversus abdominis plane block.
   C. Superior hypogastric plexus block.
   D. Splanchnic nerve block.

The correct answer is C. Patients with locally advanced cervical cancer often complain of pelvic pain that is difficult to treat with medications. Chemoradiation to treat the underlying disease can reduce tumor burden and reduce pain. This pain is primarily visceral in nature and has a sympathetically mediated component. Thus a superior hypogastric plexus block is the most appropriate intervention. This block provides analgesia to the pelvic organs by blocking afferent fibers that travel in the sympathetic chain. Pelvic splanchnic nerves (S2 to S4) provide parasympathetic innervation to the cervix and nearby structures. Postsynaptic sympathetic fibers travel through the inferior and superior hypogastric plexuses prior to reaching the pelvic viscera. A pudendal nerve block would provide blockade of somatic nerve fibers to the vagina and perineum, but would not affect pain in the cervix. Similarly, a transversus abdominis plane block would block somatic fibers to the abdomen, but not the cervix. A splanchnic nerve block would block sympathetically mediated pain in the upper abdominal viscera.

Your patient is interested in the superior hypogastric plexus block. She asks what other conditions this intervention can be used for.

2. Which of the following options is another indication for superior hypogastric plexus block?

    A. Chronic pain from bladder cancer.
    B. Lower extremity CRPS.
    C. Pain from gastric cancer.
    D. Postincisional pain from herniorrhaphy.

The correct answer is A. Superior hypogastric plexus block can be utilized for a variety of malignant and nonmalignant painful pelvic conditions, including pain from cervical, bladder, and uterine malignancies; endometriosis; pelvic inflammatory disease; dyspareunia; cystitis; prostatitis; and dysmenorrhea. Lower extremity CRPS is treated with a lumbar sympathetic block. Pain from gastric cancer would be best treated with a splanchnic nerve or celiac plexus block. Postincisional pain is somatic in nature and therefore would not be treated with sympathetic blockade, but with blockade of the somatic nerves in the affected area instead.

The patient asks about risks of the procedure and if there are any reasons not to have it performed.

3. Which of the following is a relative contraindication for superior hypogastric plexus block?

    A. History of urinary tract infection treated 2 weeks ago.
    B. Extension of the mass around the iliac vessels.

C. Rivaroxaban treatment for deep vein thrombosis held 5 days prior.
D. Concurrent radiation treatment.

The correct answer is B. Superior hypogastric plexus block is a generally safe procedure when using image guidance. The two primary approaches for the block are the medial paraspinous approach and the transdiscal approach. The medial paraspinous approach can be difficult due to the location of the plexus—anterior to the L5-S1 disc—and due to the location of bony structures in this area, such as the L5 transverse process. The transdiscal approach carries with it the risk of discitis, and prophylactic IV antibiotics are usually given for this technique, with some authors also recommending intradiscal antibiotics when the needle is withdrawn. During needle positioning, contact with the iliac vessels is a distinct possibility. Therefore, extension of the mass around these vessels could lead to significant bleeding and subsequent complications, making this a relative contraindication. A urinary tract infection that has been treated is not a contraindication to the procedure. Rivaroxaban is also not a contraindication, as holding it for 5 days will allow more than three half-lives of this anticoagulant to elapse. Concurrent radiation treatment is also not a contraindication, although certain types of chemotherapy can be, depending on their effect on the coagulation system.

Your patient experiences nearly complete pain relief with the diagnostic superior hypogastric plexus block. However, 2 weeks later, her pain returns to baseline. She asks what else can be done to control her pain.

4. What is the next appropriate action?

    A. Perform alcohol neurolysis at the superior hypogastric plexus.
    B. Repeat superior hypogastric plexus block with local anesthetic.
    C. Perform intrathecal morphine trial.
    D. Begin an extended-release oxycodone formulation.

The correct answer is A. Since this patient experienced near total pain relief with the diagnostic superior hypogastric plexus block, she is now a candidate for a repeat block with neurolysis. Neurolytic options include alcohol, phenol, radiofrequency ablation, and pulsed radiofrequency lesioning. Ethyl alcohol has a tendency to spread more widely than phenol due to its relatively low viscosity and is used in concentrations of 50% to 100%. Phenol has greater affinity for vascular tissue than alcohol and is used in concentrations of 7% to 12%. In this case, with the proximity of the iliac vessels, alcohol may be the more appropriate choice. Radiofrequency lesioning is another option. Pulsed radiofrequency lesions are performed in short, high-voltage bursts. The time between bursts allows tissue temperature to remain lower relative to conventional continuous radiofrequency lesioning.

DID YOU LEARN?

- Neuroanatomy of the cervix.
- Indications and contraindications for superior hypogastric plexus block.
- Differences between neurolytic options, including alcohol, phenol, continuous radiofrequency lesioning, and pulsed radiofrequency lesioning.

Recommended Readings

Benzon H, Rathmell J, Wu C, Turk D, Argoff C, Hurley W. *Practical Management of Pain*, 5th ed. Philadelphia, PA: Mosby; 2014.

Fishman S, Ballantyne J, Rathmell J, eds. *Bonica's Management of Pain*, 5th ed. Philadelphia, PA: Wolters Kluwer/Lippincott, Williams and Wilkins; 2018.

Nagpal AS, Moody EL. Interventional management for pelvic pain. *Phys Med Rehabil Clin N Am*. 2017;28(3):621-646.

Sabia M, Mathur R. *Interventional Pain Procedures Handbook and Video Guide*. Demos Medical; 2019.

| CASE 6 | A Construction Worker with Low Back Pain |

Anish I. Doshi, MD, and Salahadin Abdi, MD, PhD

You are caring for a 55-year-old construction worker with a 3-month history of low back pain that radiates down his left leg. He describes his back pain as a constant dull ache exacerbated by prolonged periods of standing and walking. He describes his left leg pain as an intermittent burning and shooting sensation that travels down the posterior aspect of his leg to his left ankle. Ibuprofen helps decrease the intensity of his back pain from 10/10 to 6/10 but has no effect on his left leg pain. He denies recent trauma, fevers, urinary or fecal incontinence, lower extremity weakness, or numbness.

1. Your next action is to:

A. Obtain an emergent magnetic resonance imaging (MRI) of the lumbar spine for further evaluation.

B. Perform a thorough physical examination.

C. Consult neurosurgical services for emergent surgical decompression.

D. Discharge the patient with a prescription of opioids for immediate pain relief.

The correct answer is B. The patient's history suggests a multifactorial etiology, and a thorough physical examination will facilitate an accurate diagnosis, which is critical for providing the patient with an effective treatment plan. The physical examination should include inspection of the back, posture and gait, range of motion, palpation of the axial spine and paraspinal musculature, a straight leg test, a neurological examination, peripheral pulse assessment, and the presence or absence of nonorganic signs. Bowel or bladder dysfunction and bilateral leg weakness suggest compression of the spinal cord or cauda equina, which is a medical emergency and warrants emergent MRI and prompt surgical decompression. Common conditions that cause spinal cord compression include spinal injury, tumor, infection, or an epidural hematoma. Given that our patient lacks bowel or bladder dysfunction, bilateral leg weakness, or loss of sensation, an emergent MRI study or neurosurgical consultation is not warranted. The treatment options for back pain vary significantly, based on the presumed diagnosis. A physical examination should be conducted as the next appropriate step in order to establish the proper diagnosis.

You perform a thorough physical examination on the patient. His lower back appears normal, with benign spinal curvature. He has a positive left-sided straight leg raise test, 3/5 muscle strength with left-sided plantar flexion, decreased sensation over the lateral aspect of his left foot, hyporeflexia of his left ankle, and difficulty with walking on his toes. He has some axial spine tenderness upon palpation and does not have tenderness upon palpation of his lumbosacral paraspinal muscles. However, pain is also elicited by manually extending and rotating his spine bilaterally. His left leg pain is also reproduced with forward flexion of his spine. His distal pulses are 2+ bilaterally.

2. Based on the patient's history and physical examination, you hypothesize that the etiology and nature of the patient's pain are likely:

   A. Facetogenic.
   B. Discogenic.
   C. Psychosomatic.
   D. Myofascial.
   E. Both A and B.

The correct answer is E. The patient presents with low back pain with both discogenic and facetogenic features. Back pain is the second most common symptom leading to clinician visits in the United States, with total associated health care costs exceeding $100 billion per year. Back pain has a major negative impact on quality of life, so physicians must understand the common causes and clinical features of various low back pain etiologies. Unilateral sharp, shooting, or burning lower extremity pain that radiates down the leg, and especially radiating below the knee, with decreased sensation and changes in severity with certain physical positions, is characterized as radiculopathy/radiculitis. It is often due to intervertebral disc herniation with or without disc degeneration, causing mechanical and/ or chemical nerve root irritation. The pain is reproduced on physical examination with forward flexion of the spine and unilateral straight leg raise. Neurological compromise may be evident at the level of the specific spinal nerve root(s) involved. The patient's clinical presentation suggests that the left S1 nerve root is likely affected by an L5/S1 disc herniation.

Facetogenic low back pain is characterized as nonradiating lumbar spinal pain as a result of repetitive stress and/or cumulative low-level trauma associated with the degeneration and/or inflammation of the zygapophysial joints ("facet joints"), which are formed by the superior and inferior articulating processes of each vertebra. Facet joints at each level of the spine provide the necessary support, particularly with back extension and rotation. These joints are innervated by the medial branch nerves of the dorsal rami, which convey a painful stimulus when the joint is injured or irritated. Given that the patient experiences lower back pain with prolonged periods of standing and exhibits reproducible pain with bilateral "facet loading" on examination, the etiology of his back pain is likely facetogenic in nature as well.

Myofascial pain is caused by muscular taut bands or "trigger points" and fascial constrictions, with focal point tenderness on examination. Psychosomatic pain involves symptom exaggeration, which is related to internal psychological processes or environmental contingencies and typically present with nonorganic physical findings and inconsistencies.

3. Based on the history and physical examination, your next step would be:

A. Order an x-ray of lumbar spine.
B. Order a CT study of the lumbar spine.
C. Order an MRI study of the lumbar spine.
D. Order electromyogram of right lower extremity.
E. No further testing indicated.

The correct answer is E. The patient's history and physical examination establish the probable diagnosis, and a targeted treatment plan can now be initiated without further testing. Most patients with low back pain have a favorable prognosis, and imaging studies are typically unnecessary when a thorough history and physical examination are sufficient to establish an accurate diagnosis. Unnecessary imaging studies can expose patients and physicians to high levels of radiation, produce false-positive results, drive unnecessary interventions, and significantly raise health care costs. Advanced imaging should be reserved for those patients for whom systemic disease or severe neurological compromise is strongly suspected. As discussed previously, if the patient presented with "red flag" symptoms, emergent imaging would be warranted to rule out a more deleterious cause of back pain. Plain radiographs of the lumbosacral spine may help the clinician rule out spondyloarthropathy and spondylolisthesis. CT or MRI may be indicated for progressively worsening neurological deficits or for an increased suspicion of cancer, fracture, bleeding, or infection.

The patient claimed that he has recently read about epidural steroid injections and inquires about the potential benefit of such an injection for his pain.

4. Which of the following conditions would benefit the greatest with an epidural steroid injection?

A. Left lower extremity pain due to complex regional pain syndrome (CRPS) type II.
B. Unilateral lower extremity radicular pain caused by disc herniation.
C. Back pain caused by bilateral lumbosacral facet joint arthropathy.
D. Nonradiating axial back pain associated with acute vertebral compression fracture.
E. Pain elicited at bilateral sacroiliac joints.

The correct answer is B. Epidural steroid injections (ESIs) are the most commonly performed pain clinic intervention. ESIs can provide both diagnostic and short-term pain relief for radicular lower extremity pain caused by disc herniation, degenerative disc disease, or other structural pathologies that involve compression of nerve roots or the epidural space. CRPS is a complex pain disorder for which a stellate ganglion block for upper extremity pain and a lumbar sympathetic block for lower extremity pain can be beneficial. Lumbosacral back pain caused by facet joint arthropathy is most effectively treated with physical therapy, core-strengthening exercises, and/or facet joint injections or medial branch nerve blocks. Patients who suffer an acute vertebral compression fracture typically present with tenderness upon palpation at the fracture site. Many of these patients benefit from a vertebroplasty or kyphoplasty, which involves percutaneously injecting cement into the fractured vertebra to alleviate pain and restore bone integrity. Sacroiliac joint pain is typically a result of inflammation that could be reproduced with flexion, abduction, and external rotation of the ipsilateral hip. It could be relieved with a localized intraarticular injection of local anesthetic and steroids or by blocking the nerves that innervate the joint.

DID YOU LEARN?

- The diagnostic approach to low back pain.
- How to differentiate among various etiologies of low back pain.
- The rationale and indications for performing diagnostic testing in the evaluation of low back pain.
- The roles of epidural steroid injections and other procedural interventions in treating various presentations of lower back pain.

Recommended Reading

Vrooman BM, Rosenquist RW. Chronic pain management. In: Butterworth IV JF, Mackey DC, Wasnick JD, eds. *Morgan & Mikhail's Clinical Anesthesiology*, 6th ed. New York, NY: McGraw-Hill; 2018:1047-1110.

References

Abdi S, Lucas LF, Datta S. Role of epidural steroids in the management of chronic spinal pain: A systematic review of effectiveness and complications. *Pain Physician.* 2005;8:127-143.

Barreto TW, Lin KW. Noninvasive treatments for low back pain. *Am Fam Physician.* 2017;96(5):324-327.

Benzon HT, Raja SN, Liu S, Fishman SM, Cohen SP. *Essentials of Pain Medicine,* 4th ed. Philadelphia, PA: Saunders Elsevier; 2018.

Chou R, Qaseem A, Owens DK, et al. Diagnostic imaging for low back pain: Advice for high-value health care from the American College of Physicians. *Ann Intern Med.* 2011;154:181.

Cohen SP, Raja SN. Pathogenesis, diagnosis, and treatment of lumbar zygapophysial (facet) joint pain. *Anesthesiology.* 2007;106:591-614.

Robinson Y, Olerud C. Vertebroplasty and kyphoplasty: A systematic review of cement augmentation techniques for osteoporotic vertebral compression fractures compared to standard medical therapy. *Maturitas.* 2012;72(1):42-49.

Srinivas SV, Deyo RA, Berger ZD. Application of "less is more" to low back pain. *Arch Intern Med.* 2012;172:1016.

Van der Windt DA, Simons E, Riphagen II, et al. Physical examination for lumbar radiculopathy due to disc herniation in patients with low-back pain. *Cochrane Database Syst Rev.* 2010;2:CD007431.

CHAPTER 39
Enhanced Recovery Protocols & Optimization of Perioperative Outcomes

CASE 1	Optimal Preoperative Preparation Before Colorectal Surgery

John F. Butterworth IV, MD

A 45-year-old, 98-kg man with a body mass index (BMI) of 34 kg/m^2 is posted for a laparoscopic sigmoid colon resection for an adenocarcinoma in 2 weeks. His comorbidities include type 2 diabetes, hypertension, and obstructive sleep apnea (for which he uses bilevel positive airway pressure [BiPAP] every night). He reports a functional status of 7 METs, measured using stationary rowing and elliptical machines. His medications include metoprolol, metformin, lisinopril, gabapentin, aspirin 81 mg, and PRN acetaminophen and alprazolam. His labs are significant for a hemoglobin of 13.2 g/dL, creatinine of 1.1 mg/dL, HbA1C of 6.7%, HCO$_3$ of 26, and albumin of 2.1 mg/dL.

1. Which of the following is indicated to optimize his preoperative preparation?

   A. Referral for preoperative intravenous iron supplementation.
   B. Optimization of his antihyperglycemic medications.
   C. Titration of his BiPAP treatment.
   D. Preoperative protein supplementation.
   E. Resting and stress echocardiography.

The correct answer is D. The patient's history provides reassuring levels of total hemoglobin, glycosylated hemoglobin, serum bicarbonate, and physical activity. The albumin of 2.1 is below the normal range, suggesting that this patient would benefit from preoperative protein supplementation.

2. Following appropriate optimization, which of the following instructions should he *not* follow prior to his planned 10:00 a.m. surgery?

A. Hold metformin the evening before and the morning of surgery.
B. Hold lisinopril the evening before and the morning of surgery.
C. Continue gabapentin and acetaminophen doses as scheduled, including doses the morning of surgery.
D. Refrain from all liquid intake apart from medications after midnight.
E. All of the above

The correct answer is D. Each of these instructions encourages normal homeostasis of blood pressure, blood glucose, and fluid balance during the expected stresses of anesthesia and operation. Encouraging oral fluid intake while avoiding the fluid and electrolyte swings resulting from the bowel prep that the patient most likely received encourages euvolemia and normal gastrointestinal function following surgery.

3. After arrival in the preoperative area, which of the following interventions should be avoided?

A. Continued oral water intake until 2 h prior to surgery start.
B. Prewarming of the patient with blankets, forced air warmers, and adjusting the room temperature.
C. Preoperative oral acetaminophen and gabapentin, assuming no other recent doses.
D. Heparin 5000 units subcutaneously (SC), just prior to induction.
E. Treatment of a fingerstick glucose of 182 mg/dL with short-acting SC insulin.

The correct answer is E. Most interventions listed encourage gastrointestinal motility, reduce the risk of deep venous thromboses, promote early return of mental function, and maintain normothermia. Treatment of a glucose level of 182 mg/dL in a preoperative patient has not been shown to reduce preoperative complications; rather, treatment at that level may increase the risk of dangerous and unrecognized hypoglycemic episodes.

4. After an uneventful intravenous (IV) induction with propofol 1.5 mg/kg and lido-caine 2 mg/kg, which of the following IV infusions is *least* indicated?

A. Ringer's lactate solution based on a goal-directed hemodynamic monitor.
B. Lidocaine 2 mg/kg/h.
C. Sufentanil at 0.25 mcg/kg/h.
D. Dexmedetomidine at 0.25 mcg/kg/h.
E. Ketamine at 0.25 mg/kg/h.

The correct answer is C. Goal-directed fluid therapy has been shown to reduce the risks of inadequate and excessive fluid resuscitation. Lidocaine, ketamine, and dexmedetomidine have each been shown to provide analgesia and support other opioid-sparing techniques. Sufentanil and other opioids have been associated with an increased risk of ileus as well as increased risk of postoperative respiratory complications in patients with obstructive sleep apnea.

DID YOU LEARN?

- Appropriate fasting interval for liquids before colorectal surgery.
- Opioid-sparing strategies useful in an enhanced recovery protocol.

Recommended Reading

Baldini G, Miller T. Enhanced recovery protocols & optimization of perioperative out-comes. In: Butterworth IV JF, Mackey DC, Wasnick JD, eds. *Morgan & Mikhail's Clinical Anesthesiology*, 6th ed. New York, NY: McGraw-Hill; 2018:1111-1132.

References

Ban KA, Gibbons MM, Ko CY, et al. Evidence review conducted for the agency for health-care research and quality safety program for improving surgical care and recovery: Focus on anesthesiology for colorectal surgery. *Anesth Analg.* 2019;128(5):879-889.
Gustafsson UO, Scott MJ, Hubner M, et al. Guidelines for perioperative care in elective colorectal surgery: Enhanced Recovery After Surgery (ERAS®) Society Recommenda-tions: 2018. *World J Surg.* 2019;43(3):659-695.
Ljungqvist O, Scott M, Fearon KC. Enhanced recovery after surgery: A review. *JAMA Surg.* 2017;152(3):292-298.

SECTION V

Perioperative & Critical Care Medicine

CHAPTER 40

Management of Patients with Fluid & Electrolyte Disturbances

CASE 1 | Hyponatremia During Transurethral Resection of the Prostate (TURP)

Lori Dangler, MD

A 72-year-old man with no significant medical problems other than benign prostatic hypertrophy presented for transurethral resection of the prostate (TURP), and an uneventful isobaric lidocaine spinal anesthesia was administered, producing a T10 sensory level block. Two hours later during the procedure, the patient complains of pelvic pain. In response, general anesthesia is initiated with propofol, and a laryngeal mask airway is placed. The surgeon reports difficulty with the procedure and states he expects it to continue for an additional 2 h. At this point, approximately 20 L of sterile bladder irrigation fluid has been administered. The patient is afebrile, heart rate is 88 beats/min, blood pressure is 150/89 mm Hg, and SpO$_2$ is 96%. The patient's spontaneous respirations are unlabored, with a rate of 14 breaths/min.

You are concerned about the volume of hypotonic bladder irrigation that has been administered. Point-of-care electrolyte evaluation reveals serum sodium concentration of 118 mEq/L (mmol/L), and you conclude that the patient is severely hyponatremic.

1. What is considered the *best* definition of hyponatremia in an adult?

    A. <140 mEq/L
    B. <135 mEq/L
    C. <130 mEq/L
    D. <115 mEq/L

The correct answer is B. Hyponatremia is usually defined as a serum sodium concentration below 135 mEq/L, significant hyponatremia as below 130 mEq/L, and severe hyponatremia as below 120 mEq/L.

Physical manifestations of moderate to severe hyponatremia in the conscious patient depend upon its severity and its acuity of onset and are primarily neurological: headache, confusion, and nausea/vomiting, which may progress to encephalopathy, seizures, or coma—all of which will be masked by general anesthesia—or death.

The differential diagnosis of hyponatremia requires a detailed history and physical examination in addition to verification of serum sodium concentration of less than 135 mEq/L. The patient's fluid volume status may be utilized to classify hyponatremia as *hypovolemic, euvolemic,* or *hypervolemic.* In this case, the prolonged TURP procedure using a large volume of bladder irrigation is highly suggestive of excessive water absorption and fluid overload.

Your concern here is that systemic absorption of hypoosmolar bladder irrigation fluid is dependent upon both the duration of the resection and the pressure of the irrigation fluid, and excessive absorption can result in hyponatremia, circulatory overload, and water intoxication (*TURP syndrome*). Manifestations of TURP syndrome include hyponatremia, hypoosmolality, fluid overload (congestive heart failure, pulmonary edema, hypotension), hemolysis, and solute toxicity (hyperglycinemia [glycine], hyperammonemia [glycine], hyperglycemia [sorbitol], intravascular volume expansion [mannitol]).

2. What is the *best* next step?

   A. Administer hypertonic saline intravenously (IV).
   B. Request a change to an alternate bladder irrigation fluid.
   C. Place a central venous catheter for fluid volume assessment.
   D. Restrict IV fluids and administer furosemide (Lasix) IV.

The correct answer is D. Operative cystoscopic procedures typically require continuous irrigation with a transparent, nonconductive fluid to allow the surgeon to see and to use electrocautery for tissue resection. Similar considerations apply for operative hysteroscopic procedures. Irrigating fluids may include distilled water and dilute solutions of glycine, mannitol, and/or sorbitol. The patient has absorbed several liters of hypoosmotic irrigating solution, resulting in volume overload and hyponatremia. Administration of furosemide to initiate diuresis is the appropriate response to the volume overload and excess free water.

When moderate-to-severe hyponatremia is diagnosed, the appropriate clinical response will depend upon the patient's actual condition and should take account the time line or chronicity of the disease. When hyponatremia is of rapid onset, an osmotic shift of free water into the brain occurs, leading to varying degrees of cerebral edema. When hyponatremia occurs more gradually, over 48 h or longer, brain cells have more time to adapt to osmotic fluid shifts and clinically significant cerebral edema is less likely.

For your TURP scenario, consider:

- Cessation of the procedure.
- Examination for signs of circulatory overload, and administration of appropriate respiratory and circulatory support, as indicated.
- Administration of furosemide.
- Cautious administration of hypertonic saline if acute physiological deterioration requires faster correction of hyponatremia.

You can use the following guidelines to replace sodium in a patient with hyponatremia: In the absence of signs of severe physiological distress, the optimal approach is to restrict fluid administration and promote gentle diuresis, allowing for gradual correction of the hyponatremia. Administration of normal saline or hypertonic saline with diuresis must be approached with caution, as overly rapid correction of hyponatremia has been associated with demyelination lesions in both pontine and extrapontine central nervous system areas, resulting in both temporary and permanent neurological sequelae (*osmotic demyelination syndrome*).

DID YOU LEARN?

- The definition of hyponatremia.
- General approach to assessing a patient with hyponatremia.
- Differential diagnosis of hyponatremia.
- Guidelines for sodium replacement.

References

Aylwin S, Burst V, Peri A, et al. 'Dos and don'ts' in the management of hyponatremia. *Curr Med Res Opin*. 2015;31:1755-1761.

Butterworth IV JF, Mackey DC, Wasnick JD, eds. Anesthesia for patients with kidney disease. In: *Morgan & Mikhail's Clinical Anesthesiology*, 6th ed. New York, NY: McGraw-Hill; 2018:675-694.

Cuesta M, Thompson CJ. The syndrome of inappropriate antidiuresis (SIAD). *Best Pract Res Clin Endocrinol Metabol*. 2016;30:175-187.

Filippatos TD, Liamis G, Christopoulou F, et al. Ten common pitfalls in the evaluation of patients with hyponatremia. *Eur J Int Med*. 2016;29:22-25.

Giordano M, Ciarambino T, Lo Priore E, et al. Serum sodium correction rate and the outcome in severe hyponatremia. *Am J Emerg Med*. 2017;35(11):1691-1694.

Hawary A, Mukhtar K, Sinclair A, et al. Transurethral resection of the prostate syndrome: Almost gone but not forgotten. *J Endourol*. 2009;12:2013-2020.

Leung AA, McAlester FA, Rogers SO Jr, et al. Preoperative hyponatremia and perioperative complications. *Arch Intern Med*. 2012;172:1474-1481.

Marino PL. *The ICU Book*, 4th ed. Chapter 35. Philadelphia, PA: Lippincott Williams & Wilkins; 2013.

Sterns RH. Treatment of severe hyponatremia. *Clin J Am Soc Nephrol*. 2018;13(4):641-649.

Tan SC, Freebairn R. Electrolyte disorders in the critically ill. *Anaesth Intens Care Med*. 2017;18:133-137.

CASE 2   Hyperkalemia in a Hospitalized Patient Scheduled for Wound Debridement

Benjamin Arnold, MD

You are called to evaluate a hospitalized 70-year-old, 76-kg man who is scheduled for wound debridement after colon resection for diverticulitis. His medical history includes hypertension, chronic kidney disease, and type 2 diabetes mellitus. His serum potassium is 6.2 mEq/L, and his serum creatinine is 3.1 mg/dL.

1. At what serum potassium level do the effects of hyperkalemia become life-threatening?

    A. 5.5 mEq/L.
    B. 6.0 mEq/L.
    C. 6.5 mEq/L.
    D. 7.0 mEq/L.

The correct answer is B. The definition of hyperkalemia is a plasma $[K^+]$ above 5.5 mEq/L. Hyperkalemia exceeding 6 mEq/L has lethal potential, especially if it has risen acutely, and should always be corrected prior to an elective anesthetic. Effects on skeletal and cardiac muscle are the most important effects of hyperkalemia. Skeletal muscle weakness is generally seen when plasma $[K^+]$ is greater than 8 mEq/L. Cardiac manifestations are typically seen when plasma $[K^+]$ is greater than 7 mEq/L, and electrocardiographic changes progress sequentially. Keep in mind that hypocalcemia, acidosis, and hyponatremia accentuate the cardiac effects of hyperkalemia.

Causes of Hyperkalemia

Pseudohyperkalemia
- Red cell hemolysis
- Marked leukocytosis/thrombocytosis

Intercompartmental shifts
- Acidosis
- Hypertonicity
- Rhabdomyolysis
- Excessive exercise
- Periodic paralysis
- Succinylcholine

Decreased renal potassium excretion
- Renal failure
- Decreased mineralocorticoid activity and impaired Na^+ reabsorption
- Acquired immunodeficiency syndrome

(continued)

Causes of Hyperkalemia *(Continued)*

- Potassium-sparing diuretics
  - Spironolactone
  - Eplerenone
  - Amiloride
  - Triamterene
- ACE[1] inhibitors
- Nonsteroidal anti-inflammatory drugs
- Pentamidine
- Trimethoprim

Enhanced Cl⁻ reabsorption
- Gordon syndrome
- Cyclosporine

Increased potassium intake
- Salt substitutes

---

[1]ACE, angiotensin-converting enzyme.
Reproduced with permission from Butterworth JF, Mackey DC, Wasnick JD: *Morgan and Mikhail's Clinical Anesthesiology*, 6th ed. New York, NY: McGraw-Hill Education; 2018.

2. What is the most likely cause of this patient's hyperkalemia?

    A. Intercompartmental shift of potassium ions.
    B. Decreased urinary excretion of potassium.
    C. An increased potassium intake.
    D. Drug treatment of diabetes.

The correct answer is B. Hyperkalemia can result from (1) an intercompartmental shift of potassium ions, (2) decreased urinary excretion of potassium, or (3) an increased potassium intake (see the table above). With the patient's history of chronic kidney disease, the hyperkalemia is likely due to a decreased urinary excretion of potassium.

    Decreased renal excretion of potassium can result from (1) reductions in glomerular filtration rate, (2) decreased aldosterone activity, or (3) a defect in potassium secretion in the distal nephron. Hyperkalemia is reliably seen with glomerular filtration rates less than 5 mL/min, and increased potassium loads can lead to hyperkalemia in patients with less severe kidney impairment. Decreased aldosterone activity can result from a primary defect in adrenal hormone synthesis (Addison disease) or a defect in the renin–aldosterone system. Drugs that interfere with the renin–aldosterone system include nonsteroidal anti-inflammatory drugs (NSAIDs), angiotensin-converting enzyme inhibitors, large doses of heparin, and spironolactone. A defect in distal nephron potassium secretion can be intrinsic (pseudohypoaldosteronism) or acquired (eg, systemic lupus erythematosus, sickle cell anemia, obstructive uropathies, and cyclosporine nephropathy).

    Intercompartmental shift of potassium ions is seen when K^+ moves out of cells as a result of acidosis, hemolysis, cell lysis due to chemotherapy, rhabdomyolysis, massive tissue trauma, hyperosmolality, digitalis overdoses, and administration of succinylcholine, β-adrenergic blockers, and arginine hydrochloride. Increased potassium intake rarely causes hyperkalemia because of the kidney's ability to excrete large potassium loads. Hyperkalemia may be seen when potassium intake is increased in patients with kidney impairment or receiving β-blockers. Potassium penicillin, sodium substitutes, and transfusion of whole blood are often unrecognized sources of significant potassium.

3. The surgeon would like to proceed as soon as possible. What is the most appropriate course of action?

A. Agree to go ahead with the case under monitored anesthesia care (MAC).
B. Consult nephrology service and arrange hemodialysis.
C. Agree to go ahead with the case under general anesthesia.
D. Treat and correct the hyperkalemia prior to starting the procedure.

The correct answer is D. The patient has a potentially lethal hyperkalemia, which should be corrected prior to administration of a nonemergent anesthetic. MAC runs the risk of sedation-related hypoventilation and respiratory acidosis, and there is no current indication for hemodialysis. Treatment is directed at restoration of normal plasma [K^+]. In addition to appropriate pharmacological treatment, it is essential to ensure adequate hydration, address any other electrolyte abnormalities, identify and discontinue any drugs contributing to hyperkalemia, and confirm that any avoidable sources of increased potassium intake have been stopped.

4. As you discuss the need to delay the case with the patient and his family, you note that the QRS complex is widening on the cardiac monitor. What is the most appropriate initial treatment?

A. Sodium bicarbonate 45 mEq IV.
B. 30–50 g glucose with insulin 10 units IV.
C. 10% calcium chloride 3–5 mL IV or 10% calcium gluconate 5–10 mL IV.
D. Sodium polystyrene sulfonate (SPS, Kayexalate) emulsion 50 g per rectum.

The correct answer is C. Calcium chloride or calcium gluconate is the best choice to rapidly antagonize the cardiac effects of hyperkalemia. Sodium bicarbonate is a good choice when metabolic acidosis is present, promoting cellular uptake of potassium and taking effect within 15 min. An IV infusion of glucose and insulin is effective in promoting cellular uptake of potassium, but may take up to 1 h for maximum effect. SPS is a cation-exchange resin that binds potassium; however, its efficacy in lowering serum potassium is increasingly questioned, and any effect that it does have will occur over several hours at a minimum. Thus, SPS administration is inappropriate for urgent or emergent treatment of hyperkalemia. For patients with more than minimal kidney function, IV administration of furosemide may increase urinary excretion of potassium. However, this effect will also be too gradual for urgent or emergent correction of hyperkalemia.

DID YOU LEARN?

- The clinical implications of perioperative hyperkalemia.
- The differential diagnosis of hyperkalemia.
- The most appropriate urgent or emergent treatment options for hyperkalemia.

Reference

Butterworth IV JF, Mackey DC, Wasnick JD, eds. Acid-base management. *Morgan & Mikhail's Clinical Anesthesiology*, 6th ed. New York, NY: McGraw-Hill; 2018:1169-1187.

CASE 3 — An Elderly Woman with Hypomagnesemia

Ravish Kapoor, MD, and Pascal Owusu-Agyemang, MD

A 73-year-old woman is seen for preoperative evaluation 1 week prior to scheduled repair of a large ventral hernia. Her medical history includes gastroesophageal reflux disease and daily consumption of a bottle of wine for over a decade since being widowed. She describes being chronically fatigued. Her only medication is omeprazole, which she has been using for over a year. Her vital signs are normal. ECG reveals prolonged QTc. A complete blood count and chemistry panel including magnesium level are obtained in evaluation of her fatigue complaint. The magnesium level comes back first as 1.3 mEq/L.

1. What associated electrolyte abnormality could be seen on the chemistry panel?

   A. Hyperkalemia.
   B. Hypocalcemia.
   C. Hypercalcemia.
   D. Hypernatremia.

The correct answer is B. Mild hypomagnesemia is often seen in hospitalized patients, particularly those in the ICU setting. Normal magnesium levels are between 1.7 and 2.1 mEq/L (0.7–1 mmol/L, or 1.7–2.4 mg/dL). This patient has a history of alcohol abuse and chronic proton pump inhibitor use, both of which can cause hypomagnesemia (see table on following page). Most patients with hypomagnesemia are asymptomatic, but signs and symptoms are similar to those associated with hypocalcemia and/or hypokalemia and can include arrhythmias, weakness, tetany, paresthesias, confusion, and seizures. Hypocalcemia (due to impaired parathyroid hormone secretion) and hypokalemia (due to renal K$^+$

wasting) are associated findings. Adequate magnesium levels are needed to effectively treat refractory hypocalcemia/hypokalemia.

Causes of Hypomagnesemia

Inadequate intake
- Nutritional

Reduced gastrointestinal absorption
- Malabsorption syndromes
- Small bowel or biliary fistulas
- Prolonged nasogastric tube suctioning
- Severe vomiting or diarrhea
- Chronic laxative abuse
- Proton pump inhibitors
- Acute pancreatitis

Increased renal losses
- Medications
  - Diuretics (loop and thiazide)
  - Antibiotics (aminoglycosides, amphotericin, pentamidine)
  - Cisplatin
- Diabetic ketoacidosis
- Hyperaldosteronism
- Volume expansion
- Acquired tubular dysfunction
  - Postobstructive diuresis
  - Post-renal transplant

Multifactorial
- Hyperthyroidism
- Burns

Reproduced with permission from Butterworth JF, Mackey DC, Wasnick JD: *Morgan and Mikhail's Clinical Anesthesiology*, 6th ed. New York, NY: McGraw-Hill Education; 2018.

The chemistry panel reveals borderline low calcium and potassium levels. Oral magnesium, calcium, and potassium supplements are prescribed in anticipation of her upcoming procedure. The patient has also been asked by the surgical service to take an over-the-counter polyethylene glycol laxative the day prior to her procedure. Anesthesia is induced, and the surgical procedure is started without obtaining repeat blood chemistry studies. Well into the procedure, the patient develops periodic episodes of the rhythm shown in the next figure, but remains hemodynamically stable.

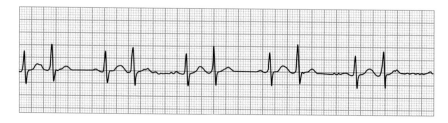

2. What is your next step?

    A. Request a chemistry panel with magnesium level.
    B. Get a 12-lead ECG.
    C. Administer glycopyrrolate.
    D. Administer calcium chloride.

The correct answer is A. Considering that the patient is hemodynamically stable and has a history of hypomagnesemia and recent laxative use, it would be prudent to obtain electrolyte levels to determine the etiology of the patient's nonsustained bigeminy. Atrial and ventricular dysrhythmias can be expected with significant hypomagnesemia, and the need for treatment should be anticipated.

Labs are remarkable for a magnesium level of 1.0 mEq/L and a potassium level of 3.0 mEq/L. You initiate an infusion of magnesium sulfate 2 g IV, but do not put the infusion on a programmable pump. Ten minutes later, gradually decreasing blood pressure is noted, and the patient is now borderline hypotensive.

3. How do you initially react to this fall in blood pressure?

    A. Administer ephedrine 20 mg IV.
    B. Request a hemoglobin level.
    C. Administer phenylephrine 200 mcg IV.
    D. Slow down the magnesium sulfate infusion.

The correct answer is D. Asymptomatic hypomagnesemia can be treated via oral or intramuscular replacement; IV administration is usually reserved for symptomatic patients. Serious manifestations of hypomagnesemia, such as seizures and dysrhythmias, are initially treated with magnesium sulfate 2 g IV for an adult patient (25–50 mg/kg, or 0.2–0.4 mEq/kg IV for children) and repeated until symptoms subside. Hypotension can be seen with rapid administration due to potentiation of vasodilatory and negative ionotropic properties of general anesthetic agents. Unless treating life-threatening symptoms, magnesium should be infused slowly over 30 to 60 min. Other complications of aggressive treatment of hypomagnesemia and resultant hypermagnesemia include loss of deep tendon reflexes, facial flushing, sedation, and potentiation of nondepolarizing neuromuscular blockade. Therefore, as always, muscle relaxation and reversal should be guided by peripheral nerve stimulation assessment. Additionally, anesthetic implications of the underlying etiology causing the hypomagnesemia must be kept in mind.

DID YOU LEARN?

- The causes of hypomagnesemia.
- The signs and symptoms of hypomagnesemia.
- The treatment of hypomagnesemia.
- The anesthetic management considerations of hypomagnesemia.

Recommended Reading

Butterworth IV JF, Mackey DC, Wasnick JD, eds. Management of patients with fluid & electrolyte disturbances. In: *Morgan & Mikhail's Clinical Anesthesiology*, 6th ed. New York, NY: McGraw-Hill; 2018:1133-1168.

References

Agus ZS. Mechanisms and causes of hypomagnesemia. *Curr Opin Nephrol Hypertens.* 2016;25(4):301-307.

Hansen BA, Bruserud Ø. Hypomagnesemia in critically ill patients. *J Intensive Care.* 2018;6:21.

Yu ASL. Evaluation and treatment of hypomagnesemia. In: Post TW, Goldfarb S, Lam AQ, eds. UpToDate. Waltham, MA; 2016.

CHAPTER 41

Fluid Management & Blood Component Therapy

CASE 1 | Acute Hemolytic Transfusion Reaction

Jagtar Singh Heir, DO, and Javier Lasala, MD

A 55-year-old man is scheduled for video-assisted thoracoscopic right upper lobectomy for a newly diagnosed small-cell carcinoma of the lung. His past medical history includes hypertension, hyperlipidemia, and coronary artery disease. During mediastinal exploration, the surgeon accidentally lacerates the right pulmonary artery (RPA) and massive hemorrhage ensues. The surgeon extends the skin incision and abandons the minimally invasive technique. Packed red blood cells (PRBCs) are rapidly transfused. The RPA is clamped and repaired. The patient's vital signs return to normal as adequate supportive measures are taken. Twenty minutes later, the patient has become tachycardic and hypotensive, and the urine is now pink. The surgeon describes the ongoing diffuse bleeding observed in the wound as coagulopathic and "nonsurgical." You believe that the patient is experiencing an acute hemolytic transfusion reaction.

1. What is the most likely cause of an acute transfusion reaction?

   A. Clerical error.
   B. Prior HLA antigen exposure.
   C. Administration of fresh-frozen plasma (FFP) in combination with PRBCs.
   D. Alloantibody from prior exposure.

The correct answer is A. In this case, the patient is exhibiting tachycardia and hypotension following administration of PRBCs. There is no evident surgical bleeding to explain the sudden decrease in blood pressure and the resultant tachycardia. The most common cause of a hemolytic transfusion reaction is clerical error. For example, the sample sent to the blood bank may have been mislabeled or misread, or the patient or blood may have not have been correctly identified by the anesthesia team at the time of transfusion. This type of error is more likely to occur in emergencies, when blood products are quickly called for and rapidly delivered to the patient. Platelets contain HLA antigens; therefore, previous exposure to non-self HLA antigens from white blood cell contamination of red cell products may lead to antibody formation that may make future platelet transfusions ineffective. The use of products such as FFP, more than PRBCs, can lead to an immune reaction such as transfusion-related acute lung injury (TRALI).

2. What is the reported frequency of acute intravascular hemolysis due to ABO blood incompatibility?

A. 1:1000.
B. 1:38,000.
C. 1:75,000.
D. 1:100,000.

The correct answer is B. Acute intravascular hemolysis is usually due to ABO incompatibility, and the reported occurrence rate is between 1:6000 and 1:50,000 transfusions. Most commonly, acute intravascular hemolysis is due to misidentification of a patient, a blood specimen, or a unit of blood being transfused. The reported frequency of a fatal hemolytic reaction is 1:100,000. The likelihood of having a hemolytic reaction from administration of blood that has a negative antibody screen ("type and screen"), but without a crossmatch, is less than 1:10,000. Crossmatching of blood takes 45 min and adds expense to the patient; however, if the need to transfuse is high, the patient has a positive antibody screen, or the risk for alloimmunization exists, it is recommended that that a crossmatch be performed prior to transfusion. This test assures an optimal safety profile.

3. In an anesthetized patient, all of the following are symptoms of acute intravascular hemolysis *except*:

A. Hypothermia.
B. Tachycardia.
C. Hypotension.
D. Hemoglobinuria.

The correct answer is A. Acute intravascular hemolysis under anesthesia can present with a wide spectrum of signs such as unexplained tachycardia, hypotension, overt hemoglobinuria, and diffuse oozing in the surgical field. A rise in temperature may also occur, although this is typically a later sign. Febrile reactions are typically caused by patient antibodies directed against antigens present on transfused lymphocytes or granulocytes, and additional symptoms may consist of chills accompanying a temperature rise greater than 1°C. These manifestations can rapidly progress to shock and acute kidney failure, and 30% to 50% of patients may develop disseminated intravascular coagulation. In patients who are not under general anesthesia, the most common symptoms are fever, chills, nausea, and chest and flank pain.

4. What is the pathophysiology of an acute intravascular hemolytic reaction?

A. An acute IgA-mediated anaphylactic reaction.
B. An immune extravascular reaction.
C. Complement-mediated, caused by preformed antibodies in the donor red blood cells.
D. Complement-mediated, caused by preformed antibodies in recipient's plasma to the donor red blood cells.

The correct answer is D. Acute intravascular reactions are due to complement-mediated hemolysis of the donor red blood cells due to preexisting antibodies in the recipient's plasma. The recipient's antibodies will specifically bind to, and attack, the donor red blood cells. These recipient antibodies most commonly consist of anti-A or anti-B antibodies, but can also include anti-Rh or anti-Kidd, which are known to be capable of fixing complement. The volume of administered incompatible blood often dictates the magnitude and severity of the reaction.

5. Management of an acute hemolytic reaction consists of each of the following *except*:

A. Blood should be drawn to identify hemoglobin in plasma, to repeat compatibility testing, and to obtain coagulation studies and a platelet count.
B. A urinary catheter should be inserted, and the urine checked for hemoglobin.
C. Osmotic diuresis should be initiated with mannitol, and vigorous supportive care should be should be performed.
D. Circulatory support should be initiated with extracorporeal membrane oxygenation (ECMO).

The correct answer is D. The management of hemolytic reactions can be summarized as follows: Once a reaction is suspected, transfusion should be immediately stopped and the institutional blood bank should be notified of the reaction. Unit(s) of blood administered to the patient should be rechecked against the patient's identity and unit(s) provided by the blood bank. Blood samples should be drawn from the affected patient and sent immediately (STAT) for analysis of plasma hemoglobin (direct Coombs test), repeat compatibility testing, coagulation studies, and a platelet count. A urinary catheter should be placed, if not already in place. A urine sample should also be obtained and sent for testing for the presence of hemoglobin. Mannitol should be given to promote osmotic diuresis along with

IV fluids as needed to maintain urine output and intravascular volume. The goal of supportive care is to maintain the patient's intravascular volume, urine output, heart rate, and blood pressure at normal values. Circulatory support initiated by ECMO is reserved for patients with extreme cardiopulmonary dysfunction and is rarely needed in patients with hemolytic transfusion reactions.

6. The surgical team believes a coagulation panel should be analyzed given the diffuse oozing on the surgical field. You recommend a thromboelastogram (TEG), given which of the following limitations of a coagulation panel?

A. Does not show fibrinolytic cascade; only coagulation cascade.
B. Does not monitor platelet function.
C. Done at room temperature.
D. Only helpful in retrospect.
E. All of the above.

The correct answer is E. No test exists that satisfies all desired characteristics for an ideal test of coagulation status, and coagulation panels have several limitations when compared to thromboelastography. They are performed at room temperature and not at the patient's inherent temperature, do not monitor platelet function, and do not provide any information regarding the fibrinolytic cascade. In addition, coagulation profiles usually take between 45 and 60 min to process and report, and thus are often helpful in retrospect only. As with rotational thrombelastometry (ROTEM), TEG is a viscoelastic hemostatic assay that quickly measures clot formation and breakdown from a sample of whole blood, providing the clinician with a global picture of clot development that represents in vivo hemostasis. TEG and ROTEM summarize information concerning coagulation factor levels and activity, fibrinogen level, platelet function, fibrin breakdown, and heparinazation. This enables the clinician to identify and potentially act upon the patient's coagulopathy more promptly and precisely. Hence, for the patient in this clinical scenario and with possible disseminated intravascular coagulation (DIC), a viscoelastic assay would provide the best clinical information.

DID YOU LEARN?

- Management of an acute hemolytic transfusion reaction in a patient under anesthesia.
- Frequency of acute hemolytic transfusion reactions.
- Symptoms of an acute hemolytic transfusion reaction.
- Pathophysiology of an acute hemolytic transfusion reaction.
- Difference between coagulation profile and viscoelastic coagulation studies.

References

Aubron C, Aries P, Le Niger C, Sparrow RL, Ozier Y. How clinicians can minimize transfusion-related adverse events? *Transfus Clin Biol.* 2018;25(4):257-261.

Osterman JL, Arora S. Blood product transfusions and reactions. *Hematol Oncol Clin North Am.* 2017;31(6):1159-1170.

CASE 2 — Patient with Osteosarcoma Scheduled for Hemipelvectomy

Jagtar Singh Heir, DO, and Javier Lasala, MD

A 61-year-old man with recurrent osteosarcoma presents for extended hemipelvectomy (en bloc resection of ilium and sacral ala). The patient has a history of hypertension, type 2 diabetes, and coronary artery disease. Physical examination reveals significant left hip tenderness and a palpable inguinal mass. Laboratory data include hemoglobin of 9 g/dL, platelet count of 123,000/μL, serum creatinine of 1.2 mg/dL, and an elevated serum alkaline phosphatase.

1. Three hours following surgical incision, the estimated blood loss is 1600 mL, and as a result, the patient has been transfused 4 units of PRBCs and 2 units of FFP in the past hour. The anesthesia team now decides to activate the massive transfusion protocol (MTP). All of the following are components of an MTP *except*:

   A. Notifying transfusion service and laboratory medicine about initiation of MTP.
   B. Making arrangements for preparation and delivery of predetermined transfusion products.
   C. Defining testing algorithms for laboratory monitoring during resuscitation, eg, partial thromboplastin time (PTT), prothrombin time (PT), fibrinogen level, arterial blood gas determination, point-of-care devices.
   D. Coordinating additional patient care needs (nursing staff, blood warmers, rapid transfusing devices).
   E. Posthospital discharge planning.

The correct answer is E. Maintenance of adequate circulation and hemostasis in the setting of massive hemorrhage can be quite challenging. MTPs have been shown to improve patient survival and reduce the incidence of trauma-related complications such as major organ failure. Although the elements of an MTP may vary from institution to institution, effective preparation for MTPs includes a predefined communication protocol and optimized care coordination between anesthesiology, surgery, laboratory medicine, and the transfusion service. Additional elements of an MTP include defined roles regarding who may initiate an MTP and when it should be initiated; how laboratory and transfusion services are to be notified regarding commencement and cessation of the MTP; and institution-specific laboratory algorithms for various tests such as PTT, PT, fibrinogen level, serum electrolytes, arterial blood gas determinations, and complete blood count. Lastly, rapid blood product preparation and delivery, as well as coordination of other patient care needs such as blood warmers, additional staff, and rapid transfusing equipment, are all critical organizational components. Although MTPs may vary among institutions in the numbers and timing of blood component therapy, all MTPs include RBC, plasma, and platelet administration.

2. The patient has now received 10 RBC units, 5 plasma units, and 2 units of platelets, and the blood loss continues. Which next step is most likely to improve the situation?

A. Order a STAT hemoglobin and serum calcium level.
B. Increase the ratio of product units to 1:1:1 (RBCs:plasma:platelets).
C. Administer cryoprecipitate.
D. Administer recombinant activated factor VII.
E. All of the above are appropriate steps.

The correct answer is B. Caution should be taken with interpretation of a single hemoglobin level determination in the massively hemorrhaging patient; instead, the hemoglobin concentration should be interpreted in the context of hemodynamic status, ongoing blood losses, end-organ perfusion, and tissue oxygenation. Although the hemoglobin level can provide additional information, it should not be used as the sole transfusion trigger. For example, the hemoglobin level can be falsely concentrated with dehydration; conversely, it can be falsely low if the patient has been overhydrated.

Massive resuscitation best practices continue to evolve due to their complexity and to the fact that prospective, randomized clinical trials are fraught with logistic, clinical, and ethical challenges. Therefore, many aspects of MTPs remain empiric rather than based upon clinical evidence. The administration of RBCs:plasma:platelets in a ratio of 1:1:1 has been supported by military combat trauma studies showing reduced mortality with this practice. In addition, the recent Prospective Observation Multicenter Major Trauma Transfusion (PROMMTT) study showed reduced in-hospital mortality with ratios of 1:1:1 or higher in the first 6 h. However, national advisory committees have been reluctant to adopt the recommendation of higher transfusion ratios for FFP and platelets until the potential for adverse outcomes has been fully explored. For example, patients with intracoronary stents or certain hypercoagulable-state cancers may be at increased risk from receiving higher ratios of procoagulant blood products.

Cryoprecipitate is useful when the fibrinogen level is low; for example, neurology and cardiac surgery studies have found increased hemorrhage risk when the fibrinogen level is below 150 to 200 mg/dL, and military trauma studies have shown that an increased fibrinogen:RBCs administration ratio is associated with improved hospital survival due to decreased hemorrhage.

Although recombinant activated factor VII (rFVIIa) was approved for patients with congenital factor VII deficiency and for patients with hemophilia A or B, it has also been used off-label in many clinical situations. Some physicians empirically advocate its use when conventional measures such as surgical hemostasis and conventional procoagulant component therapy have failed to control critical hemorrhage. However, consideration should be given to the risk-versus-benefit profile in this circumstance, as rFVIIa has also been associated with increased risk of pathological thrombosis.

3. All of the following may typically worsen acute coagulopathy during surgery *except*:

   A. Uremia.
   B. Transfusion of blood products.
   C. Infusion of crystalloids.
   D. Hyperthermia.
   E. Acidosis.

The correct answer is D. Severe hemorrhage often leads to severe anemia, which impacts primary hemostasis through platelet loss, consumption, and reduced platelet adhesion and aggregation; however, metabolic derangements including uremia can also lead to platelet dysfunction, thus exacerbating coagulopathy. Administration of excessive crystalloid or colloid solution can promote coagulopathy through dilution of platelets and clotting factors.

Similarly, administration of RBCs without additional clotting factors and/or platelets during massive transfusion can impair coagulation by hemodilution and metabolic derangement. Acidosis and hypocalcemia may occur secondary to the citrate in the RBC storage solution. Hyperkalemia may arise from administration of RBCs stored for a prolonged period of time, and hypothermia may occur if RBCs are administered without adequate warming. The potentially lethal triad of refractory coagulopathy, hypothermia, and metabolic acidosis can promote a vicious cycle of progressively worsening coagulopathy.

4. Tranexamic acid (TXA) works to improve blood loss and treat hemorrhage by which mechanism?

   A. By activating factors II, VII, IX, and X.
   B. By raising the levels of protein C and protein S.
   C. By competitively inhibiting the activation of plasminogen.
   D. By decreasing endothelial cell permeability.
   E. By improving platelet aggregation.

The correct answer is C. Antifibrinolytic agents such as tranexamic acid work by competitively inhibiting the activation of plasminogen, thus reducing the conversion of plasminogen to plasmin. Plasmin is an enzyme responsible for degrading fibrin clots, fibrinogen, and other plasma proteins, including the procoagulant factors V and VIII. In addition, tranexamic acid also directly inhibits plasmin activity, but only at higher doses than are required to reduce plasmin formation. Tranexamic does not impact platelet aggregation or endothelial permeability. Studies have shown benefit with tranexamic usage, through reduction of mortality, reducing blood loss, and/or reduction of risk of progression to severe postpartum hemorrhage.

DID YOU LEARN?

- Essential components of MTP.
- The complex nature of massive hemorrhage resuscitation, and considerations anesthesia providers must initially evaluate and continuously monitor when utilizing an MTP.
- Factors contributing to acute perioperative coagulopathy.
- Mechanism of action of tranexamic acid and its role in control of hemorrhage.

Recommended Reading

Butterworth IV JF, Mackey DC, Wasnick JD, eds. Fluid management & blood component therapy. In: *Morgan & Mikhail's Clinical Anesthesiology*, 6th ed. New York, NY: McGraw-Hill; 2018:1189-1212.

References

Flint AWJ, McQuilten ZK, Wood EM. Massive transfusions for critical bleeding: Is everything old new again? *Transfus Med.* 2018;28(2):140-149.

Foster JC, Sappenfield JW, Smith RS, Kiley SP. Initiation and termination of massive transfusion protocols: Current strategies and future prospects. *Anesth Analg.* 2017;125(6):2045-2205.

Holcomb JB, del Junco DJ, Fox EE, et al. The prospective, observational, multicenter, major trauma transfusion (PROMMTT) study: Comparative effectiveness of a time-varying treatment with competing risks. *JAMA Surg.* 2013;148:127-136.

Maw G, Furyk C. Pediatric massive transfusion: A systematic review. *Pediatr Emerg Care.* 2018;34(8):594-598.

McQuilten ZK, Crighton G, Brunskill S, et al. Optimal dose, timing, and ratio of blood products in massive transfusion: Results from a systematic review. *Transfus Med Rev.* 2018;32(1):6-15.

CHAPTER 42

Nutrition in Perioperative & Critical Care

CASE 1 | Fluid and Nutrition for a Young Burn Victim

Christin Kim, MD

A 26-year-old, 60-kg woman is brought to the emergency room after sustaining 65% total body surface area (TBSA) burns. She is obtunded and disoriented. Her past medical history is unknown. Initial vital signs include a body temperature of 35.6°C, heart rate of 113 beats/min, blood pressure of 110/65 mm Hg, and respiratory rate of 19 breaths/min. Her arterial oxygen saturation was 100% while she received 2 L/min oxygen through a nasal cannula. On physical examination, she is noted to have soot around her nares.

1. According to the Parkland formula, over the next 24 h, the patient should receive approximately:

   A. 15 L of 0.9% normal saline.
   B. 15 L of lactated Ringer's solution.
   C. 7.5 L of 0.9% normal saline.
   D. 7.5 L of lactated Ringer's solution.
   E. 3.8 L of 5% albumin.

The correct answer is B. The Parkland formula is used as a guide to fluid resuscitation within the first 24 h after a patient has sustained a severe burn injury. The amount of fluid to be administered is calculated by 4 mL/kg multiplied by the percentage of TBSA burns. Crystalloids, particularly lactated Ringer's solution, are preferred over colloids in the Parkland calculation.

2. During resuscitation, the patient becomes increasingly agitated and obtunded. Despite 2 L/min of oxygen via nasal cannula, an arterial blood gas reveals a pH of 7.19, PCO_2 of 51 mm Hg, PO_2 of 94 mm Hg, and bicarbonate of 11 mEq/L. The patient's oxygen saturation on pulse oximetry is 100%. The best next step in the management of this patient would be:

A. Noninvasive positive-pressure ventilation (NIPPV).
B. 100% nonrebreather.
C. Intubation and mechanical ventilation.
D. Hyperbaric oxygen therapy.
E. No intervention.

The correct answer is C. Obtundation and agitation are relative contraindications for NIPPV and may also herald respiratory failure. Therefore, the patient should be intubated and mechanically ventilated, especially in the setting of possible inhalational injury as suggest by the soot around her nares noted in her physical examination. Hyperbaric oxygen therapy could be indicated if the patient were found to have an elevated carboxyhemoglobin level. Significant amounts of carboxyhemoglobin could account for a falsely elevated oxygen saturation measured by pulse oximetry.

3. The arterial blood gas represents which acid–base disorder?

A. Respiratory acidosis with metabolic compensation.
B. Metabolic acidosis with respiratory compensation.
C. Mixed respiratory and metabolic acidosis.
D. Respiratory acidosis with metabolic alkalosis.
E. Metabolic acidosis with respiratory alkalosis.

The correct answer is C. The increased $PaCO_2$ and decreased bicarbonate level suggest that the patient has a mixed respiratory and metabolic acidosis.

4. On co-oximetry, the patient is found to have a carboxyhemoglobin concentration of 35%. Which of the following is an absolute contraindication to hyperbaric oxygen therapy?

A. Untreated pneumothorax.
B. Pacemaker.
C. Pregnancy.
D. Asthma.
E. Congenital spherocytosis.

The correct answer is A. An untreated pneumothorax is an absolute contraindication for hyperbaric oxygen therapy, as it poses the risk for development of a tension pneumothorax, pneumomediastinum, and gas emboli. Another absolute contraindication for hyperbaric oxygen therapy is bleomycin therapy, as it may lead to interstitial pneumonitis. The other answer choices are considered relative contraindications to hyperbaric oxygen therapy.

5. On hospital day 2, the patient is taken to the operating room for burn debridement. The patient remains intubated and mechanically ventilated. She is receiving enteral nutrition via a postpyloric feeding tube. Which of the following statements about management of the patient's tube feeds is true?

   A. Tube feeds should be held 6 h prior to surgery, as the patient is at high risk for aspiration.
   B. The feeds should be held 6 h prior to surgery, as burn injuries decrease basal metabolic rate and daily caloric requirements.
   C. Tube feeds should be continued only if gastric residual volumes are less than 200 mL/d.
   D. Tube feeds may safely be continued prior to and during surgery.

The correct answer is D. Following a significant burn injury, the patient enters a highly catabolic state, where metabolic demands increase significantly. High caloric intake is recommended (30–40 kcal/kg/d). An immediate concern with regard to abrupt discontinuation of enteral feeds is hypoglycemia. Long-term malnutrition may lead to increased risk of morbidity and mortality from infection and impaired wound healing.

6. On postoperative day 1, the patient develops a fever of 39°C, as well as a white blood cell count of 27,000. A chest radiograph is obtained that demonstrates a new right middle lobe infiltrate. Presuming a diagnosis of pneumonia, the most likely pathogen is:

   A. *Pseudomonas aeruginosa.*
   B. *Citrobacter freundii.*
   C. *Acinetobacter baumannii.*
   D. *Candida albicans.*
   E. *Staphylococcus aureus.*

The correct answer is E. The patient has a ventilator-associated pneumonia (VAP), which is suggested by a new infiltrate on chest x-ray, fever, and elevated white blood cell count. VAP that presents within 5 days of hospital admission is more often caused by non-multidrug-resistant (MDR) pathogens such as methicillin-sensitive *Staphylococcus aureus*, *Haemophilus influenzae*, and nonextended β-lactamase-producing *Escherichia coli*. *Candida* pneumonia is associated with severely immunocompromised hosts. The remaining answer choices represent multidrug-resistant pathogens.

7. Over the next 24 h, the patient develops worsening respiratory failure, with a chest radiograph demonstrating bilateral fluffy infiltrates. Despite receiving 100% oxygen, her arterial blood gas reveals a PaO_2 of 61 mm Hg. The most appropriate ventilation strategy would be:

A. Tidal volumes of 6 mL/kg based on absolute body weight.
B. Tidal volumes of 6 mL/kg based on predicted body weight.
C. Tidal volumes of 10 mL/kg based on absolute body weight.
D. Tidal volumes of 10 mL/kg based on predicted body weight.

The correct answer is B. The patient likely has acute respiratory distress syndrome (ARDS), as demonstrated by a PaO_2 to FiO_2 ratio of less than 200, relatively acute onset of respiratory failure, and characteristic radiological findings. According to current recommendations, the patient should be ventilated with a lung-protective strategy (6 mL/kg tidal volume based on ideal body weight). Predicted body weight (in kg) is calculated as 50 + 2.3 (height in inches – 60) in males, and 45.5 + 2.3 (height in inches – 60) in females.

DID YOU LEARN?

- Fluid resuscitation for patients with severe burn injuries.
- Contraindications for NIPPV.
- Acid–base analysis.
- Contraindications for hyperbaric oxygen therapy.
- Management of enteral nutrition in a critically ill patient.
- Common pathogens associated with early VAP.
- Lung-protective ventilation strategy.

Recommended Reading

Butterworth IV JF, Mackey DC, Wasnick JD, eds. Nutrition in perioperative & critical care. In: *Morgan & Mikhail's Clinical Anesthesiology*, 6th ed. New York, NY: McGraw-Hill; 2018:1223-1228.

References

Butterworth IV JF, Mackey DC, Wasnick JD, eds. Inhalation therapy & mechanical ventilation in the PACU & ICU. In: *Morgan & Mikhail's Clinical Anesthesiology*, 6th ed. New York, NY: McGraw-Hill; 2018:1329-1352.

Cartotto R, Greenhalgh DG, Cancio C. Burn state of the science: Fluid resuscitation. *J Burn Care Res.* 2017;38(3):e596-e604.

Foster KN, Holmes JH 4th. Inhalation injury: State of the science 2016. *J Burn Care Res.* 2017;38(3):137-141.

Harrington DT. Complicated burn resuscitation. *Crit Care Clin.* 2016;32(4):577-586.

McGlinch BP. Anesthesia for trauma & emergency surgery. In: Butterworth IV JF, Mackey DC, Wasnick JD, eds. *Morgan & Mikhail's Clinical Anesthesiology*, 6th ed. New York, NY: McGraw-Hill; 2018:819-842.

CHAPTER 43

Postanesthesia Care

CASE 1 | Hypotension Following Laparoscopic Splenectomy

Shreyas Bhavsar, MD

You are called to the postanesthesia care unit (PACU) to evaluate a 69-year-old, 58-kg man who has undergone laparoscopic splenectomy. His blood pressure is 83/51 mm Hg, heart rate is 111 beats/min, and SpO_2 is 94% on 2 L of nasal cannula oxygen.

1. What would be the next most appropriate course of action?

    A. Send a complete blood count.

    B. Transfuse O-positive blood.

    C. Review the anesthetic record.

    D. Conduct a rapid and focused history and physical exam.

The correct answer is D. When addressing hypotension in the PACU, the principal objective is to rapidly diagnose and treat any potential morbidity. In this situation, an organized, systems-based physical examination should focus on end-organ perfusion in the setting of low blood pressure. A brief review of the patient's medical and surgical history should be made, and key facts such as baseline blood pressure, rapidity of drop of blood pressure in the recovery area, recent drug administration, and allergies are all prudent pieces of information to obtain. The patient should be assessed for level of consciousness and queried for symptoms. Bilateral breath sounds without crackles (which could indicate possible congestive heart failure) should be verified. The cardiovascular examination should include inspection of the skin for cyanosis, palpation of the peripheral pulses, determination of the capillary refill time, and auscultation of the heart sounds. The most important indication of kidney function in this setting is urine output. Bedside ultrasonography can quickly establish whether the patient is hypovolemic and whether left ventricular function is normal. The heart rhythm should be reviewed, and the 12-lead ECG, if available, should be examined. Reviewing the anesthetic record and measuring hemoglobin and/or hematocrit are also important steps in the management of postsurgical hypotension, but only after initial assessment of the patient. Transfusion of O-positive blood should be considered when severe and progressive hypotension due to uncontrolled bleeding is present and no type-specific blood is available.

2. What is the most common cause of hypotension in the recovery area?

A. Lingering effects of sedative drugs.
B. Excessive arterial vasodilation.
C. Hypovolemia.
D. Sepsis.

The correct answer is C. In addition to the possibilities listed above, other causes of postoperative hypotension include manifestations of coronary artery disease, allergic reactions, cardiac tamponade, and tension pneumothorax. Although the etiology may be multifactorial, the differential diagnosis can be narrowed when considering causes most applicable to the clinical scenario. For example, sepsis would be less likely in a penetrating trauma patient with low blood pressure. In this situation, the most likely cause of the low blood pressure is inadequate intravascular volume. Another mechanism responsible for hypotension is the impaired cardiac output secondary to cardiac tamponade or tension pneumothorax.

Hypovolemia can be considered in absolute or relative terms. *Absolute* hypovolemia is the under-resuscitation of surgical hemorrhage or wound drainage. *Third spacing*, or fluid sequestration by tissues, is a controversial concept although it may contribute to hypovolemia. *Relative* hypovolemia is related to tone of the vasculature. The patient might be euvolemic under normal conditions, but relaxation of perivascular smooth muscle causes vasodilation and, in turn, hypotension. This can be seen with epidural or spinal anesthesia, venodilators, or α-adrenergic blockers.

Your evaluation reveals that the patient is slow to respond to verbal stimuli but appropriately tells you his name. His baseline preoperative blood pressure was 105/69 mm Hg, and his current blood pressure is 82/47 mm Hg. His heart rate is 113 beats/min. His skin feels warm, but mucous membranes are dry. Urine output in the past hour has been 20 mL.

3. What is the estimated fluid deficit in this patient?

A. <5%.
B. 10%.
C. 20%.
D. >20%.

The correct answer is B. Determining volume status in the recovery area is crucial in the evaluation of postoperative hypotension. This patient exhibits physical signs of mild-to-moderate hypovolemia. The table below provides guidance on estimated fluid loss.

The severity of the signs and symptoms guides further diagnostic and therapeutic intervention. For example, a mild decrease in blood pressure may warrant observation or a trial of intravenous (IV) fluids, whereas severe hypotension requires immediate fluids, vasopressors, and/or transfusion of blood products. Any intervention must be followed up with a reassessment of the clinical scenario to determine any benefit and suggest potential next steps. Bedside ultrasonography is an ideal way to make the diagnosis of hypovolemia and assess the response to treatment.

Signs of Fluid Loss (Hypovolemia)

Sign	Fluid Loss (Expressed as Percentage of Body Weight)		
	5%	10%	15%
Mucous membranes	Dry	Very dry	Parched
Sensorium	Normal	Lethargic	Obtunded
Orthostatic changes	None	Present	Marked
In heart rate			>15 bpm ↑[1]
In blood pressure			>10 mm ↓
Urinary flow rate	Mildly decreased	Decreased	Markedly decreased
Pulse rate	Normal or increased	Increased >100 bpm	Markedly increased >120 bpm
Blood pressure	Normal	Mildly decreased with respiratory variation	Decreased

[1]bpm, beats per minute.
Reproduced with permission from Butterworth JF, Mackey DC, Wasnick JD: *Morgan and Mikhail's Clinical Anesthesiology*, 6th ed. New York, NY: McGraw-Hill Education; 2018.

The patient initially responded to your treatment. Seventy-two hours later, you are again called to the bedside for hypotension, now accompanied by a productive cough. After a 500-mL IV fluid bolus, the blood pressure remains 84/50 mm Hg. The heart rate is 114 beats/min. The temperature is now 38.8°C.

4. Which of the following would be the most likely diagnosis in this patient?

   A. Postsplenectomy sepsis.
   B. Venous air embolism.
   C. Allergic reaction.
   D. Pneumothorax.

The correct answer is A. Evaluation and treatment of the postoperative patient encompasses not only the management of hemodynamic parameters, but also requires knowledge of the indications for surgery and the procedure—especially potential surgical complications. It is helpful to know the indications for the splenectomy, as they may contribute to postoperative morbidity. For example, splenectomy for hematologic disorders may contribute to postoperative hemorrhage due to thrombocytopenia. Splenectomy increases the risk for bacterial sepsis, and hypersplenism increases the difficulty of vascular ligation, which may contribute to postoperative hemorrhage. Complications that can occur from laparoscopic surgery itself include respiratory acidosis from carbon dioxide pneumoperitoneum, port-site abdominal wall hematoma, injury to major blood vessels or bowel, pneumothorax, or referred shoulder pain from insufflated gas. Venous air embolism usually presents as a sudden decline in blood pressure and a decrease in end-tidal carbon dioxide measurement. A mild allergic reaction can present as urticaria and pruritus, whereas anaphylaxis may result in respiratory and circulatory collapse. Pneumothorax in the PACU typically presents with sharp, pleuritic chest pain, shortness of breath, and tachycardia, and if sufficiently severe, with signs of hypoxemia and decreased or absent breath sounds in the involved hemithorax.

DID YOU LEARN?

- An initial diagnostic and therapeutic approach to hypotensive patients in the recovery room.
- How hypovolemia can be classified.
- How to estimate volume depletion based on physical exam.
- The importance of bedside ultrasonography in immediate, objective assessment of volume status.
- An appreciation of how indications for surgery can contribute to postoperative evaluation of the patient.

References

Bhandarkar DS, Katara AN, Mittal G, Shah R, Udwadia TE. Prevention and management of complications of laparoscopic splenectomy. *Indian J Surg.* 2011;73(5):324-330.

Butterworth IV JF, Mackey DC, Wasnick JD, eds. Fluid management & blood component therapy. *Morgan & Mikhail's Clinical Anesthesiology*, 6th ed. New York, NY: McGraw-Hill; 2018: 1189-1212.

Misiakos EP, Bagias G, Liakakos T, Machairas A. Laparoscopic splenectomy: Current concepts. *World J Gastrointest Endosc.* 2017;9(9):428-437.

CASE 2 Hypertension Following Cystoscopy

Benjamin Arnold, MD

You are called to the PACU to evaluate hypertension in a 77-year-old, 83-kg man who has undergone cystoscopy under general anesthesia. The patient is awake, alert, and resting comfortably. His blood pressure is 188/95 mm Hg, heart rate is 78 beats/min, and SpO_2 is 99% on 2 L/min nasal cannula oxygen.

1. How fast does postoperative hypertension typically manifest after admission to the PACU?

    A. Within 30 min.
    B. Within 60 min.
    C. Within 5 min.
    D. Within 45 min.

The correct answer is A. Postoperative hypertension is commonly seen in the PACU and typically first occurs within 30 min of arrival. The differential diagnosis of hypertension in this setting includes pain, bladder distention, hypoxemia, hypercapnia, endotracheal intubation, and excessive intravascular fluid volume. Patients with a history of hypertension often develop it in the PACU without an identifiable cause. Preexisting hypertension is present in more than one-half of the patients who develop it in the PACU and is made worse if antihypertensive medications have been withdrawn preoperatively. Marked hypertension can lead to left-ventricular failure, myocardial infarction, postoperative bleeding, or intracranial hemorrhage.

2. What is the most likely cause of hypertension in this patient?

    A. Noxious stimulation from incisional pain.
    B. Noxious stimulation from bladder distention.
    C. Noxious stimulation from endotracheal intubation.
    D. Noxious stimulation from IV placement

The correct answer is B. Because of the short duration (15–20 min) and outpatient setting of most cystoscopies, general anesthesia is usually chosen, using a laryngeal mask airway. Irrigation fluid is instilled into the bladder during the procedure to allow a thorough examination of the bladder wall, and bladder distention is a relatively common postoperative finding. Bladder perforation is a far less common (<1%), but more serious, complication and must be considered.

3. What is the end point for treatment?

   A. Systolic blood pressure <170 mm Hg.
   B. Diastolic blood pressure <110 mm Hg.
   C. Mean blood pressure consistent with the patient's own normal blood pressure.
   D. Blood pressure of 120/80 mm Hg.

The correct answer is C. Decisions to treat hypertension should be individualized, and mild hypertension does not always require treatment. In this case, the available medical records should be reviewed to find the patient's normal range. Patients often follow their own blood pressure readings at home and can report their usual range. History from the patient and the medical record will indicate what antihypertensive medications the patient may be on and if they were withheld preoperatively. Elevations in blood pressure are generally treated if they are greater than 20% to 30% of the patient's baseline, or if any adverse symptoms or signs are present that may be related to hypertension.

4. You discover that the patient suffered a myocardial infarction 3 years ago. Because of this history, which of the following is the least attractive antihypertensive agent?

   A. Labetalol.
   B. Hydralazine.
   C. Enalapril.
   D. Nicardipine.

The correct answer is B. Even though most myocardial infarctions are caused by plaque rupture and thrombosis and are not related to increased myocardial oxygen consumption per se, hydralazine may cause a reflex tachycardia that could lead to myocardial ischemia and infarction. This is more likely to occur in patients not receiving β-blockers. Labetalol, a combined α- and β-blocker, is a good option and is commonly used in the PACU. It can be given in incremental bolus injections, and its effects are apparent a few minutes after administration. When used for the treatment of postoperative hypertension, its beta effects predominate. Other β-blockers (esmolol and metoprolol), angiotensin-converting enzyme inhibitors (enalapril), and calcium channel blockers (nicardipine) are all excellent options for treating mild-to-moderate hypertension, and selecting the appropriate medication should be individualized. Severe hypertension is often treated with an intravenous infusion of nitroprusside, nitroglycerin, nicardipine, clevidipine, or fenoldopam, and in patients with limited cardiac reserve, these medications should be given with the guidance of direct intraarterial pressure monitoring.

DID YOU LEARN?

- The clinical implications of postoperative hypertension.
- The most common causes of postoperative hypertension.
- Proper evaluation of hypertension in the PACU setting.
- Appropriate hypertension treatment options in the PACU.

Recommended Reading

Butterworth IV JF, Mackey DC, Wasnick JD, eds. Postanesthesia care. In: *Morgan & Mikhail's Clinical Anesthesiology*, 6th ed. New York, NY: McGraw-Hill; 2018:1285-1304.

References

Butterworth IV JF, Mackey DC, Wasnick JD, eds. Anesthesia for genitourinary surgery. In: *Morgan & Mikhail's Clinical Anesthesiology*, 6th ed. New York, NY: McGraw-Hill; 2018:695-714.

Butterworth IV JF, Mackey DC, Wasnick JD, eds. Hypotensive agents. In: *Morgan & Mikhail's Clinical Anesthesiology*, 6th ed. New York, NY: McGraw-Hill; 2018:253-260.

Hartle A, McCormack T, Carlisle J, et al. The measurement of adult blood pressure and management of hypertension before elective surgery: Joint Guidelines from the Association of Anaesthetists of Great Britain and Ireland and the British Hypertension Society. *Anaesthesia*. 2016;71(3):326-337.

Plante A, Ro E, Rowbottom JR. Hemodynamic and related challenges: Monitoring and regulation in the postoperative period. *Anesthesiol Clin*. 2012;30(3):527-554.

CHAPTER 44

Common Clinical Concerns in Critical Care Medicine

CASE 1 — Patient with Heart Block

John D. Wasnick, MD, MPH

A 76-year-old male patient with ischemic bowel and impaired left-ventricular systolic and diastolic function (ejection fraction 18%) is awaiting urgent surgery. Preoperative vital signs include: temperature 39°C, heart rate 120 beats/min, blood pressure 85/ 55 mm Hg, and respiratory rate 30 beats/min. The patient has respiratory distress and is sitting upright on the stretcher. His abdomen is rigid.

Rapid-sequence induction of anesthesia is completed with propofol, succinyl-choline, and fentanyl. The patient's blood pressure decreases to 50/30 mm Hg, and the rhythm strip below is noted.

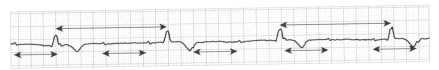

1. The rhythm disturbance noted is:

   A. First-degree atrioventricular (AV) block.

   B. Second-degree AV block (Mobitz 1).

   C. Second-degree AV block (Mobitz 2).

   D. Third-degree AV block.

   E. Ventricular tachycardia.

The correct answer is D. This patient was tachycardic and mildly hypotensive preoperatively. Impairment of the conduction system may occur secondary to ischemia, electrolyte disorders, or injury to the conduction system from surgical or catheter manipulation. First-degree heart block occurs when there is a prolongation in the AV interval beyond 200 ms, as shown below.

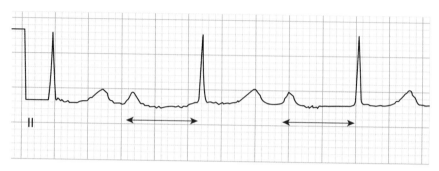

Second-degree heart block is present when not all of the atrial beats are conducted through the AV node to the ventricle, as shown below.

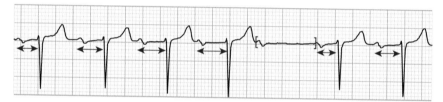

Mobitz 1 heart block is associated with gradual prolongation of the AV interval until a ventricular beat fails to occur. Mobitz 2 block has a propensity to deteriorate to third-degree block. See the following rhythm strip.

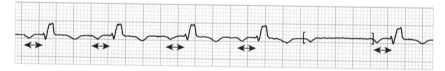

In this patient, third-degree heart block has developed. Treatment for third-degree heart block includes correction of any precipitating factors, temporary pacing, and the administration of atropine and inotrope infusion (eg, epinephrine).

2. As part of your management you obtained a blood gas at the time of induction of anesthesia. Based upon the patient's preoperative presentation, a likely finding would be:

A. Metabolic acidosis.
B. Respiratory acidosis.
C. Metabolic acidosis with respiratory compensation.
D. Respiratory acidosis with metabolic compensation.
E. pH of 7.4.

The correct answer is C. Preoperatively this patient was tachypneic with ischemic bowel. Ischemia results in an increase in lactic acid, leading to metabolic acidosis. While awake, the patient attempts to compensate for the acidemia through hyperventilation, producing a partial compensatory respiratory alkalosis. Acidosis is associated with hyperkalemia, which may have increased with the administration of succinylcholine at the time of induction. Electrolyte abnormalities such as hyperkalemia could contribute to the development of cardiac conduction defects. Myocardial ischemia should also be suspected in this elderly, previously tachycardic, and mildly hypotensive patient. Treatment includes restoration of normal sinus or paced rhythm, correction of hypovolemia, and correction of any electrolyte or acid–base abnormalities. Often patients with ischemic bowel have significant lactic acid accumulation and require extensive volume resuscitation.

3. Using pulse contour analysis of the arterial waveform, the stroke volume is determined to be 45 mL/beat. The cardiac output prior to induction was:

A. 3 L/min.
B. 5.4 L/min.
C. 5.0 L/min.
D. 4.5 L/min.
E. 2.5 L/min.

The correct answer is B. Cardiac output is the product of stroke volume (SV) and heart rate. The SV is influenced by three primary determinants. First among these is the patient's volume status. The patient with ischemic bowel is generally hypovolemic, resulting in decreased SV. The SV represents the difference between left-ventricular end-diastolic volume and left-ventricular end-systolic volume (normal SV 60–100 mL/beat). In addition to conditions that render the patient hypovolemic (eg, blood loss, dehydration), conditions that impede the venous return of blood to the heart (eg, pericardial tamponade, positive-pressure ventilation, and tension pneumothorax) can also reduce SV.

SV may also affected by systemic vascular resistance. As the resistance against which the heart pumps increases beyond the normal range, SV will decrease. Conversely, in vasodilated states (eg, systemic inflammatory syndrome), the SV may increase while blood pressure (blood pressure = cardiac output × systemic vascular resistance) decreases secondary to reduction in vascular tone.

Lastly, myocardial contractility affects the SV. Myocardial ischemia, myocardial infarction, heart failure, and valvular heart disease can all affect the ability to contract and to relax, potentially reducing the SV.

DID YOU LEARN?

- The different types of AV conduction defects.
- Acid–base status of patients with ischemic bowel.
- Determinants of SV.

Recommended Reading

Butterworth IV JF, Mackey DC, Wasnick JD, eds. Common clinical concerns in critical care medicine. In: *Morgan & Mikhail's Clinical Anesthesiology*, 6th ed. New York, NY: McGraw-Hill; 2018:1305-1328.

References

Butterworth IV JF, Mackey DC, Wasnick JD, eds. Anesthesia for patients with cardiovascular disease. *Morgan & Mikhail's Clinical Anesthesiology*, 6th ed. New York, NY: McGraw-Hill; 2018:381-440.

Butterworth IV JF, Mackey DC, Wasnick JD, eds. Cardiopulmonary resuscitation. *Morgan & Mikhail's Clinical Anesthesiology*, 6th ed. New York, NY: McGraw-Hill; 2018:1259-1284.

Butterworth IV JF, Mackey DC, Wasnick JD, eds. Cardiovascular monitoring. *Morgan & Mikhail's Clinical Anesthesiology*, 6th ed. New York, NY: McGraw-Hill; 2018:81-118.

CHAPTER 45

Inhalation Therapy & Mechanical Ventilation in the PACU & ICU

CASE 1	Ischemic Cardiomyopathy Complicated by Respiratory Distress

Christin Kim, MD

A 64-year-old man is brought to the intensive care unit (ICU) in respiratory distress. His past medical history includes ischemic cardiomyopathy, with an ejection fraction (EF) of 28%. Initial vital signs include: temperature 37.0°C; blood pressure 101/54 mm Hg; heart rate 134 beats/min (with an irregularly irregular rhythm); respiratory rate 31 breaths/min; and oxygen saturation 88% (the patient was receiving 6 L/min oxygen via a nasal cannula). On auscultation, bilateral crackles are heard. The chest radiograph demonstrates pulmonary edema.

1. According to the Starling equation, which of the following values is likely elevated in this patient?

    A. K.
    B. Pc′.
    C. σ.
    D. πc′.

The correct answer is B. The Starling equation ($Q = K \times [(Pc' - Pi) - \sigma(\pi c' - \pi i)]$) describes flow of water across the pulmonary capillary. Q equals net flow across the capillary; Pc′ and Pi represent capillary and interstitial hydrostatic pressures, respectively; πc′ and πi are capillary and interstitial oncotic pressures, respectively; K is a filtration coefficient related to effective capillary surface area per mass of tissue; and σ is a reflection coefficient that expresses the permeability of the capillary endothelium to albumin. The cause of pulmonary edema in this patient is likely cardiogenic, which will result in an increase in net hydrostatic pressure across the capillary.

2. What is the fraction of inspired oxygen (FiO_2) that most likely is being delivered to the patient?

A. 0.21.

B. 0.26.

C. 0.30.

D. 0.34.

The correct answer is D. The maximum FiO_2 that can be delivered by use of a nasal cannula is 0.44. The following table illustrates the oxygen delivery with low-flow devices.

Oxygen Delivery Devices and Systems

Device/System	Oxygen Flow Rate (L/min)	FiO_2 Range
Nasal cannula	1	0.21–0.24
	2	0.23–0.28
	3	0.27–0.34
	4	0.31–0.38
	5–6	0.32–0.44
Simple mask	5–6	0.30–0.45
	7–8	0.40–0.60
Mask with reservoir	5	0.35–0.50
Partial rebreathing mask-bag	7	0.35–0.75
	15	0.65–1.00
Nonrebreathing mask-bag	7–15	0.40–1.00
Venturi mask and jet nebulizer	4–6 (total flow = 15)	0.24
	4–6 (total flow = 45)	0.28
	8–10 (total flow = 45)	0.35
	8–10 (total flow = 33)	0.40
	8–12 (total flow = 33)	0.50

Reproduced with permission from Butterworth JF, Mackey DC, Wasnick JD: *Morgan and Mikhail's Clinical Anesthesiology*, 6th ed. New York, NY: McGraw-Hill Education; 2018.

3. The patient becomes unresponsive and subsequently undergoes tracheal intubation and mechanical ventilation. Positive-pressure ventilation has which of the following effects on cardiac afterload?

A. Afterload will increase due to increased intrathoracic pressure.

B. Afterload will decrease due to increased aortic transmural pressure.

C. Afterload will decrease due to decreased venous return.

D. Afterload will decrease due to decreased left ventricular transmural pressure.

The correct answer is D. Positive-pressure ventilation reduces afterload by causing a decrease in left-ventricular transmural pressure, which is the gradient between intraventricular pressure and intrapleural pressure. This may lead to an improvement in left-ventricular function.

4 to 11. Match the following airway pressure waveforms with their corresponding ventilator modes.

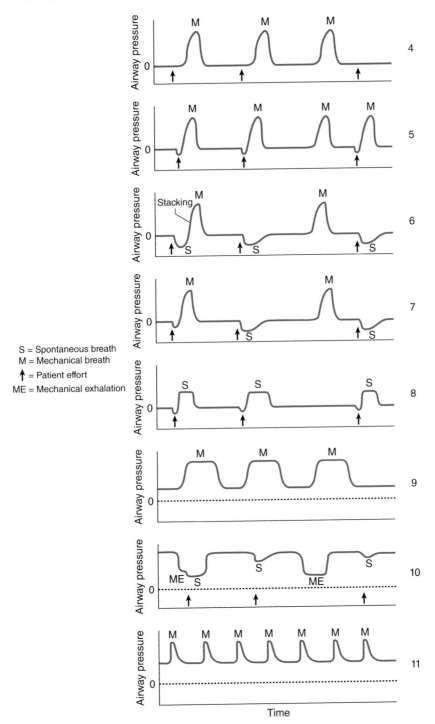

S = Spontaneous breath
M = Mechanical breath
↑ = Patient effort
ME = Mechanical exhalation

A. Airway pressure release ventilation (APRV).
B. Assist control (AC).
C. Pressure support ventilation.
D. High-frequency jet ventilation.
E. Intermittent mandatory ventilation (IMV).
F. Continuous mandatory ventilation.
G. Inverse ratio ventilation.
H. Synchronized intermittent mandatory ventilation (SIMV).

The correct answers are: 4 → F; 5 → B; 6 → E; 7 → H; 8 → C; 9 → G; 10 → A; 11 → D. In the critically ill patient, clinicians are often faced with the challenge of choosing the appropriate mode of ventilation to meet the patient's needs. At the most basic level, modes of ventilation are categorized as either volume-limited or pressure-limited ventilation, which describes the trigger for cycling from inspiration to expiration. Several modes of mechanical ventilation permit spontaneous ventilation (as in the case of IMV, AC, and SIMV) or may augment spontaneous respiratory effort (as in the case of pressure support ventilation). The duration of inspiration and expiration may be adjusted, as in the case of inverse ratio ventilation, to improve oxygenation. Modes of ventilation such as APRV and high-frequency jet ventilation may also be employed to improve oxygenation.

DID YOU LEARN?

- Applying the Starling equation to pulmonary edema.
- Oxygen support with low-flow devices.
- The effect of positive-pressure ventilation on afterload.
- Recognizing the airway pressure waveforms for different modes of mechanical ventilation.

Recommended Reading

Butterworth IV JF, Mackey DC, Wasnick JD, eds. Inhalation therapy & mechanical ventilation in the PACU & ICU. In: *Morgan & Mikhail's Clinical Anesthesiology*, 6th ed. New York, NY: McGraw-Hill; 2018:1329-1352.

Reference

Pham T, Brochard LJ, Slutsky AS. Mechanical ventilation: State of the art. *Mayo Clin Proc.* 2017;92(9):1382-1400.

CHAPTER 46

Safety, Quality, & Performance Improvement

Eliminating Unnecessary Variation Improves Quality

John F. Butterworth IV, MD

A new colorectal surgeon has joined your hospital's medical staff, recruited for her particular expertise and research. In preparation for her first surgeries, her personal preferences and care pathways were submitted to the operating room leadership for review. Her preferences and pathways are quite different from the preferences and care pathways of the other colorectal surgeons who are already on the medical staff.

1. What is the best way for the hospital leadership to handle the differences between the various surgeons' preferences and care pathways?

    A. As surgeon familiarity and comfort always provide the best results, allow each surgeon to operate and direct perioperative care as that person prefers.

    B. Ask the new surgeon to adopt the preferences and care pathways of the most senior of the existing surgeons.

    C. Ask the existing surgeons to adopt the preferences and care pathways of the newly recruited surgeon.

    D. Invite the surgeons to discuss similarities and differences, with the goal of creating shared preferences and care pathways for each operation rather than for each surgeon.

The correct answer is D. Although each training program and person has distinct preferences for various procedures, reducing unnecessary variation reduces errors and tends to improve outcomes. Forcing one member of the staff to rigidly adopt the preferences of another robs the team of an opportunity to build consensus and combine experiences. Moreover, it may indeed be the new surgeon whose techniques and preferences are best suited to a patient-oriented enhanced recovery program.

2. After the new surgeon had completed 6 months of operations, a review of all cases within the department identifies a threefold increase in surgical site infections. How should this finding be handled?

   A. Review the cases individually, searching for patient, surgical, anesthetic, or postoperative team risk factors.
   B. Blame it on the existing surgeons, as the new surgeon was recruited specifically for her expertise.
   C. Blame it on bad luck, since these things happen. Do nothing for another 6 months, and then see if the trend remains.
   D. Blame it on the new surgeon, as that person is the only variable in the established system.

The correct answer is A. Although it may be simple to blame a spate of complications on the new person, the older staff, or just a run of bad luck, the best answer for the team, the system, and the patients is to review the cases and search for risk factors.

3. After the surgical site infection rate returns to an acceptably low level, one of the surgeons returns from a national meeting and suggests significant changes in the hospital's established care pathway. How should this be handled?

   A. Rapid adoption, as the recommendations were presented at a national meeting.
   B. Maintain the current pathway, as it has been well established at your center and would be dangerous to change.
   C. Ask various perioperative leaders to evaluate the pathway, and consider testing the pathway on a series of 10 patients and then evaluating the outcomes.
   D. Quietly randomize patients between the old pathway and the new pathway, and then compare the results.

The correct answer is C. Blind adoption of any new proposal is not wise, nor is refusal to adapt to new findings. Nevertheless, all care pathways should be considered ongoing continuous quality improvement exercises; therefore, changes should be expected. However, randomizing patients between two pathways is considered research and requires open announcement, approval by an institutional review board, and a formal informed consent process. But changing a care pathway using variations of accepted clinical practice without randomization is not considered research. Evaluating clinical care in this way is considered quality improvement and is an excellent means of evaluating changes in practice on a smaller and more rapid scale. In any quality or performance improvement exercise, we favor the plan-do-study-act (PDSA) approach, reflecting the continuing influence of Dr. W. Edwards Deming on the science and practice of process improvement.

Recommended Reading

Butterworth IV JF, Mackey DC, Wasnick JD, eds. Safety, quality, & performance improvement. In: *Morgan & Mikhail's Clinical Anesthesiology*, 6th ed. New York, NY: McGraw-Hill; 2018:1353-1359.

INDEX

Page references followed by *f* indicate figures; those followed by *t* indicate tables.

hemodynamic instability and, 139–142, 145–149

hypertrophic cardiomyopathy and, 139–141, 148–149

preoperative assessment in, 119–120

preoperative electrocardiography changes and, 150–152

recent revascularization for, 120–121

cardiovascular surgery, 153–160. *See also* cardiopulmonary bypass (CPB)

cardioplegia and, 153–154

hyperglycemia during, 240

cardioversion, in Wolff–Parkinson–White syndrome, 151

catheters, multiorifice, for central venous access, positioning, 185

CBF. *See* cerebral blood flow (CBF)

central sensitization, neurogenic expression of, myofascial pain syndrome as, 354

cerebellar infarction, intraoperative, 186

cerebral artery vasospasm, 189

cerebral blood flow (CBF), posterior fossa mass lesion removal and, 186–187

cerebral ischemia, delayed, 189

cerebral oximetry, 46–47

cerebral oxygen saturation, fall in, 47

cerebral perfusion pressure, in traumatic brain injury, 191

cervical cerclage placement, 289–292

anesthetic choice for, 290

hypertension with, 290–291

pain management following, 291

cervical instability, airway management with, 43

cesarean section

aspiration during, 285

with HIV infection, 296–297

intravenous access for volume resuscitation and, 273–274

low-molecular-weight heparin following, 281–282

maternal cardiac arrest and, 276–279

in obesity

anesthetic choice for, 300

intravenous access for, 299–300

postoperative pain management for, 301

for umbilical cord prolapse, 285

children. *See* pediatric anesthesia

Child–Turcotte–Pugh (CTP) score, 228

cholinesterase antagonists, contraindication to, 68

chronic obstructive pulmonary disease (COPD)

capnography in, 39–40

electrocardiography in, 41

ventilator management in, 42

Chvostek's sign, following parathyroid surgery, 253

circle breathing systems, advantages of Mapleson breathing circuits over, 14

closing capacity, 162

CO. *See* cardiac output (CO)

CO_2 absorbers, exhausted, 17–18

coagulation status, in end-stage liver disease, 237

coagulopathy

in end-stage liver disease, 229

factors worsening, 391

cognitive dysfunction, with general vs. regional anesthesia, 344–345

colorectal surgery, optimal preoperative preparation before, 369–370

communication, with family, 10–11

competency, determining, 260–262

complex regional pain syndrome (CRPS), 359–361

Compound A, nephrotoxicity of, 19

conscious sedation, practitioners administering, 96–97

COPD. *See* chronic obstructive pulmonary disease (COPD)

coronary artery bypass grafting (CABG), with elevated creatinine, 240

coronary artery disease (CAD), following heart transplantation, 142

coronary artery stent thrombosis, prevention of, 212–213

CPB. *See* cardiopulmonary bypass (CPB)

CPR. *See* cardiopulmonary resuscitation (CPR)

cranial nerves, upper airway sensory supply from, 105

creatinine, elevated, coronary artery bypass grafting and, 240

cricothyrotomy, in angioedema, 104

croup, treatment of, 180

CRPS. *See* complex regional pain syndrome (CRPS)

cryoprecipitate, for massive hemorrhage, 390–391

CTP score. *See* Child–Turcotte–Pugh (CTP) score

Cushing reflex, 307

cyanosis, in tricuspid atresia, 133

cyclosporine A, mechanism of action of, 144

D

dead space ventilation, increased, venous air embolism and, 188

deep vein thrombosis (DVT), following orthopedic procedures, 270

delirium, postoperative, 270–271

factors predisposing to, 321

in geriatric patient, 320–321

prevention of, 322

procedures associated with, 321

delirium tremens, 321

INDEX

INDEX

SSRIs. *See* selective serotonin reuptake inhibitors (SSRIs)
Stauffer syndrome, 212
strabismus surgery, oculocardiac reflex and, 306–308
stress-induced cardiomyopathy, 189–190
stroke volume (SV), 37
subarachnoid hemorrhage (SAH)
Fisher grading scale for, 189
Hunt and Hess grading scale for, 188
succinylcholine
dosing of, 52
in myasthenia gravis, 205
sufentanil, for colorectal surgery, 371
sugammadex, 68
superior hypogastric block, 361–364
contraindications to, 362–363
indications for, 361–362
repeat, with hydrolysis, 363
superior laryngeal nerve (SLN), 105, 301
anesthetizing, 106, 107
postextubation respiratory stridor and, 250–251
supraclavicular blocks, 326, 328, 339, 346–347
supraglottic airway devices
to reduce risk of fire, 10
second-generation, 107
surgeon, as "captain of the ship," 1–2
SV. *See* stroke volume (SV)
systemic vascular resistance (SVR), regional anesthesia and, 281

T
tachycardia, in oliguria, 208
TBI. *See* traumatic brain injury (TBI)
TCAs. *See* tricyclic antidepressants (TCAs)
TEE. *See* transesophageal echocardiography (TEE)
TEG. *See* thromboelastography (TEG)
tension pneumocephalus, 186
tetralogy of Fallot, 135–136
thiazide diuretics, actions of, 252–253
thromboelastography (TEG), 23
in acute hemolytic transfusion reaction, 388
for hemorrhage following cardiopulmonary bypass, 156
thromboprophylaxis, post–cesarean section, 281–282
thyroid storm, 250
tissue hypoperfusion, 23
tonsillectomy, hemorrhage following, 309–312
total hip arthroplasty, choice of anesthesia for, 267–269
total shoulder arthroplasty, neurological complications with, avoiding, 256–257
tourniquet pain, 328, 338–339
tracheal resection, 177–180

tracheal stenosis
flow-volume loops in, 178–179
treatment of, 179
tracheostomy
in angioedema, 104
for epiglottitis, 180
tranexamic acid, for blood loss and hemorrhage, 391–392
transesophageal echocardiography (TEE), 27–31
in aortic insufficiency, 30
cardiac output estimation using, 37–38
cardiopulmonary bypass and, 214–215
intraoperative, with hypotension or hypoxemia, 213–214
systolic heart failure on, 27–28
for venous air embolism detection, 184–185
venous air embolism monitoring using, 187–188
transurethral resection of the prostate (TURP)
anesthetic technique for, 219
TURP syndrome and, 220–221
traumatic brain injury (TBI), 190–192
Trendelenburg position, steep, respiratory distress and, 218
tricuspid atresia
cyanosis in, 133
Fontan procedure for, 130–133
tricuspid valve, 35
tricyclic antidepressants (TCAs), for diabetic neuropathy, 351
trigeminal nerve, 105
trigeminocardiac reflex, 307
trigger point injections, for myofascial pain syndrome, 355
Trousseau's sign, following parathyroid surgery, 253
tube feedings, for burn injury patient, 395
tumor embolism, cardiopulmonary bypass for, 215
TURP. *See* transurethral resection of the prostate (TURP)
TURP syndrome, 220–221
minimizing risk of, 221

U
umbilical cord prolapse, 283–286
umbilical hernias, in end-stage liver disease patients, 227–228

V
VAE. *See* venous air embolism (VAE)
vagus nerve, 105
VAP. *See* ventilator-associated pneumonia (VAP)
variation, unnecessary, eliminating, 413–414
vascular insufficiency, lumbar sympathetic block for, 360

INDEX